Third Edit

The **E**arly

Intervention

Dictionary

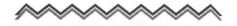

A Multidisciplinary
Guide to Terminology

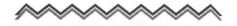

Jeanine G. Coleman, M. Ed.

Woodbine House ■ **2006**

All rights reserved under International and Pan-American copyright conventions. Published in the United States of America by Woodbine House, Inc., 6510 Bells Mill Rd., Bethesda, MD 20817. 800-843-7323. www.woodbinehouse.com

Cover illustration: Liz Wolf

Library of Congress Cataloging-in-Publication Data

Coleman, Jeanine G.
    The early intervention dictionary : a multidisciplinary guide to terminology / Jeanine G. Coleman. — 3rd ed.
p.   cm.
    ISBN-13: 978-1-890627-63-8
    ISBN-10: 1-890627-63-1
    1. Developmentally disabled children--Terminology. 2. Early childhood educa-tion--Terminology. I. Title.
HV891.C63 2006
362.1'968--dc22   2006028557
                                                                          CIP

Manufactured in the United States of America

Second Edition
10 9 8 7 6 5 4 3 2 1

DEDICATION

*This book is dedicated with love to
Jacob Charlie, my miracle.
And to the memory of my mom,
Lillian C. Tancredi,
who understood the magic of children
and made me feel magical.*

Table of Contents

Advisory Board

Thomas Roccapalumbo, D.O. earned a degree of Doctor of Osteopathic Medicine from Western University of Health Sciences, Pomona, California. He completed his internship at Pacific Hospital in Long Beach, California and is Board Certified in family practice. Presently, Dr. Roccapalumbo practices industrial medicine in the City of Commerce, California, and is Regional Medical Director for Immediate Medical Care Centers.

Karen Ezaki, PT, ATP, M.Ed. earned a Bachelor of Science degree in Physical Therapy from the University of California, San Francisco Medical Center and a Master's degree in Education from California Polytechnic University, Pomona, California. Ms. Ezaki is a RESNA certified Assistive Technology Practitioner and listed as a National Consultant in the Early Head Start Directory. Currently, she is the only full-time School Physical Therapist attached to the Assistive Technology Program for the Los Angeles Unified School District, the second largest school district in the U.S. She is also an adjunct professor at Citrus Community College in Glendora, California on subjects related to the child with special needs and early childhood education.

Brandi Buchanan, OTD, OTR/L received her Bachelor's degree in Spanish from Pacific University in Forest Grove, Oregon and received her graduate level training in Occupational Therapy at the University of Southern California in Los Angeles. Her doctoral residency was completed in the area of public policy and disability advocacy at which time she co-authored "Saving Lives: Including People with Disabilities in Emergency Planning," a report sponsored by the National Council on Disability. Dr. Buchanan is currently the coordinator of Pediatric and NICU Rehabilitation at a southern California hospital where she enjoys working in areas of early intervention and child/family advocacy. She lives in Monrovia, California with her husband and her English bulldog, Harley.

Stephanie Renee Booth, M.D. earned a degree of Doctor of Medicine from the University of Southern California, School of Medicine. She completed her internship and residency in pediatrics through the University of California at Irvine Medical Center. Currently, Dr. Booth is practicing general pediatrics in Long Beach, California.

Acknowledgements

There are many people who influence our lives, who in gentle and strong ways contribute to who we are and who we become. I am blessed with some very special people who have enhanced my life and who encourage me to believe in myself and to follow my dreams. This book and its creation have benefited from the encouragement I have received over the years. I now have the unique opportunity and privilege to thank the people who directly and indirectly helped make this project a reality.

Thank you to my sister, Michelle T. Vergara, B.A., for countless hours of research, writing, typing, and reviewing; for your thoughtful advice, dedication, encouragement, intelligence, and skill for teaching young children who have special needs; and for being my partner on this and so many other projects. You deserve so much credit for the completion of our book, and I truly could not have done it without you! Jacob and I are so fortunate to have your loving care.

Thank you to my brother-in-law Derek Vergara, Ed.D., for so generously sharing your time and talents with me. You brought this project up to speed and I will always appreciate your help.

Thank you to my sister, Julie T. Basiago, B.A., for all your help with proofreading, researching, and reviewing, and for your thoughtful suggestions and encouragement. Your keen eye and commitment to this and all my projects give me so much peace of mind. Caring for and loving me and Jacob has made it possible to complete this book.

Thank you to Dale, my husband, for your endless words of encouragement, for easing my mind with your sound advice and objectivity, for your sensitive understanding of what this book means to me, and most of all for being the love of my life and for the treasures your friendship brings me.

Thank you to my son Jacob Charlie, for being my inspiration, my joy, and my dream come true. Your snuggles are the best gifts I'll ever receive.

Thank you to my nephew Jonathan Basiago, my sister, Gina Moore, and to Kendahl Moore, for the many hours of research you provided. I really appreciate your conscientious effort.

Thank you to my brother Tom Tancredi for all your hard work and encouraging words. I'll always appreciate the way you, Julie, and Michelle care about me, believe in me, and dream with me.

Thank you to Mom and Dad for always believing in me and making me feel special. And to Jonathan, Kevin, and Jared for the joy and inspiration you naturally give – you guys, along with Jacob, are the best teachers, and help me in ways you'll never know! Thank you to my Tancredi/Basiago/Vergara and Coleman/Conover families and to my friends for your enthusiasm and support — how fortunate I am to have your love and encouragement as we embrace this adventure called life!

Thank you to Tom Roccapalumbo, D.O.; Karen Ezaki, PT, ATP, M.Ed., Brandi Buchanan, OTD, OTR/L; Joan Altvater; Karen Tancredi; Stephanie Booth, M.D.; Chris Basiago, D.D.S.; Diane Hinds, M.S.; Kathryn Harris; and Sheila James for your time and effort, and for the care and expertise you gave to this book.

Thank you to Sister Mary Dennis Peters, OSB, MLS, and to all the very helpful staff members of Wilson Library at the University of La Verne, California. Your knowledge, assistance, and consideration made my research environment feel like a "home away from home."

Thank you to the team at Woodbine House for your commitment to *The Early Intervention Dictionary.* Especially, I would like to thank Susan Stokes for the many ways this book has benefited from your skill and talent. Thank you to Nancy Gray Paul for your dedication to making sure this third edition is as helpful and reader-friendly as possible. Your writing style and keen eye for detail are amazing and appreciated!

Finally, I would like to express my thanks to God for the many ways He has guided and blessed my life.

Introduction

The field of early intervention, much like the young children who benefit from it, is evolving and optimistic, with unlimited potential for growth. It is an expansive, multidisciplinary field comprised of a host of medical, therapeutic, and educational professionals who join in a collaborative effort to deliver the most effective programs for young children (ages zero to three). It is well documented that infants and young children with disabilities, and their families, need comprehensive services delivered by well-trained interventionists. One of the challenges of implementing such a comprehensive multidisciplinary service delivery system is to develop a better understanding of the various disciplines, each with its own system of unique and specialized interventions. It is vital that early interventionists understand the terminology of the various disciplines so we can support each other's efforts and truly provide effective and comprehensive programs to infants and young children with special needs.

My goal in writing the first edition of *The Early Intervention Dictionary* was to identify and comprehensively define early intervention terminology, making it accessible and understandable to parents and all professionals. My goal has remained the same for this third, revised edition. More than ever, infants and toddlers with special needs are included in the same child development and preschool programs as their peers who do not have disabilities. Often, the staff members of inclusive programs are challenged to quickly learn about disabilities in order to provide quality care and education. My hope is that the third edition of *The Early Intervention Dictionary* will provide the information needed to gain an understanding of many of the disabilities and at-risk factors that can affect the development of infants and toddlers.

Furthermore, this edition has been expanded to include more than 400 new entries and thoroughly revised to reflect what we've learned through research in the past several years about many syndromes and disorders, such as autism spectrum disorder (ASD). How these advances have affected the early intervention field and our attitudes is echoed in the changes in favored terminology. New educational approaches and treatments as well as transition-related terms have also been added to help parents prepare for the preschool years ahead.

As with any dictionary, this one is not intended to provide the level of in-depth information that some parents or early interventionists may seek about the various medical, therapeutic, educational, or psychological terms that are defined. Rather, the intent of *The Early Intervention Dictionary* is to clarify many of the more frequently used terms, to provide a starting point in the search for more in-depth information, and to provide readers with a better foundation for understanding the early intervention process.

The entries included in this dictionary were culled from current articles and literature; medical, therapeutic, educational, and psychological reports on individual children; and from discussions with students and professionals working with infants and toddlers in early intervention programs. I've chosen to include some very common terms, such as "jumping," which need definition in order to accurately assess and maintain appropriate expectations for young children with special needs. Certainly, there are other terms (for conditions, evaluation tools, drugs, etc.) that pertain to early intervention that are not included. The disciplines represented in the dictionary include pediatric medicine, child development, early childhood education, early childhood special education, physical therapy (PT), occupational therapy (OT), speech and language therapy, audiology, counseling, social work, child life, education of the hearing impaired and visually impaired, and special education.

It is a rare individual who joins an early intervention team already trained and fully knowledgeable about all areas of early intervention. And even someone this qualified must continuously strive to keep up with the growth of the field. The majority of us do have room for expansion of our knowledge base. It is my hope that *The Early Intervention Dictionary* will help the committed early intervention practitioner acquire the information necessary to provide compassionate and effective early intervention services and to help connect professionals of varying disciplines. As with any type of learning, the more knowledgeable and comfortable we are with the "tools of our trade," the more capable we are of utilizing our resources and integrating our learning into concrete practices that will benefit the young children and families we endeavor to serve.

Finally, as we explore and respond to some of the more challenging aspects of our work as early interventionists, it is my hope that we always appreciate the amazing children who inspire and motivate us to reach our potential.

Notes to the Reader

◆ The definitions in this dictionary are written as they apply to early intervention or to the care and development of infants and young children in general. Many words have other, equally accurate, definitions that are not included because they do not pertain to early intervention. For the same reason, not all available information about a condition, drug, evaluation tool, etc., is included. (The reader will note that some terms that pertain to special education of children above five years of age are included, as these terms may be encountered in helping children make the transition from early intervention to special education.)

◆ In order to accurately describe the children who are in early intervention programs, I have alternated the use of masculine and feminine pronouns by letter (i.e., masculine pronouns are used in definitions of words beginning with A, feminine pronouns for words beginning with B, etc.).

◆ Within definitions, I have used terminology that emphasizes that children with special needs are children first, not their conditions. While it is important to understand a child's diagnosis, it is equally important to avoid labeling children. First of all, a diagnosis does not fully describe a child and capture his or her unique capacities and potential; nor is a diagnosis always accurate and/or comprehensive. Secondly, our focus of time and energy must be on children, not on their labels. We teach Michael and Beth, who have Down syndrome, not two Down's kids named Michael and Beth.

◆ Entries are alphabetized by the letter-by-letter method; that is, disregarding spaces and punctuation. For example:
> IAC
> IAL
> I and O
> -iasis
> iatr-

◆ All but the most common words used within a definition are also defined in the book. The definition for a word is provided in the following manner:

—defined in full at its own entry (it is also likely printed in italics within a definition of another word as a reminder to the reader that additional information is available)
or
—defined briefly in parentheses within the definition of another word if it is integral to comprehension of that definition.

♦ The causes of medical and developmental conditions are provided if they are known. Sometimes the only information regarding how a disorder occurs is the pattern of inheritance (and this is not always known, either).

♦ The ages provided at entries describing acquisition of skills and emergence of behaviors are only approximations (and then only for typically developing children).

♦ Drugs are defined at the generic (official) names of the drugs. Brand names are indicated by the notation of ™ (trademark) after the name.

♦ The instruction "*Refer to*" at the end of some listings indicates either that information on this topic is given under a different term or that there are other entries that contain information on related topics. For example, at "**State**," I have suggested "*Refer to Arousal Level.*"

♦ "*Compare*" is used to indicate terms that are opposites of, or otherwise contrasting to, the word defined, or one of several in a sequence of related terms. For example, at **Ductus Arteriosus**, I have suggested "*Compare Patent Ductus Arteriosus*" and at **Scoliosis**, I have suggested "*Compare Kyphosis and Lordosis*" (other types of spinal curvature).

♦ "*Also known as*" points out additional formal and/or informal names of conditions, supplies, agencies, etc. For example, at **Down Syndrome**, I have listed, "*Also known as Trisomy 21.*"

Pronunciation Key

—/a/ as in "pat"
—/ay/ as in "baby"
—/ah/ as in "ahh"
—/ar/ as in "car"
—/b/ as in "boy"
—/ch/ as in "chew"
—/d/ as in "dog"
—/e/ as in "pet"
—/ee/ as in "feet"
—/f/ as in "finger"
—/g/ as in "gag"
—/h/ as in "hot"
—/i/ as in "infant"
—/ie/ as in "tie"
—/j/ as in "jabber"
—/k/ as in "kiss"
—/kw/ as in "quick"
—/l/ as in "learn"
—/m/ as in "mom"
—/n/ as in "new"
—/ng/ as in "thing"
—/o/ as in "pot"

—/oe/ as in "go"
—/oi/ as in "toy"
—/oo/ as in "boot"
—/or/ as in "more"
—/ou/ as in "out"
—/p/ as in "papa"
—/r/ as in "run"
—/s/ as in "sand"
—/sh/ as in "shoe"
—/t/ as in "toddler"
—/th/ as in "throw"
—/u/ as in "cup"
—/yoo/ as in "use"
—/uh/ as in "about"
—/ur/ as in "turn"
—/v/ as in "voice"
—/w/ as in "win"
—/x/ as in "x-ray"
—/y/ as in "you"
—/z/ as in "zoo"
—/zh/ as in "vision"

09/25/07

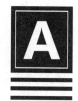

ā
The abbreviation for before.

a-
A prefix meaning away from, not, without, or lack.

AAC
The abbreviation for Augmentative and Alternative Communication.

AAMD
The abbreviation for American Association on Mental Deficiency (now known as American Association on Mental Retardation).

AAMR
The abbreviation for American Association on Mental Retardation, formerly known as American Association on Mental Deficiency.

AAP
The abbreviation for American Academy of Pediatrics.

ab-
A prefix meaning away from.

Ab
The abbreviation for antibody.

ABA
The abbreviation for Applied Behavior Analysis.

Abdomen (AB-doe-men or ab-DOE-men)
The area of the body located between the chest and the *pelvis*.

Abdominal (ab-DOM-i-nuhl)
Referring to the *stomach* area, the area of the body between the chest and *pelvis*.

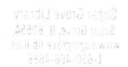

Abdominal Thrust
>*Refer to* **Heimlich Maneuver**.

Abduct (ab-DUKT)
To move away from the *midline* of the body.
>*Compare* **Adduct**.

Abduction
The act of moving apart, as in moving leg or arm muscles away from the *midline* of the body.
>*Compare* **Adduction**.

Abductor
One of several muscles that pulls a part of the body away from *midline*. For example, abductor muscles pull the thumb away from the other fingers.
>*Compare* **Adductor**.

Abnormal/Abnormality
Describing a condition that differs from the typical, usual, or average standards.

ABO Incompatibility
The differences in *blood type* (O, A, B, or AB) between mother and baby. This incompatibility can result in *anemia* and *jaundice* in the baby.

Abortion
The delivery of an *embryo* or *fetus* with no chance of survival. Spontaneous abortion refers to a *miscarriage* and elective abortion refers to a deliberate, medically induced termination of pregnancy.

Abortus (uh-BOR-tus)
A *fetus* with no chance of survival.
>*Refer to* **Abortion**.

ABR
The abbreviation for Auditory Brainstem Response.

Abrachia (uh-BRAY-kee-uh)
Congenital absence of arms.

Abruptio Placenta (uh-BRUP-shee-oe pluh-SEN-tuh)
A life-threatening condition in which the *placenta* separates prematurely from the wall of a pregnant woman's *uterus*. Severe bleeding can result, making it dangerous for both the mother and the *fetus*.
>*Also known as* **Placenta Abruptio**.

Absence Seizure (AB-sens or uhb-SAHNS SEE-zhur)
A form of *generalized seizure* that causes a brief (less than 20 seconds) clouding or loss of consciousness. The child stares blankly, and sometimes his eyes blink

or roll upward. The child recovers quickly from this type of seizure. Absence seizures may occur many times a day and can be brought on by *hyperventilation*.
> *Formerly known as a* **Petit Mal Seizure.**
> *Refer to* **Generalized Seizure** *and* **Epilepsy.**

Absorption
The process by which substances pass into body *tissues*, such as when digested food is absorbed into the walls of the intestines.
> *Compare* **Malabsorption** *and* **Reabsorption.**
> *Refer to* **Nutrition.**

Abstract Thinking
The ability to grasp concepts, principles, or processes that cannot be experienced directly through the senses; to draw relationships (such as between like and unlike things); and to derive meaning from symbols.

ac
The abbreviation for the Latin words meaning before meals.

ACC
The abbreviation for Agenesis of Corpus Callosum.

Accommodation
1. The ability of the eye to adjust its shape for *vision*. (The eye adjusts to variations in distance.)
2. An adaptation of the environment, format, or situation made to suit the needs of those participating.

Accutane™ (AK-yoo-tayn)
> *Refer to* **Retinoic Acid.**

Acetabular Dysplasia (as-uh-TAB-yuh-luhr dis-PLAY-zee-uh)
Underdevelopment of the hip socket.

Acetabulum (as-i-TAB-yuh-luhm)
The hip socket holding the head of the *femur* (thigh bone).

Acetaminophen (uh-see-tuh-MIN-uh-fen)
A drug used to relieve pain and reduce fever. Tylenol™ is the brand name of this drug.

Acetazolamide (as-et-uh-ZOL-uh-mied)
A drug used to treat *edema*, to reduce eye pressure in *glaucoma*, and to treat certain *seizure disorders*. Diamox™ is the brand name of this drug.

Acetylcholine (as-e-til-KOE-leen)
A *neurotransmitter*, or chemical in the body that transmits messages from one *nerve cell* to another, or between nerve and muscle cells.

Achilles Tendon (uh-KIL-eez)
The *tendon* of the calf muscles.
> *Also known as* **Calcaneal Tendon** *or* **Heel Cord.**

Achilles Tendon Lengthening
A surgical procedure in which the *Achilles tendon* is cut to lengthen the *tendon* and to correct *contractures*. The procedure helps the child place his foot in a *neutral position* (toes forward, foot flexed), and to walk on his whole foot rather than on his toes.
> *Also known as* **Heel Cord Lengthening** *or* **Tendo-Achilles Lengthening.**

Achondroplasia (uh-kon-droe-PLAY-zee-uh)
A sometimes *autosomal dominant disorder* in which bones fail to grow normally due to *abnormal* conversion of *cartilage* to bone. This causes extreme shortness of the arms and legs, resulting in *short stature*. Achondroplasia is also characterized by *macrocephaly*, mild *hypotonia*, *lordosis*, and, usually, *normal intelligence*. Achondroplasia is a type of *Chondrodystrophy*.
> *Refer to* **Chondrodystrophy.**

Acidemia (as-i-DEE-mee-uh)
An excess of acid in the blood.
> *Refer to* **Acidosis.**

Acidosis (as-i-DOE-sis)
An excess of acid in the blood and body *tissues*, which can lead to disruption of the chemical processes within the body. There are two types of acidosis: *metabolic acidosis* and *respiratory acidosis*.
> *Refer to* **Metabolic Acidosis** *and* **Respiratory Acidosis.**

Acoustic Nerve
> *Refer to* **Auditory Nerve.**

Acoustic Neuroma
A *benign tumor* of the *auditory nerve* (located within the *auditory canal*) that may cause *auditory impairment*, headache, *balance* disturbance, pain or numbness of the face, and a ringing or buzzing noise within the ear or ears.

Acquired (uh-KWIE-uhrd)
Referring to a feature, *state*, or *disease* that happens after birth. (Acquired conditions are not *inherited*, but rather a response to the environment.)
> *Compare* **Congenital** *and* **Inherited.**
> *Refer to* **Adventitious.**

Acquired Childhood Epileptic Aphasia (ep-i-LEP-tik uh-FAY-zee-uh)
> *Refer to* **Landau-Kleffner Syndrome.**

Acquired Epileptic Aphasia
> *Refer to* **Landau-Kleffner Syndrome.**

Acquired Immune Deficiency Syndrome (AIDS)

A *disorder* caused by the *human immunodeficiency virus* (*HIV*). *Symptoms* in children include damaged *immune system*, recurrent *infections*, poor growth, and possibly *brain disease* resulting in *developmental delay*. AIDS is usually fatal.

Acrocephalopolysyndactyly (ak-roe-sef-uh-loe-pol-ee-sin-DAK-ti-lee)

A group of very rare *genetic disorders* in which the *infant* is born with *craniostenosis* (premature closure of *sutures* of the *cranium*), causing *oxycephaly* (a long, narrow head that appears pointed at the top), extra fingers and/or toes, and *syndactyly* (*webbing*, or fusion, of fingers and/or toes). There are several types of acrocephalopolysyndactyly, describing different genetic disorders.

> *Compare* **Acrocephalosyndactyly.**
> *Refer to* **Carpenter Syndrome, Goodman Syndrome, Noack Syndrome,** *and* **Sakati-Nyhan Syndrome.**

Acrocephalopolysyndactyly, Type I

> *Refer to* **Noack Syndrome.**

Acrocephalopolysyndactyly, Type II

> *Refer to* **Carpenter Syndrome.**

Acrocephalopolysyndactyly, Type III

> *Refer to* **Sakati-Nyhan Syndrome.**

Acrocephalopolysyndactyly, Type IV

> *Refer to* **Goodman Syndrome.**

Acrocephalosyndactyly (ak-roe-sef-uh-loe-sin-DAK-ti-lee)

A group of very rare *genetic disorders* in which the infant is born with *craniostenosis* (premature closure of *sutures* of the *cranium*), causing *oxycephaly* (a long narrow head that appears pointed at the top) and *syndactyly* (*webbing*, or fusion, of fingers and/or toes). There are several types of acrocephalosyndactyly, describing different genetic disorders.

> *Compare* **Acrocephalopolysyndactyly.**
> *Refer to* **Apert Syndrome, Pfeiffer Syndrome,** *and* **Saethre-Chotzen Syndrome.**

Acrocephalosyndactyly, Type I

> *Refer to* **Apert Syndrome.**

Acrocephalosyndactyly, Type III

> *Refer to* **Saethre-Chotzen Syndrome.**

Acrocephalosyndactyly, Type V

> *Refer to* **Pfeiffer Syndrome.**

Acrocephaly (ak-roe-SEF-uh-lee)

> *Refer to* **Oxycephaly.**

Acrocyanosis (ak-roe-sie-uh-NOE-sis)
Bluish discoloration around the mouth, nose, ears, or *extremities* (fingers or toes) that occurs when the *nerves* and small *blood vessels* of the skin over-respond to cold temperature. The condition is more common in newborns but may persist in children with *heart disease*. Acrocyanosis can also occur due to emotional *stimuli*.

Acrofacial Dysostosis, Nager Type
(ak-roe-FAY-shuhl dis-os-TOE-sis, NAY-guhr)
> *Refer to* **Nager Acrofacial Dysostosis.**

ACTH
The abbreviation for Adrenocorticotropic hormone.

Active Learner
> *Refer to* **Kinesthetic Learner.**

Active Range of Motion (AROM)
The range of movement through which a child can move a *joint* without assistance.
> *Compare* **Passive Range of Motion.**
> *Refer to* **Range of Motion.**

Activities of Daily Living (ADL)
Normal, everyday actions, such as eating, dressing, or brushing the teeth.
> *Refer to* **Self-Help.**

Activity Schedules
A teaching technique used to promote independent (or less *prompt-dependent*) action from children with *developmental disabilities*. It involves creating a visual sequence (either written or pictorial) that depicts what activities should be done in what order, such as for brushing teeth or completing a puzzle.

Acuity (uh-KYOO-i-tee)
The level at which a child can accurately see images or hear sounds.
> *Refer to* **Visual Acuity.**

Acute Illness
Referring to a condition that occurs suddenly and is usually short in duration.
> *Compare* **Chronic Illness.**

ad-
A prefix meaning to or toward.

AD
1. The abbreviation for the Latin words meaning right ear.
2. The abbreviation for Asperger's Disorder.
3. The abbreviation for Autistic Disorder.

ADA
The abbreviation for Americans with Disabilities Act of 1990.

Adactyly (ay-DAK-ti-lee)
A *congenital anomaly* in which one or more fingers or toes are missing.
  Compare **Polydactyly.**

Adaptive
Normal or useful.

Adaptive Behavior/Skill
The ability to adjust to new situations and to apply familiar or new skills to those situations. Adaptive behaviors are required to perform everyday activities, such as communicating, dressing, and helping with household tasks. For example, a 2-year-old is displaying his ability to adapt when he says, "Mine!" to the child who is attempting to take his toy. A 5-year-old shows adaptive behavior when he is able to use the same table manners he uses at home at a friend's house.

Adaptive Equipment/Device
A commercially made piece of equipment or product system, such as an adaptive eating device or a powered mobility toy, used to maintain or improve the functional capacities of a child with *special needs*.

Adaptive Skill
  Refer to **Adaptive Behavior.**

Adaptive Switch
A device that can be added to an electronic or battery-operated toy, a computer, a *communication* or *mobility aid*, or an appliance (such as a light or a television) to allow the child with a *disability* to access (activate or control the functions of) the object. Since activating an adaptive switch does not require precise *motor skills*, the child with a *motor disability* is able to better control his environment.
  Refer to **Assistive Technology** and **Augmentative and Alternative Communication.**

ADD
The abbreviation for Attention Deficit Disorder.
  Refer to **Attention-Deficit/Hyperactivity Disorder, Predominantly Inattentive Type.**

Adderall™ (AD-ur-ahl)
An *amphetamine* (a *nervous system stimulant drug*) mixture sometimes used to treat certain *behaviors* associated with *attention-deficit/hyperactivity disorder*.

Adduct (uh-DUKT or a-DUKT)
To move toward the *midline* of the body.
  Compare **Abduct.**

Adduction
The act of moving a *limb* toward the *midline*, as in the arm or leg *muscles* toward the middle of the body.
    Compare **Abduction.**

Adductor
One of several *muscles* that pulls a part of the body toward *midline*. For example, adductor muscles pull the thigh toward the midline of the body.
    Compare **Abductor.**

adeno-
A prefix meaning *gland*.

Adenoid (AD-e-noid)
One of two masses of *lymph tissue* high on the back wall of the throat, behind the nose.

Adenoidectomy (ad-e-noid-EK-toe-mee)
Surgical removal of the *adenoids*.

Adenoma Sebaceum (ad-uh-NOE-muh se-BAY-see-uhm)
Usually *benign* skin *lesions* on the faces of individuals with *tuberous sclerosis*.

Adenopathy (ad-e-NOP-uh-thee)
Swelling of *lymph nodes*.

Adenosis (ad-e-NOE-sis)
A *disease* or *abnormal* growth in a *gland*, especially a *lymph* gland.

AD/HD
The abbreviation for Attention-Deficit/Hyperactivity Disorder.

Adhesion (ad-HEE-zhun)
A formation of scar *tissue* that binds together two surfaces that are normally apart. Adhesions develop most commonly in the *abdomen* as a result of *inflammation* or surgery.

adip-
A prefix meaning fat.

Adipose (AD-i-poes)
Fatty.

ADI-R
The abbreviation for Autism Diagnostic Interview-Revised.

Adjusted Age
    Refer to **Corrected Age.**

ADL
The abbreviation for Activities of Daily Living.

ADOS-R
The abbreviation for Autism Diagnostic Observation Schedule-Revised.

Adrenal Gland (uh-DREE-nuhl)
The organ that sits on top of each *kidney* and produces *hormones* that assist with body *metabolism*, chemical balance, *immune system* functioning, and response to stress. The adrenal glands also produce male sex hormones, and to a lesser degree, female sex hormones. The adrenal glands are essential to life.

Adrenaline (uh-DREN-uh-leen or uh-DREN-uh-lin)
Refer to **Epinephrine.**

Adrenergic (ad-ren-ER-jik)
Referring to *nerves* that release *epinephrine* or *norepinephrine* at *synapses* (the junctional regions between two *nerve cells*—the place across which a *nerve impulse* is transmitted from one nerve cell to another), or relating to drugs that mimic the action of epinephrine or norepinephrine.

Adrenocorticotropic Hormone (ACTH) (ad-ree-noe-kor-ti-koe-TROP-ik)
A *hormone* made by the *pituitary gland* to stimulate growth and function of the adrenal *cortex* (the outer layer of the *adrenal glands*). ACTH is also commercially made and is used to treat *endocrine* and *rheumatic disorders* and *infantile spasms*.
Also known as **Corticotropin.**

Adrenoleukodystrophy (ALD) (uh-dree-noe-loo-koe-DIS-troe-fee)
A rare, *X-linked recessive disorder* of *metabolism*. It is characterized by wasting away of the *adrenal glands* and loss of *myelin* in the *cerebrum*. This results in mental deterioration, *aphasia*, *apraxia*, *blindness*, *quadriplegia*, and *seizures*. It is a progressive *disease* usually resulting in death within 1 to 5 years. ALD mainly affects males with onset between 5 and 8 years of age.

Adult-Directed Instruction
Instruction consisting of adult-directed activities in which the infant or young child is expected to participate. The value of adult-directed activities depends heavily on the adult's skill and on a correct *assessment* of the interests and *developmental* level of the individual child so that participation occurs and objectives are met. A greater emphasis on *child-directed instruction* over adult-directed instruction is appropriate with the infant or young child.
Compare **Child-Directed Instruction.**

Adventitious (ad-ven-TISH-uhs)
A condition that is *acquired* through illness or accident, such as adventitious *deafness*.
Refer to **Acquired.**

Advocate
An individual who represents or speaks out on behalf of another person's interests (as in a parent with his/her child).

AEP
The abbreviation for Auditory Evoked Potential.
> *Refer to* **Auditory Brainstem Response.**

AER
The abbreviation for Auditory Evoked Response.
> *Refer to* **Auditory Brainstem Response.**

Aeration (er-AY-shuhn)
1. The exposure of blood to air and *oxygen*, such as takes place in the *lungs*. (*Carbon dioxide* is exchanged with oxygen.)
2. The charging of a liquid substance with air, oxygen, or carbon dioxide.

af-
A prefix meaning to.

AFDC
The abbreviation for Aid to Families with Dependent Children.

Afebrile (a-FEB-ril or ay-FEB-ril)
Without a fever.
> *Compare* **Febrile.**

Affect (AF-fekt)
The outward signs of a child's emotion, intent, or desire, such as a smile, grimace, or *tone* of voice. The *brain* imprints information more efficiently when learning occurs along with increased affect.
> *Compare* **Flat Affect.**

Affective Exchanges
Reciprocal (back and forth) verbal and/or nonverbal exchanges (i.e., using words, facial expression, body language, and *gestures*) between two people emotionally engaged with intention and purpose.

Afferent (AF-er-ent)
Moving from the surface of a body organ to the center, as in *veins* that carry blood to the *heart*, or *nerves* that carry impulses to the *central nervous system*.
> *Compare* **Efferent.**

Affricate (AF-ri-kit)
A speech sound produced when the breath stream is completely stopped and then released at articulation. The /ch/, /g/, and /j/ sounds are affricates.

AFO
The abbreviation for ankle-foot orthosis.

AFP
The abbreviation for Alpha-fetoprotein.

Afterbirth
Refer to **Placenta.**

AGA
The abbreviation for appropriate (or average) for gestational age.

Aganglionic Megacolon (uh-gang-lee-ON-ik MEG-uh-koe-luhn))
Refer to **Hirschsprung Disease.**

Age-Equivalent Score
The age (in years and months) that a child's performance is typical of in the non-disabled population. For example, if a child's ability to understand words is age equivalent to 2-10, this means he can understand the same vocabulary that a typically-developing 2-year, 10-month-old child can.
Compare **Standard Score.**

Agenesia Corticalis (uh-je-NEE-see-uh kor-ti-KAL-is)
A condition in which some of the *embryo's brain cells* do not grow, causing loss of *motor* function and *severe mental retardation* in the infant.

Agenesis (uh-JEN-e-sis)
The complete or partial absence of an *organ* or body part at birth, due to a lack of *embryonic* development.

Agenesis of Corpus Callosum (ACC)
(uh-JEN-e-sis of KOR-pus ka-LOE-sum)
A condition in which the *corpus callosum* of the *brain* fails to form (leaving the two *cerebral hemispheres* unjoined) or forms incompletely. A child with this defect may have difficulty transferring information from one cerebral hemisphere to the other, affecting language ability. Since the two hemispheres of the brain are capable of functioning independently of each other, agenesis of the corpus callosum alone does not seriously impair intellectual abilities. However, ACC can occur in combination with other brain malformations, which may then result in *mental retardation, seizures,* or other *central nervous system* problems.
Also known as **Corpus Callosum Agenesis.**

Ages and Stages Questionnaires® (ASQ): A Parent-Completed, Child Monitoring System, Second Edition
A tool to screen for *developmental delay* in infants and young children up to 5 years of age. *Intervention* activities are included.

Ages and Stages Questionnaires®: Social-Emotional (ASQ:SE): A Parent-Completed, Child Monitoring System for Social-Emotional Behaviors
A companion tool to the *Ages and Stages Questionnaires* that identifies 6- to 60-month-olds at risk for *social/emotional* difficulties. *Intervention* activities are included.

Agnosia (ag-NOE-zhuh)
Loss of the ability to interpret visual, *auditory*, or other sensations even though the sight, *hearing*, or other *sensory* organs are intact. This type of *sensory impairment* is caused by damage to the *brain*.
> *Refer to* **Auditory Agnosia** *and* **Verbal Auditory Agnosia**.

Agonist Muscle (AG-uh-nist)
A muscle that is opposed by an *antagonist muscle* as it contracts to move a part of the body. Muscles work as both agonists and antagonists, contracting to bring about an action, and stretching in the opposite direction for reverse movements, such as in *flexion* and *extension*.
> *Compare* **Antagonist Muscle**.

AGS
The abbreviation for Alagille Syndrome.

Agyria (uh-JIE-ree-uh)
> *Refer to* **Lissencephaly**.

Aicardi Syndrome
A rare X-*linked dominant disorder* (occurring primarily in females) characterized by *agenesis of corpus callosum*, *vertebral* and eye *anomalies*, *infantile spasms* (a form of *seizures*), and *mental retardation*.

AIDS
The abbreviation for Acquired Immune Deficiency Syndrome.

Aid to Families with Dependent Children (AFDC)
A federally and state funded financial assistance program that provides money to qualified needy individuals who have children under age 19. An AFDC check is sometimes referred to as a "welfare" check.
> *Refer to* **Department of Public Social Services**.

AIT
The abbreviation for Auditory Integration Training/Therapy.

Akinetic Seizure (ay-kin-ET-ik)
A *generalized* minor *motor seizure*.
> *Refer to* **Atonic Seizure**.

Alagille Syndrome (AGS) (ah-la-ZHEEL)
An *autosomal dominant disorder* in which there are too few *bile* ducts in the liver. It is characterized by newborn *jaundice*; *cholestasis*; *pulmonary stenosis* (that can cause *heart murmurs*) and occasionally other *heart anomalies*; unusual *facies* (a prominent forehead, nasal bridge, and ears; deep set eyes that are sometimes widely spaced apart; and a small chin); and eye, *spinal column*, and *nervous system abnormalities*.
> *Also known as* **Arteriohepatic Dysplasia**.

Albinism (AL-bin-izm)

A *congenital* condition characterized by partial or total lack of pigment (color) in the skin, hair, and eyes. Certain eye *disorders* (*astigmatism, photophobia,* and *nystagmus*) may be associated with albinism.

Albumin (al-BYOO-min)

A *protein* that expands the volume of blood and is used for treating *hyperbilirubinemia* and other *disorders*.

Albuterol (al-BYOO-ter-ol)

A *bronchodilator drug* used to treat *asthma* and *bronchitis*. Proventil™ is the brand name of this drug.

Alcohol-Related Neurodevelopmental Disorder (ARND)

A combination of *congenital abnormalities* caused by *maternal* consumption of alcohol during pregnancy. The effects of alcohol on the infant include growth retardation and *central nervous system neurodevelopmental abnormalities*—the same as those present in a child with *fetal alcohol spectrum disorder (FASD.)* However, the characteristic facial features of a child with FASD are not required for the ARND *diagnosis*. Research shows that children with such *fetal alcohol effects* may be just as affected (have as difficult a time functioning and adapting) as children with FASD or *prenatal exposure to drugs*.

> *Formerly known as* **Fetal Alcohol Effects.**
> *Compare* **Partial Fetal Alcohol Syndrome.**
> *Refer to* **Fetal Alcohol Spectrum Disorder (FASD)** *and* **Fetal Alcohol Syndrome (FAS).**

ALD

The abbreviation for Adrenoleukodystrophy.

Aldactone™ (al-DAK-toen)

> *Refer to* **Spironolactone.**

-algia

A suffix meaning pain.

Alimentary (al-e-MEN-tar-ee)

Pertaining to food or a nutritive substance, or to the organs of *digestion*.

Allen Cards

A *visual acuity* test in which the preschooler (as young as 2½ years of age) is asked to name pictures at a distance of 20 feet.

Allergen (AL-er-jen)

A foreign substance that can cause an *allergic* response in susceptible people. Examples of allergens include airborne pollens, molds, and animal dander; and foods such as dairy products, cereals, and strawberries.

Allergenic (al-er-JEN-ik)
Capable of causing an *allergic* response in susceptible people.
    Refer to **Allergy/Allergic.**

Allergy/Allergic
A sensitivity to a generally harmless substance. Exposure to an *allergen* causes *symptoms* of allergic reaction (an adverse physical reaction) in susceptible people, but causes no response in others, and may be mild in some (such as a runny nose), and severe in others (such as *shock*).
    Refer to **Antihistamine Drug** and **Epinephrine.**

Alopecia Areata (al-uh-PEE-shuh er-ee-AY-tuh)
Patchy hair loss possibly caused by *disease* affecting the *immune system*. The most common cause of hair loss in children, alopecia areata often clears without treatment in 6 to 12 months.

Alpern-Boll Developmental Profile
    Refer to **Developmental Profile II.**

Alpha-fetoprotein (AFP) (AL-fuh fee-toe-PROE-teen)
A *protein* produced by the *fetus* that flows from the *amniotic fluid* to the mother's blood. An unusually low level of AFP has been found in women who gave birth to children with *Down syndrome*. An unusually high level of AFP has been associated with *neural tube defects, twin* pregnancies, or threatened or actual *miscarriages*.

Alpha Wave (AL-fuh)
One of the four types of *brain waves* creating the rhythm of electrical activity as seen on an *EEG*. Alpha waves are normally seen when a child is awake but relaxed (not alert) and with the eyes closed. Alpha waves are characterized by a relatively high voltage and a *frequency* of 8 to 13 *Hz*.
    Compare **Beta Wave, Delta Wave,** *and* **Theta Wave.**
    Refer to **Brain Wave.**

Alport Syndrome
A *genetic disorder* characterized by *congenital*, progressive *sensorineural hearing impairment*, *kidney* malfunction, and occasionally eye defects. Alport syndrome can be *inherited* as an *autosomal dominant disorder*, but is most commonly an X-linked disorder resulting from *mutations* of the type IV *collagen gene*.

Alprostadil (al-PROS-tuh-dil)
A drug given to newborns who have certain types of *heart defects* to help with blood flow.

Alternative Communication
    Refer to **Augmentative and Alternative Communication.**

Alupent™ (AL-yoo-pent)
    Refer to **Metaproterenol Sulfate.**

alve-
A prefix meaning channel or cavity.

Alveolar Ridge
The ridge of the *hard palate* just behind the upper teeth.
> *Refer to* **Hard Palate.**

Alveolars
Speech sounds produced when the tongue touches or approximates the *alveolar ridge*. The /t/ and /d/ sounds are examples of alveolar speech sounds.

Alveoli (al-VEE-oe-lie)
1. Tiny air sacs in the *lungs* where *carbon dioxide* leaves the blood and *oxygen* enters the bloodstream.
2. Tiny sacs in the milk *glands* of the breast where nutrients from the mother's bloodstream are converted to milk.

Alveolus (al-VEE-oe-lus)
Singular of *alveoli*.

Amblyopia (am-blee-OE-pee-uh)
A condition affecting *visual acuity* that can lead to loss of vision in an eye that is structurally capable of seeing. Amblyopia develops when corresponding images are not formed on the *retinas* of both eyes. The *brain* suppresses vision in one eye to prevent blurred or double vision. Over time, this suppression causes permanent *visual impairment* in that eye. Vision can be maintained if the underlying cause (usually *strabismus*, a *cataract*, or *astigmatism*) is corrected while the child is young (before 8 years of age). Treatment may include eyeglasses, *patching*, or surgery.

Ambulate/Ambulatory
Able to walk or move about.
> *Compare* **Nonambulatory.**

Amelioration (uh-meel-yoe-RAY-shuhn)
The process of lessening pain or improving *symptoms*.

American Academy of Pediatrics (AAP)
A professional organization for physicians with specialty training in the diseases and disorders of childhood.

American Association on Mental Deficiency (AAMD)
> *Refer to* **American Association on Mental Retardation.**

American Association on Mental Retardation (AAMR)
A professional organization established to promote research in *mental retardation* and development of services for individuals with mental retardation. Information regarding the prevention of mental retardation is available through the AAMR.
> *Formerly known as* **American Association on Mental Deficiency.**

American Psychiatric Association (APA)

An organization for *psychiatrists*, other *physicians*, mental health professionals, and other professionals that promotes research and education, and provides information to the public. The APA works to improve the treatment and rehabilitation of children and adults with mental illness, *mental retardation*, and emotional problems. The APA publishes the *Diagnostic and Statistical Manual of Mental Disorders*.

American Sign Language (ASL)

A complex visual-spatial language used by the *Deaf* community and those with *auditory impairment* in the US. This method of communicating relies on hand signs and facial expression. Each sign represents either one word or a concept that is typically expressed with several spoken words. For words that do not have a sign, *fingerspelling* is used. In addition to the hand shape that is made, the location of the hand, its movement in a specific direction, and its placement in relation to the palm of the other hand are all components that are used to express a word or concept.

Refer to **Signed Exact English** *and* **Sign Language.**

Americans with Disabilities Act (ADA) of 1990 (Public Law 101-336)

The federal law that states that individuals with *disabilities* must be afforded the same opportunities to participate in our society and obtain the same benefit from that participation as their peers without disabilities. This law prohibits *discrimination* against people with disabilities in employment, public *accommodations*, and access to public facilities. The ADA took affect in 1992.

Amino Acids

Chemicals that, when linked together, form *proteins* essential for growth and health. The body produces some amino acids, which are called nonessential amino acids. Other amino acids, which must be obtained through diet, are called essential amino acids.

Aminoaciduria (uh-mee-noe-as-i-DYOO-ree-uh)

The excessive *excretion* of *amino acids* in the urine, often the result of an *inherited metabolic disease*. Aminoaciduria results in *failure to thrive* and is not treatable.

Aminophylline (uh-mee-noe-FIL-in)

A *bronchodilator drug*.

Amniocentesis (am-nee-oe-sen-TEE-sis)

A *prenatal* test in which a needle is inserted into the pregnant woman's *abdomen* and *uterus* and *amniotic fluid* is withdrawn. The fluid is analyzed to detect *genetic disorders* including *metabolic* and *chromosomal disorders*, and *neural tube defects*; to measure *alpha-fetoprotein* levels; to assess the maturity of the *fetus's lungs*; and to determine the fetus's age and gender.

Amniotic Band Disruption Sequence Syndrome

A condition of pregnancy in which fibrous *bands* develop within the *uterus* entangling the *fetus* and causing structural and functional *anomalies*, such as *clubfeet*, missing *limbs*, *simian creases*, and skull and internal organ defects. Amniotic band disruption sequence syndrome can be detected *prenatally* and specific medical treatments may be possible.

Also known as **Amniotic Band Syndrome.**

Amniotic Band Syndrome

Refer to **Amniotic Band Disruption Sequence Syndrome.**

Amniotic Fluid (am-nee-OT-ik)

The fluid surrounding the *fetus* in the *uterus* of the pregnant mother.

Amoxicillin (uh-moks-i-SIL-in)

A type of *penicillin* (*antibiotic*) drug used to treat *infections*. Augmentin™ is the brand name of this drug.

Amphetamine (am-FET-uh-meen)

A group of *nervous system stimulant drugs* used to help increase attention and help the child focus.

Ampicillin (am-pi-SIL-in)

A type of *penicillin* (*antibiotic*) drug used to treat *infections*.

Amplification

The process of increasing or enhancing sound.

Amygdala (a-MIG-duh-luh)

A small mass of *gray matter* (nervous *tissue*) of the *brain* believed to be involved in memory processing and in producing and responding to negative emotions (such as "learned fear").

Amyotonia (ay-mie-oe-TOE-nee-uh)

A muscle defect characterized by loss of *tone*, weakness, and wasting due to *disease* of the *nerves* that send signals from the *brain* to the muscles.

an-

A prefix meaning not, without, or lack.

Anabolic Steroid (an-uh-BOL-ik STEER-oid)

Refer to **Steroids.**

Anaclitic Depression (an-uh-KLIT-ik di-PRESH-uhn)

A *disorder* in infants that occurs after sudden separation from the mother or *primary caregiver*, characterized by tension, fear, withdrawal, incessant crying, and sleeping and eating problems. The infant who experiences this *trauma* may become extremely passive and unresponsive.

Anafranil™ (uh-NAF-ruh-nil)

Refer to **Clomipramine Hydrochloride.**

Anal Atresia (AY-huhl uh-TREE-zhuh)
Refer to **Imperforate Anus**.

Anal Fissure (FISH-uhr)
Refer to **Fissure**.

Anaphylaxis
An acute life-threatening hypersensitivity (*allergic*) reaction after exposure to a previously encountered *allergen*. Symptoms may include itching, *urticaria*, *bronchospasm*, difficult breathing, *hypotension*, *blood vessel* collapse, and *shock*.
Refer to **Allergy** *and* **EpiPen**™.

andr-, andro-
Prefixes meaning man or male.

Anemia (uh-NEE-mee-uh)
A condition in which the *hemoglobin* in the blood is too low. *Symptoms* of anemia include fatigue, dizziness, headache, pale coloring, and *heart* palpitations (rapid, strong beats). There are several types and causes of anemia, which, along with the speed of development of the anemia, can affect the severity. The most common type of anemia is caused by *iron* deficiency.
Refer to **Aplastic Anemia, Sickle Cell Anemia,** *and* **Thalassemia**.

Anencephaly (an-en-SEF-uh-lee)
A *congenital anomaly* in which all but the most primitive part of the *brain*, *spinal cord*, and overlying bones of the *skull* are absent, due to failure of the *neural tube* to close during early *fetal* development. A baby born with this anomaly will not survive the newborn period.

Anergy (AN-er-jee)
1. A lack of activity or energy.
2. A condition of the *immune system* in which the body does not mount a normal sensitivity reaction to a substance that would usually be *allergenic*. Anergy may occur in people with serious *infections*, *AIDS*, and some *malignancies*.

Anesthesia/Anesthetic (an-es-THEE-zee-uh/an-es-THET-ik)
Medication that causes loss of sensation. Local anesthesia causes loss of feeling, thereby obstructing pain, in the area where it is injected. General anesthesia can be injected into the bloodstream or inhaled prior to surgery, causing lack of consciousness and loss of feeling throughout the body.
Refer to **Nerve Block Anesthesia**.

Anesthesiologist (an-es-thee-zee-OL-oe-jist)
A doctor trained to administer *anesthesia* and to assess and monitor the lungs, *heart*, and *circulation* before and during surgery.

Angelman Syndrome (AYN-juhl-muhn)
A *chromosomal disorder* linked to the *deletion* of *genetic* material from the long arm of chromosome 15. Usually the *abnormality* is *inherited* from the

mother but can also result from a *uniparental disomy* (i.e., if the child receives two structurally normal chromosome 15s from the father and none from the mother) or from a *mutation*. Often referred to as *"Happy Puppet syndrome,"* Angelman syndrome is characterized by *severe mental retardation*; *microcephaly*; unusual *craniofacial* features, including *microbrachycephaly* (a small, short head), *occipital* groove (resulting in a flattened back of the head), *hypoplasia* of the *midface*, a protruding lower jaw, a large mouth with a large tongue, widely spaced teeth, and decreased eye pigmentation resulting in pale blue eyes; ataxic, jerky movements and stiff *gait* due to *contracture* of *proximal joints* (giving the "puppet"-like appearance); *paroxysms* of laughing (unconnected to feelings of happiness) that usually develop between 12-36 months of age; no development of speech; *hypotonia*; and occasionally, *epilepsy* that usually develops between 18-24 months of age.

angi-, angio-
Prefixes meaning *vessel*.

Angina (an-JIE-nuh or AN-ji-nuh)
Severe pain in the chest, in the area of the *heart*, caused by an inadequate supply of *oxygen* to the heart muscle.

Angiography (an-jee-OG-ruh-fee)
An *x-ray* study that involves injecting contrast materials into *blood vessels* so the vessels may be visualized. A sequence of x-rays is taken to examine the flow of blood within a particular organ.

Angioma (an-jee-OE-muh)
A harmless *tumor*, usually present at birth, made up mainly of *blood vessels* or *lymph* vessels.

Angular Movement
Movement that creates an angle of varying degree. For example, the angle between the upper and lower leg gets bigger or smaller as the leg is straightened or bent at the knee. Angular movement is one of four basic kinds of movement by the *joints* of the body.
>   Compare **Circumduction Movement, Gliding Movement,** and **Rotation Movement.**

Aniridia (an-i-RID-ee-uh)
Absence of an *iris* of the eye at birth, resulting in some degree of *visual impairment*.

Aniridia-Wilms Tumor Association (an-i-RID-ee-uh VILMS)
>   *Refer to* **WAGR Syndrome.**

Anisometropia (an-i-soe-me-TROE-pee-uh)
A condition in which there is a significant difference in the *refractive* (focusing) power between the two eyes.

Ankle-Foot Orthosis (AFO)
A short leg *brace* that provides support at the ankle.
    Refer to **Orthosis**.

ankyl-
A prefix meaning crooked or growing together, such as the stiffening of a *joint* that results in it remaining fixed in a (usually) *abnormal* position.

Ankyloglossia (ang-ki-loe-GLOS-ee-uh)
A condition in which the tongue is fused to the floor of the mouth, restricting the tongue's movement. Surgery to reconstruct the tongue and the floor of the mouth is required. Partial ankyloglossia (sometimes referred to as tongue-tie) occurs when the *lingual frenum* is too short or is attached too close to the tip of the tongue to allow adequate movement of the tongue. A simple surgical procedure can correct the condition. These conditions can negatively affect speech and possibly eating.

Ankylosis (ang-ki-LOE-sis)
The stiffening of a *joint*, usually into an *abnormal* position, resulting in loss of movement in the joint. It is caused by *degeneration* of the bone, followed by fusion of the two bone surfaces that form the joint. Ankylosis may result from injury, *infection*, or *inflammation*, or it may be the result of *arthrodesis* (a procedure in which the joint is surgically fused).

Annual Goal
A statement of the desired outcome of *early intervention* services for a specific child and his family. For example, an annual goal might be for the child to develop mobility skills. Annual goals are selected by the child's parents and early intervention *multidisciplinary team* and are stated on the *Individualized Family Service Plan* (IFSP). *Objectives*, which are more specific and measurable, such as "(child's name) will *creep* forward on his hands and knees for 10 feet" and "will walk forward with both hands held for 15 feet" may also be stated to provide *developmentally* appropriate activities and measurement of progress toward attainment of the goal.
    Also known as **Outcome**.

Annual Review
An annual report describing a child who is *at-risk* or has *disabilities*, including his health status, needs, strengths, eligibility for *early intervention* services, current functioning level, family involvement, family financial situation, rights, legal status, involvement with service providers and *physicians*, assessment of progress toward meeting the goals stated on the *Individualized Family Service Plan*, and discussion of any new areas of *intervention* from which the child would benefit. Usually, the *service coordinator* is the professional who completes the annual review.

Annular Pancreas (AN-yuh-luhr PAN-cree-uhs)
A *congenital* anatomical *anomaly*, sometimes seen in children with *Down syndrome*, in which the *pancreas* is ring-shaped and encircles the *duodenum*. This

can result in narrowing or blockage of the *small intestine*. If *bowel* obstruction occurs, surgery will be required.

Anomalies (uh-NOM-uh-leez)
Plural of *anomaly*.

Anomalous Pulmonary Venous Return
(uh-NOM-uh-luhs PUL-moe-ne-ree VEE-nuhs)
> *Refer to* **Total Anomalous Pulmonary Venous Return.**

Anomaly (uh-NOM-uh-lee)
A change or *deviation* from what is considered normal, such as a malformation of part of the body. A missing finger and an extra finger are examples of anomalies.
> *Refer to* **Congenital Anomaly.**

Anophthalmos (an-of-THAL-mos)
Absence of an eyeball, occurring either as a *congenital anomaly* or due to surgical removal.

Anorectal (ay-noe-REK-tuhl)
Referring to the *anus* and *rectum*.

Anoxia (uh-NOK-see-uh)
A condition in which there is insufficient *oxygen* to an individual *organ* or to the whole body. Anoxia can occur when there is a decreased amount of oxygen to the *lungs*, when the blood is not able to deliver oxygen to body *tissues*, or when the tissues are not able to absorb the oxygen from the blood. Anoxia can be life-threatening, such as when the *brain* receives too little oxygen. Anoxia during *fetal* development can lead to *mental retardation*.

Antagonist Muscle
A muscle that acts in opposition to the action of another muscle (an *agonist*), stretching as the agonist muscle contracts. The antagonist muscle is responsible for bringing a body part back to its resting position.
> *Compare* **Agonist Muscle.**

ante-
A prefix meaning before.

Antecedent (an-ti-SEE-duhnt)
The event or condition that immediately precedes a *behavior*. Determining the antecedent (i.e., cause) of a behavior is an important step when using *applied behavior analysis* (*ABA*).

Antepartum (an-tee-PAR-tuhm)
Before birth.
> *Compare* **Postpartum.**

Anterior
Front.
> *Also known as* **Ventral.**
> *Compare* **Posterior.**

Anteversion (an-tee-VER-zhun)
The position of an *organ* or structure that is *abnormally* tilted forward.

anti-
A prefix meaning against.

Antianxiety Drug (an-tie-ang-ZIE-uh-tee)
> *Refer to* **Anxiolytic Drug.**

Antibacterial Drug (an-ti-bak-TEE-ree-uhl)
A drug used to treat *infections* caused by *bacteria* by destroying or suppressing growth of the bacteria.

Antibiotic Drug (an-ti-bie-OT-ik)
A drug that kills *organisms* (such as *bacteria*) or halts their growth. Antibiotics are not effective for treating *viral infections*.

Antibody (Ab) (AN-ti-bod-ee)
A *protein* produced by the body that combats *antigens* (such as those found in *viruses*, *bacteria*, and other *microorganisms*).
> *Also known as* **Immune Body.**

Anticholinergic Drug (an-ti-koe-lin-ER-jik)
A drug that blocks the effect of *acetylcholine* and decreases muscle *spasms*.

Anticonvulsant Drug
> *Refer to* **Antiepileptic Drug.**

Antidepressant Drug (an-tie-dee-PRES-uhnt)
A drug used to treat *depression*.

Antidiuretic Hormone
> *Refer to* **Diabetes Insipidus.**
> *Compare* **Diuretic.**

Antiepileptic Drug (an-ti-ep-i-LEP-tik)
A drug that prevents or arrests *seizure* activity, or lessens the severity of the seizures. Antiepileptics work by quieting the *abnormally* high electrical activity in the *brain* and preventing the spread of the activity to other areas of the brain.
> *Also known as an* **Anticonvulsant Drug.**

Antifungal Drug (an-ti-FUNG-guhl)
A drug used to treat *infections* caused by *fungi* such as *candidiasis*. Antifungal drugs destroy or suppress growth of fungi.

Antigen (AN-ti-jen)
A substance that activates the body's *immune system* to produce an *antibody*.

Antigravity Activity
An activity that requires a baby to resist gravity, such as sitting up.

Antigravity Position
A position that requires a baby to resist gravity, such as an all-fours position (weight on hands and knees), sitting, and standing.

Antihistamine Drug (an-ti-HIS-tuh-meen)
A drug that decreases the effects of histamine, a chemical made by the body. (Histamines can cause *symptoms* of *allergic* reactions.)

Antipsychotic Drug (an-ti-sie-KOT-ik)
A drug used to treat *symptoms* of *psychosis*.

Antispastic Drug
A drug used to reduce *spasticity*.

Antiviral Drug (an-tie-VIE-ruhl)
A drug that is destructive to *viruses*.

antr-
A prefix meaning chamber.

Anus (AY-nus)
The opening at the *distal* (farthest from origin) end of the *rectum* through which *feces* are evacuated from the *bowel*.

Anvil (AN-vil)
    *Refer to **Incus**.*

Anxiety (ang-ZIE-uh-tee)
A feeling of unease, dread, fear, or nervousness, which can be accompanied by physical *symptoms* such as increased *heart rate* or sweating. Some degree of anxiety may be normal (for example, in new situations), but when anxiety is irrational, excessive, or causes distress or impairment, it can be part of an *anxiety disorder.*
    *Refer to **Anxiety Disorder**.*

Anxiety Disorder
A *psychiatric* illness characterized by high levels of *anxiety* that causes distress or impairment to the individual. Types of anxiety disorders include phobias (fear of some specific thing), generalized anxiety disorder, panic disorder, and post traumatic stress disorder, among others. A child under 3 years old with an anxiety disorder may exhibit *symptoms* such as persistent fearfulness, hypervigilance, agitation, avoidance, panic reactions, worries, excessive *tantrums*, distress, and *obsessions* or preoccupations.
    *Refer to **Anxiety**.*

Anxiolytic Drug (ang-zie-oe-LIT-ik)
A drug used to relieve *anxiety*.

Aorta (ay-OR-tuh)
The *artery* that carries *oxygenated* blood from the left *ventricle* of the *heart* to the rest of the body.
    Refer to **Circulation.**

Aortic Coarctation (ay-OR-tik koe-ark-TAY-shuhn)
Refer to **Coarctation of the Aorta.**

Aortic Stenosis (AS)(ay-OR-tik ste-NOE-sis)
A defect of the *heart* in which the *aortic valve* between the left *ventricle* and the *aorta* is narrowed, blocking the flow of blood at the left ventricle into the aorta. Aortic stenosis causes the ventricle to work harder to move blood past the blockage and may result in a decreased output of blood from the heart, lung congestion, and *congestive heart failure*. Surgical repair may be necessary, with frequent examinations after surgery. Children with AS are usually restricted from strenuous play.

Aortic Valve
One of four *valves* in the *heart* that open and close with each heartbeat to control the flow of blood. Blood exits each chamber of the heart through one of the valves. The aortic valve is located between the left *ventricle* and the *aorta*. The three cusps (small flaps) of the aortic valve close during each heartbeat to prevent blood from flowing back into the left ventricle from the aorta.
    Compare **Mitral Valve, Pulmonary Valve,** *and* **Tricuspid Valve.**

ap
The abbreviation for the Latin words meaning before dinner.

APA
The abbreviation for American Psychiatric Association.

Apathy
Indifference.

Apert Syndrome (AY-pert or uh-PAYR)
A *genetic disorder* characterized by irregular and premature fusion of skull bones, underdevelopment of facial bones, wide-spaced and bulging eyes, fused or *webbed* fingers and toes, and sometimes *mental retardation*. The child with Apert syndrome is often challenged by speech and language, and *cognitive* impairment as well as *conductive hearing impairment*. Apert syndrome most often results from a genetic *mutation* but it also occurs as an *autosomal dominant disorder*.
    Also known as **Acrocephalosyndactyly, Type I.**

Aperture (AP-uh-chuhr)
An opening or *orifice*.

Apex
The top or tip of a body structure.

Apgar Score (AP-gar)
The score given to a *newborn* to determine overall physical condition. The infant is tested at 1 and 5 (and sometimes 10) minutes after delivery on the following: color, *heart rate, respiratory* effort, *muscle tone*, and *reflexes*. A score of 0-2 is given in each of the five categories with a maximum total score of 10. An infant with a score of 0-3 is considered to be in severe distress and needing *cardiopulmonary resuscitation*; a score of 4-6 indicates moderate distress; and a score of 7-10 is normal, indicating a well baby.
> *Refer to the* **Apgar Chart** *in the Appendix.*

Aphakia (uh-FAY-kee-uh)
Absence of the *lens* of the eye, either at birth or due to surgical removal. Extreme *farsightedness* results without a lens.

Aphasia (uh-FAY-zee-uh)
A *communication disorder* characterized by difficulty with producing *language* (expressive aphasia) and/or with understanding language (receptive aphasia). Aphasia is caused by *brain damage* that may result from lack of *oxygen*, severe head injury, or a *stroke* that causes *nerve* damage.
> *Refer to* **Broca's Aphasia, Landau-Kleffner Syndrome, Paraphasia**, *and* **Wernicke's Aphasia.**

APIB
The abbreviation for Assessment of Pre-Term Infant Behavior.

Aplasia (uh-PLAY-zhuh)
Defective development or *congenital* absence of an *organ* or *tissue* at birth.

Aplastic Anemia (uh-PLAS-tik uh-NEE-mee-uh)
A form of *anemia* characterized by reduced *red blood cell, white blood cell*, and *platelet* cell formation caused by damage to the *bone marrow*. The bone marrow may be damaged during *radiation therapy*, or when exposed to certain drugs (including anticancer drugs) or poisonous chemicals. Sometimes the cause of aplastic anemia is not known.

Apnea (ap-NEE-uh)
A pause in breathing that lasts 20 seconds or longer, or any pause in breathing accompanied by *cyanosis* and *bradycardia*.
> *Compare* **Periodic Breathing.**

Apnea Monitor
A monitor that sounds an alarm when an infant has a period of *apnea*. The apnea monitor can be set for any time period, but is usually set at 20 seconds.

apo-
A prefix meaning detached, without, or separation from.

Appendix (uh-PEN-diks)
A projection extending from the *cecum* (a pouch that forms the first portion of the *large intestine*). The appendix itself has no known function, but it contains *lymphoid tissue* (tissue resembling *lymph*, a body fluid that plays an important role in the *immune system* and in absorbing *fats* from the intestine), which provides a defense against local *infection*.

Apperception (ap-uhr-SEP-shun)
A person's awareness and understanding of *sensory stimuli* based on his previous experiences, his thoughts, and his feelings.
> *Compare* **Perception.**

Applied Behavior Analysis (ABA)
A behavioral approach that uses research-based, highly structured teaching procedures to develop skills in individuals, particularly those with an *autism spectrum disorder*. An emphasis is placed on modifying *behavior* in a precisely measurable manner using repeated trials.
> *Refer to* **Discrete Trial Instruction.**

Appropriate for Gestational Age (AGA)
Referring to a baby whose *birth weight* is between the 10th and 90th percentiles for his *gestational age*.
> *Also known as* **Average for Gestational Age.**
> *Compare* **Large for Gestational Age** and **Small for Gestational Age.**
> *Refer to the* **CDC Growth Charts** *in the Appendix.*

Apraxia (uh-PRAK-see-uh)
A loss of the ability to perform voluntary, purposeful movements due to damage to the *brain* (although there is no actual *paralysis*). Because of this damage, the brain is unable to make the transfer between the idea of movement to an actual physical response. Examples of apraxia include the inability to perform the movements of a command (such as, "clap your hands"), to repeat words correctly, or to demonstrate understanding of the use of an object. The damage to the brain that causes apraxia may result from a head injury, a brain *tumor*, an *infection*, or a *stroke*.

Apraxic
> *Refer to* **Apraxia.**

Aqueduct of Sylvius
> *Refer to* **Cerebral Aqueduct.**

Aqueductal Stenosis (aw-kwuh-DUK-tuhl sti-NOE-sis)
A narrowing of the *cerebral aqueduct* (the canal through which *cerebrospinal fluid* passes) in the *midbrain*. It can be a *congenital* or *acquired* condition and can cause *hydrocephalus*. Aqueductal stenosis can occur with *neurofibromatosis*, or result from *tumors* or *cysts*.

Aqueous Humor (AY-kwee-us HYOO-mor)
The fluid produced in the eye.

Arachnodactyly (uh-rak-noe-DAK-ti-lee)
A *congenital* condition (seen in *Marfan syndrome*) in which a baby is born with long, thin spider-like fingers and toes.

Arachnoid (uh-RAK-noid)
The middle layer of the *meninges* (the *membranes* that surround the *brain* and *spinal cord*). The *pia mater* is the innermost layer and the *dura mater* is the outermost layer.
    Refer to **Meninges.**

ARC (The ARC of the United States)
A national organization formerly known as the Association for Retarded Citizens. It provides advocacy services to individuals with *mental retardation* and their families, and publishes and disseminates information about mental retardation. The ARC has local and state branches throughout the United States.

Arch Insole Pad
A small pad that can be placed in a child's shoe to provide arch support. A Scaphoid Pad is an example of one type.

Arginase Deficiency (AR-jin-ays)
An *autosomal recessive amino acid disorder* characterized by an enlarged *liver*, *mental retardation*, and *spastic diplegia*. Restricting the child's diet can prevent *symptoms* from progressing.

Argininosuccinic Acidemia (ar-jin-in-oe-suk-SIN-ik as-i-DEE-mee-uh)
An *inherited disorder* of *amino acid metabolism* characterized by *seizures* and *mental retardation*. Treatment mostly consists of dietary restrictions.

ARND
The abbreviation for Alcohol Related Neurodevelopmental Disorder.

Arnold-Chiari Malformation (AR-noelt KEE-a-ree)
A *congenital hernia* of the *brainstem* and *cerebellum* that can block the outflow of *cerebrospinal fluid* from the *ventricles* of the *brain*. *Hydrocephalus* is a common *symptom*. This defect often occurs with *spina bifida* or other brain and *spine disorders*.

AROM
The abbreviation for active range of motion.

Arousal Level
The degree of alertness with which an infant responds to *stimuli*. For example, when the newborn is being assessed, it is important to note the infant's arousal level, or *state* of alertness. The states of alertness include: deep sleep;

sleep with rapid eye movements; drowsiness; a quiet, alert state (the state of alertness at which the infant can best respond to and interact with people and things in his environment); an awake and active state; and a state of active, intense crying.

Arrhythmia (uh-RITH-mee-uh)
Any change in the rhythm or rate of the heartbeat. Arrhythmias occur when electrical conduction to or within the *heart* fails.

Arterial (ar-TEE-ree-uhl)
Pertaining to an *artery* or to the arteries.

Arterial Blood Gas
A sampling of blood from an *artery* that is analyzed to determine its *oxygen*, *carbon dioxide*, and acid content.
> *Also known as **Arterial Stick**.*

Arterial Catheter/Arterial Line (ar-TEE-ree-uhl KATH-uh-ter)
A *catheter* placed in an *artery* to provide continuous access to *arterial* blood so it can be withdrawn for monitoring *arterial blood gases* and *blood pressure*. In a newborn, it is usually placed in the *umbilical* artery, but may be placed in the arm or the foot.
> *Refer to **Catheter**.*
> *Also known as **Indwelling Arterial Catheter/Line**.*

Arterial Stick
> *Refer to **Arterial Blood Gas**.*

Arteriogram (ar-TIR-ee-uh-gram)
An *x-ray* film of an *artery* to show blood flow. The procedure is done by injecting dye into the blood stream that shows up on an x-ray.

Arteriohepatic Dysplasia
(ar-tir-ee-oe-he-PAT-ik dis-PLAY-zee-uh or dis-PLAY-zhuh)
> *Refer to **Alagille Syndrome**.*

Arteriole (ar-TIR-ee-oel)
The smallest of the *arteries*.

Artery
Any *blood vessel* that delivers blood from the *heart* to the rest of the body. There are two types of arteries: *systemic arteries*, which carry *oxygenated* blood to all parts of the body except the *lungs*, and *pulmonary arteries*, which carry non-oxygenated blood from the heart to the lungs.

arthro-
A prefix meaning *joint*.

Arthrodesis (ar-throe-DEE-sis)
A surgical procedure in which a *joint* is fused to correct a bone deformity, to provide support, or to relieve pain.
>   *Also known as **Artificial Ankylosis** and **Joint Fusion.***
>   *Refer to **Ankylosis.***

Arthrogryposis (ar-throe-gri-POE-sis)
A condition in which an infant is born with multiple *joint contractures* due to some interference with *fetal* movements. It may be caused by a *neuromuscular* problem, small muscle fibers, or *congenital muscular dystrophy*.

Arthrogryposis Multiplex Congenita
(ar-throe-gri-POE-sis MUHL-ti-pleks kuhn-JEN-i-tuh)
A severe form of *arthrogryposis*. The exact cause is unknown, but may result from *degenerative* changes in *motor nerve cells* or an *abnormality* of muscle possibly due to too little *amniotic fluid in utero*. In addition to the *joint contractures*, there are other bone and muscle *abnormalities*. *Intelligence* is usually unimpaired. Treatment for *motor* impairment may include *physical therapy*, surgery, or casting.
>   *Refer to **Arthrogryposis.***

Arthrosis (ar-THROE-sis)
A *joint*.

Articular
Pertaining to a *joint*.

Articulation
1. The ability to produce and connect *vowel* and *consonant* sounds. This ability is based on the coordination of movements of the lips, tongue, *palate*, and jaw and the manner in which they modify the air stream into meaningful speech sounds.
2. A *joint*, or the site of the junction between two or more bones.

Articulation Disorder
A *speech disorder* in which speech sounds are omitted or produced incorrectly. An articulation disorder may be caused by a structural defect such as *cleft lip* or *cleft palate*, *auditory impairment*, weakness or lack of coordination of the oral musculature, or language delay.
>   *Compare **Language Disorder.***

Artificial Ankylosis (ang-ki-LOE-sis)
>   *Refer to **Arthrodesis.***

Artificial Respiration
The process of breathing for a child either by mechanical means (a *ventilator*) or by *mouth-to-mouth* or mouth-to-nose *resuscitation* when the child is unable to breathe on his own.
>   *Refer to **Resuscitation.***

AS
1. The abbreviation for the Latin words meaning left ear.
2. The abbreviation for Asperger Syndrome.
3. The abbreviation for aortic stenosis.

As and Bs
The abbreviation for apnea and bradycardia spells.
> *Refer to* **Apnea** *and* **Bradycardia.**

ASD
1. The abbreviation for Atrial Septal Defect.
2. The abbreviation for Autism Spectrum Disorder.

-ase
A suffix meaning *enzyme*.

ASL
The abbreviation for American Sign Language.

Asperger's Disorder (AD) (AHS-puhr-guhrs)
An *autism spectrum disorder* (*pervasive developmental disorder*) with similar *diagnostic* criteria to *autistic disorder*, except that individuals with Asperger's Disorder tend to have average or above-average *intelligence* and typical language development. Some children may be diagnosed with autistic disorder when they are young, and then be given the diagnosis of Asperger's Disorder when they are older and show greater skill acquisition. Asperger's Disorder is diagnosed when a child frequently exhibits at least three *symptoms* listed as diagnostic criteria in the *Diagnostic and Statistical Manual of Mental Disorders* (*DSM*), including at least two involving qualitative impairment in *social skills*, and at least one symptom involving restricted and repetitive *behaviors*. The symptoms of social impairment include: 1) marked impairment in the use of multiple nonverbal behaviors such as eye-to-eye gaze, facial expression, body *postures*, and *gestures* to regulate social interaction; 2) failure to develop peer relationships appropriate to *developmental* level; 3) lack of spontaneous seeking to share enjoyment, interests, or achievements with other people; 4) lack of social or emotional *reciprocity*. The symptoms of restricted repetitive and *stereotyped* patterns of behavior, interests, and activities include: 1) encompassing preoccupation with one or more stereotyped and restricted patterns of interest that is *abnormal* either in intensity or focus; 2) apparently inflexible adherence to specific, nonfunctional routines or rituals; 3) stereotyped and repetitive *motor* mannerisms (e.g., *hand* or finger *flapping*); 4) persistent preoccupation with parts of objects. AD occurs more often in boys than girls and, although early *signs* (prior to 3 years of age) are present, AD is often not diagnosed until a child is 6 years or older. Early *developmental milestones* tend to occur at the typical times, with the exception of motor development. These *fine* and *gross motor* delays can make the child appear less coordinated.
> *Also known as* **Asperger Syndrome.**
> *Refer to* **Autism Spectrum Disorder.**

Asperger Syndrome (AS) (AHS-puhr-guhr)
Refer to **Asperger's Disorder**.

Asphyxia (as-FIK-see-uh)
Improper exchange of *oxygen* and *carbon dioxide*, resulting in blood with too little oxygen and too much carbon dioxide, and possibly *brain damage* and death. Asphyxia can be caused by many things, including the stress of *labor* on an infant, drowning, aspirating vomit, or an airway obstruction.
Also known as **Suffocation**.

Asphyxiation
Refer to **Asphyxia**.

Aspiration (as-pi-RAY-shuhn)
1. The act of inhaling.
2. Breathing a foreign material, such as *meconium*, food, or vomit, into the lungs (which may cause *aspiration pneumonia*).
3. Withdrawing blood, *mucus*, or gases from the body by *suctioning*.

Aspiration Pneumonia (as-pi-RAY-shuhn noo-MOE-nee-uh)
Inflammation of the lungs caused by inhaling a foreign material.

Aspirin (AS-pur-in)
A *nonsteroidal anti-inflammatory drug* used to alleviate pain and reduce *inflammation* in *joints* and *soft tissues* and to lower temperature. Aspirin should not be given to children with *viral* infections (such as the *flu* or chickenpox), because it has been implicated in the cause of *Reye syndrome*.

ASQ
The abbreviation for Ages and Stages Questionnaires®.

ASQ:SE
The abbreviation for Ages and Stages Questionnaires: Social-Emotional®.

Assay (AS-ay or a-SAY)
Analysis of a substance (for example, a drug or *hormone*) to determine its presence, amount, and effects on organs.

Assessment
Identification of the needs and strengths of the infant/child who is *at-risk* or has *developmental delays*, as well as those of his family. Assessment may include both formal and informal procedures to appraise the child's abilities in all areas of *development*.
Also known as **Evaluation**.

Assessment in Infancy Ordinal Scales of Psychological Development
An *evaluation* tool used to measure *cognition* in infants between 1 month and 2 years of age. This test is based on *Piaget's* stages of *cognitive development*.
Formerly known as the **Ordinal Scales of Infant Development**.

Assessment of Pre-Term Infant Behavior (APIB)

An *assessment* (adapted from the *Brazelton Neonatal Behavioral Assessment Scale*) used to evaluate the *behaviors* of the *premature infant*. The aim of the APIB is to provide an overall description of the baby, with less emphasis on a score.

Assimilation

1. The process of absorbing and incorporating new concepts or experiences into one's consciousness.
2. The bodily process of metabolizing nutrients constructively.
   Refer to **Nutrition.**

Assistive Technology (AT)

Use of a device (a commercially made piece of equipment or a product system such as an *adaptive* eating device or a powered mobility toy) or a service (such as assisting with the selection, acquisition, or use of a device) to maintain or improve the functional capacities of a child with *special needs*. Assistive technology is one of the considerations mandated on the *Individualized Education Program* (*IEP*) and *Individualized Family Service Plan* (*IFSP*).
   Refer to **Adaptive Switch** *and* **Augmentative and Alternative Communication.**

Associated Reactions

Increased muscle *tension* resulting in *abnormal* patterns of movement or *posture* in various parts of the body due to movement in other body parts. For example, when the child whose legs are affected by *cerebral palsy* attempts to maintain a sitting position, the muscle tension in his arms may increase (even though his arms do not usually appear to have increased *tone*).

Association for Retarded Citizens

The organization now known as the ARC of the United States.
   Refer to **ARC (The ARC of the United States).**

Astatic Seizure (ay-STAT-ik)

   Refer to **Atonic Seizure.**

Asthma (AZ-muh)

A chronic *respiratory disorder* characterized by coughing, *wheezing*, and difficult breathing due to *bronchospasm* (*abnormal contraction* of the *bronchi* resulting in temporarily narrowed airways). Asthmatic attacks may be caused by infection, inhaling *allergens* or irritating airborne substances, exercise, or emotional stress, but sometimes it is difficult to determine what triggers a particular attack.
   Also known as **Bronchial Asthma.**
   Refer to **Albuterol.**

Astigmatism (uh-STIG-muh-tizm)

Defective curvature of the *cornea* or *lens* of the eye. Astigmatism is a common condition that causes blurred vision and can usually be corrected with eyeglasses.

Asymmetric
Not equal on both sides.

Asymmetrical (ay-sim-MET-ri-kuhl)
Referring to parts of the body that are unequal in size or shape, or that are different in arrangement or movement patterns.
Compare **Symmetrical.**

Asymmetrical Tonic Neck Reflex (ATNR)
A normal *reflex* in infants up to 6 months in which turning the head to one side causes the arm and leg on that side to extend and the opposite arm and leg to flex.
Compare **Symmetrical Tonic Neck Reflex.**
Refer to **Primitive Reflex.**

Asymptomatic (ay-simp-toe-MAT-ik)
Without *symptoms*.
Compare **Symptomatic.**

AT
The abbreviation for Assistive Technology.

Ataxia (uh-TAK-see-uh)
Difficulty with coordinating muscles in voluntary movement that may be caused by damage to the *brain* or *spinal cord*. The damage may be the result of a *congenital disorder*, birth *trauma*, infection, *tumor*, *toxin*, or *traumatic brain injury*. Ataxia may be associated with *extrapyramidal cerebral palsy* and may cause the child to have difficulty with maintaining *balance*. It is also a common *side effect* of many *antiepileptic drugs*.

Ataxia-Telangiectasia (uh-TAK-see-uh tel-an-jee-ek-TAY-zee-uh)
A rare *autosomal recessive disorder* characterized by progressive *ataxia* and *choreoathetosis*; dilated *capillaries* visible on the whites of the eyes, the ears, the face, the neck, and the *extremities*; and a poorly functioning *immune system*. Permanent lung damage and *respiratory failure* can result if the immune system is not able to resist infection. *Cognitive* impairment is common in this fatal disorder.
Also known as **Louis-Bar Syndrome.**

Atelectasis (at-ee-LEK-ta-sis)
A condition in which part or all of the lungs is collapsed. Babies born prematurely sometimes experience this condition if their lungs do not expand completely at birth. Atelectasis is characterized by increased *respiratory* distress and may be difficult to differentiate from *pneumonia* on a chest *x-ray*.

Atenolol (a-TEN-uh-lol)
A drug sometimes used in the treatment of certain *autistic-like behaviors* and in the treatment of *angina* and *hypertension*. Tenormin™ is the brand name of this drug.

Athetoid Movements (ATH-e-toid)
Refer to **Athetosis.**

Athetosis (ath-e-TOE-sis)
Slow, involuntary, writhing movements, particularly of the wrist, fingers, face, and occasionally the feet and toes, caused by injury to the *nerves* supplying the muscles or by damage to the *brain*, as in some types of *cerebral palsy*.
Also known as **Athetoid Movements.**

Ativan™ (AT-i-van)
Refer to **Lorazepam.**

Atlantoaxial Instability (at-lan-toe-AK-see-al)
Increased space between the first 2 *vertebrae* of the *spinal column* in the neck causing weakness or instability. It can lead to *subluxation*.
Refer to **Atlantoaxial Subluxation.**

Atlantoaxial Subluxation (at-lan-toe-AK-see-al sub-luks-AY-shuhn)
Partial *dislocation* of the *joint* between the first 2 *vertebrae* in the neck (the *atlas* and the *axis*). It is particularly common in children with *Down syndrome*, most likely due to *lax ligaments*. It may lead to compression of the *spinal cord*, which can cause *paresis* or *paralysis*, and even death.

Atlas
The first *vertebra* lying just beneath the skull. It connects the *occipital* bone of the skull and the *axis* (the second vertebra in the neck).

ATNR
The abbreviation for asymmetrical tonic neck reflex.

Atonic (uh-TON-ik)
Lacking *muscle tone*.
Compare **Tonic.**

Atonic Cerebral Palsy
(uh-TON-ik suh-REE-bruhl or SER-uh-bruhl POL-zee)
A form of *extrapyramidal cerebral palsy* characterized by floppy *muscle tone*. Atonic cerebral palsy results when there is damage to the *nerve* pathways that transmit impulses for controlling movement and maintaining *posture* from the *brain* to the *spinal cord*.
Refer to **Extrapyramidal Cerebral Palsy.**

Atonic Seizure
A *generalized seizure* characterized by a sudden loss of normal *muscle tone* that causes the child to fall, drop objects, or lose consciousness. The seizure typically lasts 1 to 2 seconds and the child is usually unaware of even a brief loss of consciousness. An atonic seizure is similar to an *akinetic seizure*, and the two names are often used interchangeably.
Also known as **Astatic Seizure, Drop Seizure,** *or* **Drop Attack.**
Refer to **Generalized Seizure** *and* **Epilepsy.**

Atony (AT-oe-nee)
A lack of normal *muscle tone* or strength.

Atresia (uh-TREE-zhuh)
A condition in which a normal body opening (such as the *auditory canal* or *anus*) fails to form or closes *prenatally*.

Atresia Choanae (uh-TREE-zhuh KOE-a-nay)
Refer to **Choanal Atresis.**

Atria (AY-tree-uh)
Plural of *atrium.*

Atrial Septal Defect (ASD) (AY-tree-uhl SEP-tuhl)
A form of *congenital heart disease* in which there is a hole between the two *atria* of the heart that allows blood to pass from the left atrium to the right atrium. The blood passage that occurs with this malformation enlarges the right atrium, the right *ventricle*, and the *pulmonary artery*. Surgery to close the hole is usually recommended but postponed until later childhood unless the *anomaly* is severe. Ostium secundum defects, ostium primum defects, and sinus venosus defects are types of atrial septal defects.

Atrioventricular Canal (ay-tree-oe-ven-TRIK-yoo-luhr)
A complex *heart defect* involving holes between the right and left *atria* and the right and left ventricles. Sometimes a baby is also born with a defect of the *mitral valve* (the *valve* between the left *atrium* and the left ventricle). This defect occurs frequently in children with *Down syndrome*. The atrioventricular canal is the most severe form of *endocardial cushion defect*.
Refer to **Endocardial Cushion Defect.**

At-Risk
Referring to an infant who needs *early intervention* services to prevent or halt illness, delayed *development*, or death. A baby may be at-risk due to biological factors (such as a *genetic disorder*), environmental factors (such as *prenatal exposure to drugs*, an unstable home environment, or lack of adequate physical care as an infant or young child), or a premature birth.

Atrium (AY-tree-uhm)
A body chamber, such as the *atria* of the *heart*.

Atrophy (AT-roe-fee)
Wasting away of a *tissue* or organ. Either the number of *cells* in the body part decreases, or the size of the cells is reduced. Atrophy is often caused by *disease*, inadequate blood *circulation*, or lack of physical exercise.

Attachment
Bonding emotionally to another person.

Attachment Disorder

Refer to **Reactive Attachment Disorder of Infancy or Early Childhood.**

Attend

Refer to **Attention Span** *and* **Shared Attention and Meaning.**

Attention Deficit Disorder (ADD)

Refer to **Attention-Deficit/Hyperactivity Disorder, Predominantly Inattentive Type.**

Attention-Deficit/Hyperactivity Disorder (AD/HD)

The current blanket, or umbrella term for *Attention-Deficit/Hyperactivity Disorder, Predominantly Inattentive Type*; *Attention-Deficit/Hyperactivity Disorder, Predominantly Hyperactive-Impulsive Type*; and *Attention-Deficit/Hyperactivity Disorder, Combined Type.* A diagnosis of one type or another depends on the specific symptoms that a child has. Children with AD/HD usually have normal or above average *intelligence.* AD/HD is the most commonly *diagnosed psychiatric* disorder in children, and has been diagnosed in individuals as young as 2 years as well as in adults. AD/HD is more common in boys than in girls. Strategies to help children learn, such as by decreasing distractions and increasing awareness of body position and movement can be effective. Some children benefit from medication to reduce the symptoms of AD/HD, especially when combined with teaching the child and family *behavior* management techniques.

Refer to **Attention-Deficit/Hyperactivity Disorder, Combined Type;** **Attention-Deficit/Hyperactivity Disorder, Predominantly Hyperactive-Impulsive Type;** *and* **Attention-Deficit/Hyperactivity Disorder, Predominantly Inattentive Type.**

Attention-Deficit/Hyperactivity Disorder, Combined Type

A *neurodevelopmental disorder* believed to be caused by slight differences in *brain* structure and function. The *symptoms* include inattention, or a *developmentally* inappropriate lack of ability to *attend* (such as difficulty with listening to and following directions), *impulsivity*, distractibility, restlessness, and *hyperactivity.*

Compare **Attention-Deficit/Hyperactivity Disorder, Predominantly Inattentive Type** *and* **Attention-Deficit/Hyperactivity Disorder, Predominantly Hyperactive-Impulsive Type.**
Refer to **Attention-Deficit/Hyperactivity Disorder.**

Attention-Deficit/Hyperactivity Disorder, Predominantly Hyperactive-Impulsive Type

A *neurodevelopmental disorder* believed to be caused by slight differences in *brain* structure and function. The *symptoms* primarily include *hyperactivity*, *impulsivity*, restlessness, and fewer symptoms related to inattention (a developmentally inappropriate lack of ability to *attend*) and distractibility.

Compare **Attention-Deficit/Hyperactivity Disorder, Predominantly Inattentive Type** *and* **Attention-Deficit/Hyperactivity Disorder, Combined Type.**
Refer to **Attention-Deficit/Hyperactivity Disorder.**

Attention-Deficit/Hyperactivity Disorder, Predominantly Inattentive Type

A *neurodevelopmental disorder* believed to be caused by slight differences in *brain* structure and function. The *symptoms* primarily include inattention (a *developmentally* inappropriate lack of ability to *attend*) and distractibility, and fewer symptoms related to *impulsivity* and restlessness. *Hyperactivity* may be a feature.

> *Formerly known as* **Attention Deficit Disorder (ADD).**
> *Compare* **Attention-Deficit/Hyperactivity Disorder, Predominantly Hyperactive-Impulsive Type** *and* **Attention-Deficit/Hyperactivity Disorder, Combined Type.**
> *Refer to* **Attention-Deficit/Hyperactivity Disorder.**

Attention Span

The length of time a child is able to concentrate on an activity. *Also known as* the ability to *attend*.

> *Refer to* **Shared Attention and Meaning.**

Attenuation

The process of reducing the strength or effect of a *virus* or *bacteria*.

Atypical (ay-TIP-i-kuhl)

Unusual or *abnormal*.

AU

The abbreviation for the Latin words meaning both ears.

Audiogram (AW-dee-oe-gram)

The results of *hearing* tests, as described on a graph. An audiogram records the child's ability to hear sounds of varying *frequency* (pitch) and intensity (loudness) in each ear. Sound frequency that is measured ranges from 125 *Hz* (a low-pitched sound) to 8000 Hz (a high-pitched sound). Sound intensity that is examined ranges from quiet 10 *decibel* sounds to loud 120 decibel sounds. The softest sounds a child hears at each pitch at least 50 percent of the time are considered his hearing thresholds. Testing hearing using headphones provides "air" conduction thresholds and testing hearing using a bone-conduction vibrator (as small device that is placed on the bone behind the ear) provides bone conduction thresholds. When the two types of thresholds are compared at each pitch, it is possible to determine if an *auditory impairment* is *conductive*, *sensorineural*, or *mixed*.

> *Refer to* **Auditory Impairment** *and* **Hearing.**

Audiologist (aw-dee-OL-oe-jist)

A specialist who determines the presence and type of *auditory impairment*. An audiologist conducts *hearing* tests and makes recommendations for *hearing aids*.

Audiology (aw-dee-OL-oe-jee)

The study of *hearing* and hearing *disorders*.

Audiometric Testing (aw-dee-oe-MET-rik)

Tests to measure the ability in each ear to hear sounds of varying *frequency* (pitch) and intensity (loudness), thereby revealing any *auditory impairment*. Results are then recorded on an *audiogram*.

> *Also known as* **Audiometry.**
> *Refer to* **Audiogram.**

Audiometry (aw-dee-OM-uh-tree)

> *Refer to* **Audiometric Testing**.

Auditory (AW-di-toe-ree)

Pertaining to the sense of *hearing*.

Auditory Agnosia (AW-di-toe-ree ag-NOE-zhuh)

Loss of ability to understand sounds (for example, words or environmental sounds, such as a dog barking), although *hearing* is intact.

> *Compare* **Verbal Auditory Agnosia.**

Auditory Brainstem-Evoked Potentials (ABEPs)

> *Refer to* **Evoked Potential Studies.**

Auditory Brainstem Response (ABR)

A test to measure *hearing* and to assess the health of the ear structures from the *auditory nerve* through the *brainstem*. The ABR can be used to screen a newborn's *hearing*.

> *Also known as* **Auditory Evoked Potential** *and* **Auditory Evoked Response.**

Auditory Canal

The ear canal leading from outside the ear inward to the *tympanic membrane* (eardrum). (This is actually the external auditory canal. There is also an internal auditory canal from the opening of the *inner ear* to the *cochlea*.)

> *Refer to* **Ear.**

Auditory Defensiveness

> *Refer to* **Sensory Defensiveness.**

Auditory Discrimination

The ability to detect differences in sounds, including subtle differences between sounds in words, such as /b/ and /p/ or /d/ and /t/.

Auditory Evoked Potential (AEP)

> *Refer to* **Auditory Brainstem Response.**

Auditory Evoked Response (AER)

> *Refer to* **Auditory Brainstem Response.**

Auditory Impairment

Hearing loss resulting from problems in any part of the ear or in the *hearing* center of the *brain*. Auditory impairment refers to a decrease in the range of

perception of loudness and/or pitch, and may be described as mild, moderate, severe, or profound depending on the degree of hearing loss. Auditory impairment may be a *congenital anomaly* or it may be caused by *disease* or injury.
>*Refer to* **Bilateral Hearing Impairment, Conductive Hearing Impairment, Deafness, Sensorineural Hearing Impairment, Mixed Hearing Impairment, and Unilateral Hearing Impairment.**

Auditory Integration Training/Therapy (AIT)
A method aimed at normalizing the way the *brain* processes auditory information, including reducing hypersensitivity to particular sounds, and addressing the problems associated with disorganized *hearing*, or hearing that is different between the two ears (possibly resulting in difficulty with sound *discrimination*). The treatment involves listening through headphones to music from which certain sound frequencies have been eliminated (intensive music therapy). Research credits AIT with improving the language and *attending* skills in some children, including those with *autism spectrum disorder, attention-deficit/hyperactivity disorder, central auditory processing disorder*, and *language disorders*.
>*Refer to* **Digital Auditory Aerobics.**

Auditory Learner
A child who learns best by *hearing* rather than through other senses such as vision. For example, singing songs in which parts of the body are named and identified may be useful when teaching the auditory learner about body parts.

Auditory Nerve
The *nerve* that transmits sound impulses from each *inner ear* to the *brain*. It consists of *cochlear* (*hearing*) nerve fibers and *vestibular* (*balance*) nerve fibers.
>*Also known as* **Acoustic Nerve, Vestibulocochlear Nerve,** *and the* **Eighth Cranial Nerve.**
>*Refer to* **Ear.**

Auditory Ossicles (AW-di-toe-ree OS-i-kuhlz)
The three small bones of the *middle ear*: the *malleus, incus*, and *stapes*. They bridge the gap between the *tympanic membrane* and the *inner ear*.
>*Refer to* **Ear.**

Auditory Processing
The *brain* function that involves interpreting auditory information that is heard. Auditory processing involves the ability to *attend* to someone speaking, to *discriminate* sound differences (such as between the words "sit" and "sick"), to comprehend spoken language, and to remember what is heard.

Auditory Processing Disorder
>*Refer to* **Central Auditory Processing Disorder.**

Auditory Script
A word, phrase, or sentence provided *verbally* to a child with the intention of encouraging him to initiate and expand language use and pursue social interaction. In one method, the adult tells the child a few appropriate script-

ed comments (often reflecting the child's preferences and interests) and the child is encouraged to select one to speak about what he has done or is planning to do. In another method, scripts are recorded for the child on a mini voice recorder or card reader and he is taught through physical prompts to play the script (and later say the script) in appropriate situations. For very young children and non-readers, scripts are paired with pictures of desired objects or activities. Using scripts allows the child to engage others in his activities and to share and receive information. After the child has mastered several scripts, the process of script-fading begins. The last word of the script is removed, then the next to last, and so on, until the script is absent.
*Compare **Textual Script**.*

Auditory Training
A method of teaching children with *auditory impairments* how to listen for and localize sounds and how to *discriminate* one sound from another. The emphasis is on teaching the child to use whatever *hearing* ability he has.

Augcom (AUG-kom)
An informal term for *Augmentative Communication*.
*Refer to **Augmentative and Alternative Communication**.*

Augmentative and Alternative Communication (AAC)
Any method of communicating that utilizes an assistive technique or device, such as signs, *gestures*, picture boards, or electronic or non-electronic devices. These methods can help children who are unable to use speech or who need to supplement their speech to communicate effectively.
*Refer to **Adaptive Equipment/Device** and **Assistive Technology**.*

Augmentin™ (og-MENT-in)
*Refer to **Amoxicillin**.*

Aura (OR-uh or AW-ruh)
A "warning" feeling, such as a sensation of movement, light, or warmth, that precedes a *simple partial seizure* and that some children feel just before a *generalized seizure*. It is similar to a feeling of "deja vu."

auri-
A prefix meaning ear.

Auricle (AW-ri-kl)
*Refer to **Pinna**.*

Auscultation (aws-kul-TAY-shuhn)
Listening to sounds in the chest, *abdomen*, etc., through a stethoscope to assess the condition of the body systems, such as the *heart* and lungs.

Autism (AW-tizm)
A commonly used term to describe *autistic disorder*.
*Refer to **Autistic Disorder** and **Autism Spectrum Disorder**.*

Autism Diagnostic Interview-Revised (ADI-R)

An interview-format *assessment* used to evaluate children and adults (who demonstrate a *mental age* above 2 years, 0 months) suspected of having an *autism spectrum disorder*. The ADI-R addresses three functional *domains*: language/*communication*; *reciprocal* social interactions; and restricted, repetitive, and *stereotyped behaviors*. To administer the ADI-R, a trained clinician interviews the child's parent or caregiver. This tool is useful for treatment and educational planning.

Autism Diagnostic Observation Schedule-Revised (ADOS-R)

An *assessment* tool used to evaluate the social and *communication* skills and *behaviors* of toddlers to adults suspected of having an *autism spectrum disorder*.

Autism Spectrum Disorder (ASD)

A *neurodevelopmental* condition (a *physiological* condition that is present early in development, probably *prenatally*; is *symptomatic* in early childhood; and affects the development and function of the *brain*) characterized by a *triad* of symptoms: 1) qualitative impairments in *social skills*; 2) qualitative impairments in *communication*; and 3) the presence of restricted, repetitive, and *stereotyped* patterns of *behavior*, interests, and activities. The *Diagnostic and Statistical Manual of Mental Disorders (DSM-IV-TR)* uses "pervasive developmental disorders" when describing what are now commonly known as autism spectrum disorders. The DSM lists five subcategories of *syndromes* included within the spectrum: *autistic disorder, Asperger's Disorder, Childhood disintegrative disorder, Rett's disorder*, and *Pervasive Developmental Disorder-Not Otherwise Specified*. With the exception of Childhood disintegrative disorder, the behaviors associated with an ASD must be present prior to 3 years of age for a child to be *diagnosed*. An ASD diagnosis is behaviorally-based (i.e., there are no medical tests to diagnose the condition) and requires searching for **clusters** of behaviors (not just one or two behaviors) which, when combined, indicate whether or not a diagnosis is warranted. To make a diagnosis, a professional evaluator (usually a *psychologist* or *neurologist*) compares a child's *developmental history* and behavioral profile with the behaviors listed under the various subcategories of ASDs in the DSM-IV-TR. The skills, behaviors, and potential of children with ASDs vary greatly. The majority of children with an ASD test in the *mentally retarded* range. However, it should be noted that most *IQ* tests tend to be socially- and language-biased, and since social and communication skills are 2 areas of difficulty for children with ASDs, IQ tests may underestimate their actual intellectual abilities (particularly in children under age 6). In addition to mental retardation, other common features of ASDs include: well-developed *motor* and *visual-motor coordination* and mechanical skills (with the exception of the motor discoordination sometimes observed in people with Asperger's Disorder and poor coordination in children with Rett's disorder); special interest in letters or numbers; rote memory skills; odd responses to *sensory stimuli*; distractibility and high activity level; *mood lability* (moods that change quickly without an apparent environmental cause); insistence on sameness; limited food preferences; sleep disturbances; lack of danger awareness; depression; seizures; and *self-injurious behavior*. Not all of these features are necessarily experienced by a person with an ASD.

The exact cause of ASDs has not yet been determined, but research has identified factors that may cause a child to develop an ASD, including a *genetic predisposition* (tends to run in families) and *central nervous system* (brain) involvement, such as an excessive or depleted level of *neurotransmitters* in the brain, differences in brain structure, and rapid head growth by 18 months of age (after having a smaller than average *head circumference* at birth). Medical conditions including autoimmune *disease* within families, and environmental factors, such as exposure to heavy metals, are also being studied to see if they contribute to the potential for ASDs. As of the publication of this work, the Centers for Disease Control and Prevention (CDC) estimates the *incidence* of ASDs at between 1 in 500 to 1 in 166 children, and current evidence suggests this number is growing at a rate of 10-17 percent per year. Presently, ASDs are four times more likely to occur in males than females.

> *Refer to* **Pervasive Developmental Disorder.**

Autistic Disorder (AD) (aw-TIS-tic)
The technical term for *autism*, autistic disorder is the most common of the *autism spectrum disorders* (*pervasive developmental disorders*). It occurs in about 1 in 500 people, and 4 to 5 times as many boys as girls are diagnosed. The symptoms of autistic disorder are present prior to 3 years of age. Some research points to 3 early *signs*, detectable by age 1, that increase the probability that autistic disorder is present: the absence of 1) looking at others' faces; 2) responding to one's name; and 3) pointing. A *diagnosis* of autistic disorder is made when a child frequently exhibits 6 or more of 12 symptoms listed in the *Diagnostic and Statistical Manual of Mental Disorders*, including at least 2 involving qualitative impairment in *social skills*, at least 1 involving qualitative impairment in communication, and at least 1 involving restricted, repetitive, and stereotyped patterns of behavior, interests, and activities. Some professionals refer to children with autistic disorder as either "high-functioning" or "low-functioning." There are no clear criteria for making such a determination; however, these descriptions (based on the professional's subjective perceptions) generally relate to 1) the presence or absence of *mental retardation* (approximately 70 percent of people with autistic disorder function within the mentally retarded range); 2) whether or not the child is verbal; and 3) the degree to which challenging behaviors are present.

> *Also known as* **Early Infantile Autism, Infantile Autism,** *and* **Kanner's Syndrome.**
> *Compare* **Pervasive Developmental Disorder-Not Otherwise Specified.**
> *Refer to* **Autism Spectrum Disorder.**

Autistic-Like Behaviors/Characteristics
Behaviors that include verbal and physical *perseveration* (seemingly purposeless repeated behavior) and rituals, poor eye contact, and limited social awareness. Autistic-like behaviors are sometimes seen in individuals with *developmental disabilities* who do not have an *autism spectrum disorder*.

auto-
A prefix meaning self.

Autoimmune Disorder

One of a group of many *diseases* in which the body's *immune system* produces *antibodies* against the body's own *cells*. Nearly any cell in the body can be affected, causing disease in that *tissue* or system. For example, *Hashimoto's disease* is an autoimmune *thyroid disorder*.

Automatic Movement Reaction

Refer to **Automatic Reflex.**

Automatic Reflex

One of several involuntary *reflexes* that develop during the first 2 years of life and which develop as the *primitive reflexes* are suppressed. The automatic reflexes are necessary postural responses in the infant as he begins to assume new positions, such as sitting, and as he begins to *crawl*. The main automatic reflexes are *righting reactions*, which allow the infant to maintain an upright position (for example, the *head righting* reflex in which the infant holds his head upright even when his body is tilted); *equilibrium reactions*, which help the infant maintain *balance* (for example, the *balance reaction* of extending the arms when balance has been lost); and protective reactions, which protect the infant during a fall (for example, the *parachute reflex* in which the arms and legs extend to protect the head and body from a fall). Automatic reflexes remain throughout one's lifetime.

    Also known as **Automatic Movement Reaction, Postural Reaction, and Postural Reflex.**
    Compare **Primitive Reflex.**

Automatism (aw-TOM-uh-tizm)

Repetitive *behaviors* that occur without conscious volition. These behaviors look purposeful, although the child is not controlling the behavior on a conscious level. Automatisms are most commonly *symptoms* of a *complex partial seizure,* although they may occur with other conditions, such as certain *brain disorders* or drug intoxication. Examples of automatisms include making *chewing* motions or manipulating the buttons on a shirt.

Autonomic Nervous System (o-tuh-NOM-ik)

The part of the *nervous system* that regulates involuntary body functions, including those of the *heart* muscle, smooth muscles, and *glands*. It is comprised of the *sympathetic nervous system* and the *parasympathetic nervous system*.

    Compare **Central Nervous System** *and* **Peripheral Nervous System.**

Autonomic Seizure (aw-toe-NOM-ik)

A type of *partial seizure* characterized by a rapid heartbeat, *anxiety* or fear, paleness, sweating, or dilation of the *pupils*.

    Refer to **Partial Seizure** *and* **Epilepsy.**

Autonomy (aw-TON-oe-mee)

The ability to function independently.

Autosomal Dominant Disorder (aw-toe-SOE-muhl)
A *genetic disorder* that a child inherits (via a defective *gene*) from one of his parents, who also has the autosomal dominant disorder. (A single defective gene is all that is necessary to pass on the disorder.) The term "dominant" means that the defective gene of the gene pair (*inherited* from either the mother or the father) is able to override the normal gene. Each child born to a parent who has an autosomal dominant disorder has a 50 percent chance of inheriting the disorder and, if inherited, a 50 percent chance of passing it on to offspring. (However, if the parent has two defective genes, the child has a 100 percent chance of inheriting the disorder.) Another way a child can be affected by an autosomal dominant disorder is if the defective gene develops as the result of a *mutation* (a change in *genetic* information that occurs during early *cell* division). *Achondroplasia* is an example of an autosomal dominant disorder.
    Compare **Autosomal Recessive Disorder.**

Autosomal Recessive Disorder
A *genetic disorder* that occurs when the child inherits two defective *genes*, one from each parent. (Either each parent is a *carrier* of the defective gene that causes the disorder, or one parent is a carrier and the other parent has the autosomal recessive disorder.) The term "recessive" means that the defective gene of the parent's gene pair is hidden by the normal gene. When parents who are carriers for the same disorder have children, each child born will have a 25 percent chance of having the disorder (if each parent's defective gene is *inherited*), a 50 percent chance of being a carrier (if one parent's defective gene and the other parent's normal gene is inherited), and a 25 percent chance that the gene pair will be normal (if each parent's normal gene is inherited). When one parent has the autosomal recessive disorder and the other parent is a carrier, the offspring have a 50 percent chance of having the disorder and a 50 percent chance of being a carrier. If a child inherits only one defective gene (rather than one from each parent), he is known as a carrier. Carriers do not have the disorder but can pass it on to offspring. *Tay-Sachs disease* is an example of an autosomal recessive disorder.
    Compare **Autosomal Dominant Disorder.**

Autosome (AW-tuh-soem)
Any *chromosome* other than the *X* and *Y* (sex) chromosomes. Human beings have 44 (22 pairs) of autosomal chromosomes.
    Refer to **Chromosome.**

Average for Gestational Age (AGA)
    Refer to **Appropriate for Gestational Age.**

Aversive (uh-VUR-siv)
Referring to an avoidance *behavior*, or an unpleasant *stimulus* that causes avoidance behavior. For example, an aversive such as a medication that induces vomiting might be paired with drinking alcohol in order to eliminate the drinking.

Axilla (ak-SIL-uh)
The armpit.

Axillary (AK-si-layr-ee)
Referring to the armpit.

Axillary Temperature

The body's temperature reading when the thermometer is placed under the arm. It runs approximately ½ to 1 degree lower than the *oral temperature*.
Compare **Oral Temperature, Rectal Temperature,** *and* **Tympanic Membrane Temperature.**

Axis

The second *vertebra* in the neck, lying just below the *atlas*, or first *cervical* vertebra.

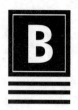

Babbling

Infant vocal play characterized by repetition of *consonant-vowel* combinations, such as "ba," "ma," or "da." Initially, babbling is non-specific in that the sounds do not have attached meaning. Later the infant babbles with more specific intent and the babbling begins to sound similar to actual speech and varies in intonation like adult speech patterns. Babbling typically begins by 6 months of age.

Compare ***Cooing, Jabbering,*** *and* ***Jargon.***

Babinski's Sign/Reflex/Response (buh-BIN-skeez)

A response that consists of *extension* of the big toe and is usually associated with *fanning* of the other toes. It is elicited when the outer side of the bottom of the foot is stroked from the heel to the ball of the foot. In the child under 12 months, a Babinski response can be normal. In an older child or an adult, this response (Babinski's sign) may indicate *brain injury*. (The normal response, i.e., a negative Babinski, in an older child or an adult would be for the toes to bend downward.)

Refer to ***Primitive Reflex.***

Baby Bird™

A type of *ventilator* used with infants.

Baby Teeth

Refer to ***Primary Teeth.***

Back Knee

Refer to ***Genu Recurvatum.***

Backward Chaining

Teaching the steps of a skill backwards, beginning with the last step. For example, in learning to wash her hands, the child turns off the faucet after it's already been turned on and she's had her hands lathered and rinsed. After she has mastered turning off the faucet, she can begin practicing rinsing. This moves the child toward independent completion of the entire task while allowing her to "finish" the task from the very beginning.

Compare ***Forward Chaining.***

Baclofen (BAK-loe-fen)
An *antispastic drug* used to relax *hypertonic* muscles. Lioresal™ is the brand name of this drug.

Bacteria (bak-TEER-ee-uh)
One-*celled microorganisms* that can cause *infection.*
　　　Also known as **Germs.**
　　　Compare **Virus.**

Bacterial Meningitis
　　　Refer to **Meningitis.**

Bacterium
Singular for *bacteria.*

BAER Test
The abbreviation for Brainstem Auditory Evoked Response.

Bag and Mask
　　　Refer to **Bagging.**

Bagging
An informal term describing a method of giving *artificial respiration* in which air and/or *oxygen* is pumped into a baby's lungs by compressing a bag attached to a mask that covers the baby's nose and mouth.
　　　Also known as **Bag and Mask.**

Balance
The ability to assume and maintain upright body position while sitting, standing, or moving.

Balance Reaction
An automatic response that occurs when *balance* has been lost in which the arms quickly extend in an attempt to regain upright balance.
　　　Refer to **Automatic Reflex.**

Band
A bundle of fibers (such as an *adhesion*), that binds two parts of the body together, or that encircles a body structure.

Bardet-Biedl Syndrome (bar-DAY BEE-dl)
An *autosomal recessive disorder* characterized by *retinitis pigmentosa, mild* to *moderate mental retardation*, extra and webbed fingers and/or toes, obesity beginning in infancy, and *hypogonadism.*

Barium Enema (BA-ree-uhm)
A procedure in which barium (a chalky contrast material) is administered into the *rectum* and *x-ray* pictures are taken as it passes through the *large intes-*

tine. The barium enema is performed to examine the *colon* and to *diagnose* the cause of *abnormalities* such as rectal bleeding or persistent diarrhea and *diseases* such as *tumors* of the colon and *celiac disease.*

Barium Swallow

A procedure in which barium (a chalky contrast material) is swallowed and *x-ray* pictures are taken as it passes through the *esophagus.* In variations of the barium swallow (the barium meal and the barium follow-through), the barium is observed as it passes through the stomach and *small intestine.* The barium swallow is performed to *diagnose* the cause of pain or difficulty in swallowing and *disorders* such as narrowing of the esophagus.

Basal (BAY-suhl or BAY-zuhl)

Referring to the fundamental or base. On an *evaluation* tool, basal refers to the highest test item passed before the child fails an item. (The child may have other "passed" items later in the test, as well.)
    Compare **Ceiling.**

Basal Ganglia (BAY-suhl or BAY-zuhl GANG-glee-uh)

The interconnected gray masses within the *cerebral hemispheres* and the *brainstem* that are involved in *motor* coordination.

Baseline

Referring to the level at which a child performs before training or *intervention.*
    Also known as **Operant Level.**

Bath Seat

A special seat placed in the bathtub that secures the child while being given a bath. There are several types of bath seats, each designed to position the child according to her abilities (i.e., sitting independently, maintaining *head control,* etc.).

Batten Disease

An *autosomal recessive disorder* in which the child develops normally until 6 months to 2 years of age, when progressive *brain disease* becomes apparent. Batten Disease is characterized by seizures, *mental retardation,* and *blindness,* and is fatal. With early onset, the disease usually progresses more quickly.
    Also known as **Neuronal Ceroid Lipofuscinosis.**

Bayley—III

The abbreviation for Bayley Scales of Infant and Toddler Development™- Third Edition.

Bayley Scales of Infant and Toddler Development™—Third Edition (Bayley – III)

A *standardized test* used to assess the *cognitive,* language, *motor, social/ emotional,* and *adaptive behavior* development of infants between 1 and 42 months of age. The Bayley – III also includes a *screening test,* caregiver report, and growth scores and charts. *Standard scores* on the Bayley have a *mean* (average) of 100 and a *standard deviation* of 15, which means that the majority of children score within 15 points above to 15 points below the average score of 100. Training on how to administer the Bayley is required. Typically the Bayley is administered by a professional who holds a doctoral degree in psychology or education and/or has significant, relevant experience and training.

B Cell
A type of *lymphocyte* that plays a major role in the body's immune response and is responsible for the production of *immunoglobulins* (*antibodies*).
>   *Compare **T Cell**.*
>   *Refer to **Lymphocyte**.*

BEAM
The abbreviation for Brain Electrical Activity Mapping.

Bear Walk
A form of *locomotion* in which the child "walks" on the hands and feet on the floor.

Becker Muscular Dystrophy
A form of *muscular dystrophy* that is milder and develops more slowly than other muscular dystrophies. (Children usually can maintain the ability to walk into adolescence or young adulthood.) Becker Muscular Dystrophy is an *X-linked recessive disease* that starts between 8 and 30 years of age.
>   *Refer to **Muscular Dystrophy**.*

Beckwith-Wiedemann Syndrome
A *disorder* characterized by *low blood sugar*, overproduction of *insulin*, an increased rate of *tumor* development, a large tongue and body, *omphalocele* (intestinal protrusion through an opening in the *abdominal* wall), eye and ear *anomalies*, and a forehead birthmark. The cause of this *syndrome* is unknown; however, the *gene* for Beckwith-Wiedemann syndrome is on *chromosome* 11.

Bedsore
>   *Refer to **Decubitus Ulcer**.*

Behavior
1. Any physical action or mental activity in which a child engages.
2. The manner in which a child acts.

Behavioral Assessment
Gathering (through direct observation and by parent report) and analyzing information about a child's *behaviors*. The information may be used to plan ways to help the child change unwanted behaviors. *When* a behavior occurs (i.e., the events, times, and situations that trigger a behavior), as well as the frequency and *duration* of the behavior, are variables that are noted.
>   *Refer to **Behavior Management Plan, Brazelton Neonatal Behavioral Assessment Scale,** and **Functional Behavior Analysis**.*

Behavioral Contract

A written agreement that defines the *behavioral* expectations of a child. This behavioral management tool can be designed with input from parents, teachers, and the child herself. Appropriate consequences (*reinforcers* or penalties usually previously agreed upon) are given to the child depending on whether or not behavioral expectations are met.

> *Refer to* **Behavior Management Plan.**

Behavior Management Plan

A plan designed to modify or reshape the *behavior* of a child with *disabilities* that addresses existing behavior, *interventions*, support, and goals.

> *Refer to* **Behavioral Contract, Behavior Modification** *and* **Behavioral Assessment.**

Behavior Modification

Systematic approaches to change *behavior* that include the concepts of using *positive reinforcement* to increase a behavior and using *negative reinforcement* to decrease a behavior.

> *Refer to* **Reinforcement.**

Belly Button

> *Refer to* **Umbilicus.**

Belly Crawl

> *Refer to* **Crawl.**

Benadryl™ (BEN-uh-dril)

> *Refer to* **Diphenhydramine Hydrochloride.**

Benign (bi-NIEN)

Referring to a condition that is not harmful or a threat to health.

> *Compare* **Malignancy.**

Benign Rolandic Epilepsy

An *epileptic syndrome* generally affecting children between 3 and 15 years of age, characterized by *partial seizures* that usually occur at night. The term is sometimes shortened to simply Rolandic Epilepsy.

Benzodiazepine (ben-zoe-die-AZ-uh-peen)

One of a group of *psychotropic drugs* such as *Diazepam* used to treat *anxiety disorders* and to produce sedation. It is sometimes used in the treatment of certain *behaviors* associated with an *autism spectrum disorder* and as an *antiepileptic drug.*

BER

The abbreviation for Brainstem Evoked Response.

> *Refer to* **Brainstem Auditory Evoked Response.**

BERA
The abbreviation for Brainstem Evoked Response Audiometry.
>*Refer to Brainstem Auditory Evoked Response.*

Best Practice
Accepted procedures that are based on the current knowledge and research.

Beta-Adrenergic Drug (BAY-tuh ad-ren-ER-jik)
A drug that may be used to try to stop *labor*.
>*Also known as a Betamimetic Drug or Betasympathomimetic Drug.*

Betamethasone (bay-tuh-METH-uh-soen)
A *corticosteroid* drug given to a pregnant woman before delivering prematurely to help the baby's lungs mature and to decrease the chance of the baby developing *respiratory distress syndrome*. Celestone™ is the brand name of this drug.

Betamimetic Drug
>*Refer to Beta-Adrenergic Drug.*

Betasympathomimetic Drug
>*Refer to Beta-Adrenergic Drug.*

Beta Wave (BAY-tuh or BEE-tuh)
One of the four types of *brain waves* creating the rhythm of electrical activity as seen on an *EEG*. Beta waves are normally seen when a child is awake and alert with the eyes open. Beta waves are characterized by a relatively low voltage and a *frequency* of more than 13 *Hz*.
>*Compare Alpha Wave, Delta Wave, and Theta Wave.*
>*Refer to Brain Wave.*

Beuren Syndrome
>*Refer to Williams Syndrome.*

bi-
A prefix meaning two.

Bicarbonate (bie-KAR-boe-nayt)
>*Refer to Sodium Bicarbonate.*

Bicuspid Valve
>*Refer to Mitral Valve.*

bid
The abbreviation for the Latin words meaning twice a day.

Bilabial (bie-LAY-bee-uhl)
Pertaining to both lips.

Bilabial Closure
Bringing the lips together, closing the mouth.

Bilabial Speech Sound
A *consonant* sound produced by specific movement or positioning of the two lips, such as the /p/ sound when a stream of air is released or the /b/ sound when voice is added.

Bilateral (bie-LAT-er-uhl)
Pertaining to, affecting, or relating to two sides of the body (such as a two-handed reach or both ears).

Bilateral Hearing Impairment
Auditory impairment in both ears.
> *Refer to* **Auditory Impairment.**

Bile
A substance *secreted* by the *liver* that removes waste products from the liver and helps break down *fats.*

Bililights (BIL-i-liets)
Bright fluorescent lights used to treat *jaundice.*
> *Also known as* **Phototherapy** *or* **Bilirubin Lights.**
> *Refer to* **Bilirubin.**

Bilirubin (bil-i-ROO-bin)
A pigment byproduct of the breakdown of *red blood cells* that causes the baby's skin to become yellow, or *jaundiced.* A very high level of bilirubin can cause *kernicterus,* which results in *brain damage* and, if untreated, death.
> *Refer to* **Bililights.**

Bilirubin Lights
> *Refer to* **Bililights.**

Binocular Fusion (bie-NOK-yuh-luhr)
The process by which both eyes send messages to the *brain* (about what is seen) and the brain integrates, or fuses, them into one 3-dimensional picture.

Binocular Vision (bi-NOK-yuh-luhr)
Normal two-eyed sight that produces a single 3-dimensional image.

Biochemical (bie-oe-KEM-i-kuhl)
Of, or related to, the structure or composition (and changes) of living things.

Biofeedback (bie-oe-FEED-bak)
A technique used to learn information about and to control one's involuntary body activity (such as *brain waves*). The child uses a recording instrument that monitors body activity and then signals the changing levels of the activity. The

signal (such as a flashing light) gives the child information (feedback) that a change has taken place within her body and, with experience, the child can become aware of how she was feeling at the time of the signal (the change) and then learn techniques in order to voluntarily bring about a change in the signal (and thus a change in her body activity).

Biological Risk
Refer to At-Risk.

Biopsy (BIE-op-see)
A procedure to remove living tissue from the body for microscopic examination and to determine a diagnosis.

Biotinidase Deficiency (bie-uh-TIN-i-days)
An autosomal recessive metabolic disorder caused by enzyme deficiency. Characteristics may include ataxia, hair loss, skin inflammation (rash), vision and auditory impairment, hypotonia, and seizures. Treatment with biotin (a B-complex vitamin) can reverse the symptoms, although vision and hearing loss may continue.

Birth Defect
Refer to Congenital Anomaly.

Birth Length
The length of an infant at birth. Fifty centimeters (about 20 inches) is the average birth length.

Birth Weight
The weight of an infant at birth. 3500 grams (about 7½ pounds) is the average birth weight. A baby weighing less than 2500 grams (5½ pounds) is considered to be a low birth-weight baby.
Refer to Extremely Low Birth Weight Infant, Low Birth Weight Infant, and Very Low Birth Weight Infant.

Bisacodyl (bis-AK-oe-dil)
A laxative drug that stimulates the intestine. Dulcolax™ is the brand name of this drug.

Bite Reflex
Jaw closure when the gums or teeth are stimulated. This reflex is noted in the 1- to 8-month-old.
Refer to Primitive Reflex.

Bivalved Cast
A removable cast used to correct foot, wrist, or elbow positioning.

Bladder (Urinary)
The organ located in the center of the lower abdomen that functions as a reservoir for urine. It receives urine from the kidneys through the ureters, then passes urine from the body through the urethra.

Bladder Tap
A procedure to withdraw urine by inserting a sterile needle through the *abdomen* and into the *bladder*. Urine obtained in this manner (as opposed to normal voiding) is sterile, and can be examined to see if infection exists.

Blalock-Taussig Shunt (BLAY-lok TAH-sig)
An operation performed on the *heart* in which two *arteries* are joined to allow more blood to flow to the lungs. This procedure manages one of the four *heart defects* of *tetralogy of Fallot* until permanent correction can be done.

Blanket Swinging
An activity (similar to swinging in a *hammock*) for *vestibular stimulation.*

blast-, blasto-
Prefixes meaning bud or *embryonic* form.

blephar-, blepharo-
Prefixes meaning eyelid.

Blepharophimosis (blef-uh-roe-fi-MOE-sis)
Narrowing of the opening between the upper and lower eyelids (the *palpebral fissure*) due to an inability to open the eye normally. It is seen in some *hereditary disorders*, such as *Dubowitz syndrome*.
    Also known as **Blepharostenosis.**

Blepharospasm (BLEF-uh-roe-spazm)
The involuntary tightening (*contraction*) of the muscles of the eyelid. It can be caused by a sore or wound of the eye, a neurologic condition, psychological stress, or fatigue.

Blepharostenosis (blef-uh-roe-sten-OE-sis)
    Refer to **Blepharophimosis.**

Blindness
A lack or loss of vision due to damage to the organs of vision or to the vision centers of the *brain*. A child is considered *legally blind* if she has corrected *visual acuity* of 20/200 (she can at best see at 20 feet what ordinarily can be seen at 200 feet) or less in the better eye, or a *visual field* of no more than 20 degrees in the better eye.

Blinking Reflex
A normal lifetime response of blinking at a bright light or object that shines on or approaches the eye.
    Refer to **Automatic Reflex.**

Blood Cell
    Refer to **Platelet, Red Blood Cell,** *and* **White Blood Cell.**

Blood Count
Refer to **Complete Blood Count.**

Blood Gas
The *oxygen, carbon dioxide*, and nitrogen gases dissolved in blood.

Blood Gas Determination
A test to measure the oxygen, *carbon dioxide*, and acid content of the blood. These measurements reflect changes in blood chemistry which indicate the severity of *respiratory* illness.

Blood Group or Type
A classification of blood according to the presence or absence of specific substances (*proteins*) on the surface of the *red blood cell*. Each person is either type O, A, B, or AB, and Rh positive or Rh negative (determined by the presence or absence of the *Rh factor*). There are many other less commonly used blood groups as well.
Refer to **ABO Incompatibility.**

Blood Pressure
The pressure exerted on the walls of the *arteries* caused by the flow of blood. The blood pressure measurement consists of 2 numbers. The systolic pressure (top number) is the measurement of the pressure exerted when the *heart* muscle contracts and blood surges to the body. The diastolic pressure (lower number) is the measurement of the pressure exerted when the ventricles relax between heartbeats when the pumping chambers are filling. Blood pressure reflects the elasticity of the *blood vessels*.

Blood Sugar
A substance in the blood that is necessary for *metabolism. Glucose*, fructose, and galactose are blood sugars. However, when measured, blood sugar usually refers to glucose in the blood. Both high and low levels of glucose in the blood are associated with certain *diseases*. For example, increased glucose concentration is associated with *diabetes mellitus* and *hyperthyroidism*. Decreased glucose concentration is associated with *hypothyroidism* and *muscular dystrophy*.

Blood Urea Nitrogen (BUN) (yoo-REE-uh)
The amount of nitrogen in the blood in the form of *urea* (bodily waste product). Testing BUN levels provides information about *liver* and *kidney* function and possibly *nutritional* status.

Blood Vessel
Any one of the network of tubes throughout the body that carry blood. The types of blood vessels are *arteries, arterioles, capillaries, veins*, and *venules*.

Blount Disease
A condition in which the *tibia* (shin bone) fails to develop normally causing the lower leg to angle inward. It resembles genuvarum (bow-leg), except Blount disease is progressive. It can be associated with obesity and early walking.

Bobath Therapy
A treatment philosophy designed by Karl and Berta Bobath that is used by *physical therapists*.
> *Refer to* **Neurodevelopmental Treatment/Therapy.**

Body Homeostasis
> *Refer to* **Homeostasis.**

Body Image
One's concept of one's own body, specifically of physical attributes. This mental picture of one's appearance may be based upon self-observation, develop from others' reactions, or reflect one's experiences. One's body image may or may not be realistic.

Body Measurements
An infant's height, weight, head, and chest measurements.
> *Also known as* **Somatic Growth Measurements.**

Body Shell
A *thoraco-lumbar-sacral orthosis* that is worn to treat a progressive spinal defect such as *neuromuscular scoliosis*.

Bolster
> *Refer to* **Roll.**

Bolus (BOE-lus)
1. A lump of chewed food or medication that is ready for swallowing.
2. An amount of *IV* fluid or IV medication that is given all at once.

Bonding
The process by which parents (or *primary caregiver*) and baby become emotionally attached.

Bone Graft
Transplantation of a section of bone from one area of the body to another.

Bone Marrow
The *soft tissue* located within bone shafts that is concerned with production of *blood cells* and *hemoglobin*.

Bonnevie-Ullrich Syndrome
> *Refer to* **Turner Syndrome.**

Booster Injection
An additional dose of *antigen*, such as a *vaccine*, to reinforce the protection provided by the original series of *immunizations*.

BOR
The abbreviation for branchio-oto-renal syndrome.

Bossing
1. A rounded projection, such as on the surface of a bone.
2. A prominence of the forehead.

Bouncing
A technique for providing *proprioceptive* and *vestibular input*, and for increasing *muscle tone*. The child is gently bounced while seated on the adult's lap or on an inflated pillow or beach ball. The child must have adequate *head control* or support, and be positioned with proper body alignment.

Bourneville Disease
> *Refer to* **Tuberous Sclerosis.**

Bowel
The *small* and *large intestines*.
> *Refer to* **Large Intestine** *and* **Small Intestine.**

Bowel Movements
> *Refer to* **Defecation** *and* **Feces/Fecal Matter.**

Bowleg (BOE-leg)
> *Refer to* **Genu Varum.**

BP
The abbreviation for blood pressure.

BPD
The abbreviation for bronchopulmonary dysplasia.

Brace
A device used to support a part of the body and hold it in position. Wearing a brace can enable the supported body part to function, such as making standing and walking possible, and can prevent *contractures* or deformities. A brace is one kind of an *orthosis*.
> *Refer to* **Orthopedic Appliance.**

brachi- (BRAYK-ee)
A prefix meaning arm.

Brachial (BRAY-kee-uhl)
Referring to the arm.

Brachial Artery
The principal *artery* of the upper arm.

Brachial Plexus
A network of *nerves* located in the neck, shoulder, and *axilla* (armpit). They supply the muscles and skin of the chest, shoulders, and arms with nervous *stimuli* and are part of the *peripheral nervous system*.

brachy- (BRAYK-ee)
A prefix meaning short.

Brachycephaly (brayk-ee-SEF-uh-lee)
A *congenital* malformation of the skull caused by premature closure of a (specific) *suture*. This results in a short, broad shape to the head. Brachycephaly alone does not necessarily indicate an *abnormality* since the range of head measurements involved falls within the range that is normal for human beings.

Brachydactyly (brayk-ee-DAK-tuh-lee)
A condition in which the fingers or toes are *abnormally* short. It can occur alone or characterize a *genetic syndrome*.

brady- (BRAYD-ee)
A prefix meaning slow.

Bradycardia (brayd-ee-KAR-dee-uh)
A steady but slower than normal heartbeat rate. In a newborn, bradycardia is a heartbeat rate below 100 beats per minute. In other children under 7 years, bradycardia is a heartbeat rate below 60 beats per minute.

Brain
The organ of *nerve tissue* located within the *cranium* that controls the activity of the nerves, and regulates the function of many processes, including *sensory*, *reflexive*, *motor*, *cognitive*, and *communication*. The main parts of the brain include the *cerebrum*, the *cerebellum*, *diencephalons*, *and brainstem*. The brain and the *spinal cord* form the *central nervous system*.

Brain Attack
  Refer to **Stroke.**

Brain Bleed
  Refer to **Intraventricular Hemorrhage.**

Brain Damage
Injury to the *brain* that can be caused by *anoxia*, *hypoxia*, *inborn errors of metabolism*, infection, problems during pregnancy or delivery, head injury, *stroke*, a brain *tumor*, or *status epilepticus*. Brain damage may result in a lack or loss of *cognitive* abilities; *epilepsy*; *motor*, language, or *sensory deficits*; or *hydrocephalus*.
  Also known as **Brain Dysfunction.**

Brain Death
An absence of *brain* function (electrical impulses from the brain) resulting in irreversible unconsciousness while the *heart* continues to beat.

Brain Dysfunction
  Refer to **Brain Damage.**

Brain Electrical Activity Mapping (BEAM)
A procedure that produces a picture of the *brain*, which distinguishes *abnormalities* from healthy areas. BEAM consists of computerized analysis of *EEG (electroencephalogram)* signals to map the electrical activity of the brain.

Brain Imaging Techniques
Procedures that produce pictures of the *brain*, such as *x-ray*, *Computerized Tomography (CT) Scanning*, *Magnetic Resonance Imaging (MRI)*, *Ultrasound Scanning*, *Brain Electrical Activity Mapping*, and *Positron Emission Tomography (PET)*.

Brain Injury
> *Refer to* **Brain Damage.**

Brainstem
The part of the *brain* that connects the *cerebral hemispheres* with the *spinal cord*. The parts of the brainstem are the *midbrain* (or *mesencephalon*), *pons,* and the *medulla oblongata*. The brainstem controls basic body functions such as breathing and *blood pressure*, and contains *nerves* which control *sensory, reflex,* and *motor* functions. The brainstem functions on a *reflexive* (involuntary) level.

Brainstem Auditory Evoked Response (BAER Test)
A newborn *hearing* screening tool in which electrodes are placed on the scalp and ears. The electrical activity of the *brainstem* auditory tracts are recorded when stimulated by sound (clicks). The BAER test can determine if there is *hearing impairment* caused by *middle ear, inner ear,* or *nerve disorder*.

Brainstem Evoked Response (BER)
> *Refer to* **Brainstem Auditory Evoked Response.**

Brainstem Evoked Response Audiometry (BERA)
> *Refer to* **Brainstem Auditory Evoked Response.**

Brain Wave
The pattern of electrical impulses activated by *neurotransmitters* as they move from one *brain cell* to the next. There are 4 types of brain waves: *alpha waves, beta waves, delta waves,* and *theta waves*. Brain waves are detectable by *electroencephalograph*.

Branched-Chain Ketoaciduria (kee-toe-as-i-DYOO-ree-uh)
An *autosomal recessive disorder* in which an infant is unable to metabolize 3 *amino acids*: valine, leucine, and isoleucine. (This causes *central nervous system* dysfunction including *coma* and *seizures*, and urine smelling of maple syrup.) Without early *diagnosis* (before about 10 days of age) and treatment (restricting dietary intake of the listed amino acids), this *disorder* will result in death. *Prenatal diagnosis* is possible.
> *Also known as* **Maple Syrup Urine Disease.**

Branchial Arch (BRANG-kee-uhl)
Arched structures in the *embryonic* throat and neck area that, when development is disrupted, can result in *anomalies* of a baby's ear, neck, and throat areas. These branchial arch anomalies may be associated with *syndromes* such as *Treacher Collins syndrome* or *branchio-oto-renal syndrome.*

Branchio-Oto-Renal Syndrome (BOR)
(BRANG-kee-oe OE-toe REE-nuhl)
A rare *autosomal dominant disorder* characterized by *branchial arch anomalies* (*abnormal* passages from the throat to the outside surface of the neck, *cysts*, and ear pits or tags in front of the *outer ear*), *auditory impairment*, and abnormal development of the *kidneys. Melnick-Fraser syndrome* is similar to BOR, with the addition of eye and vision problems.

Brazelton Neonatal Behavioral Assessment Scale (NBAS)
A test used to evaluate the newborn's *reflexes, behavior*, and interactions with her environment. The infant is observed for her responses to various tasks as she makes the transition from sleep to alert *states*. Although a score is determined, the aim of the assessment is to provide an overall description of the baby. The *pediatrician* typically administers the NBAS.

Breech Delivery
> *Refer to* **Breech Presentation.**

Breech Presentation
Birth (delivery) of a baby with the buttocks, knees, or feet appearing first in the mother's *pelvis.*
> *Also known as* **Breech Delivery.**
> *Refer to* **Fetal Presentation.**

Brethine™ (breth-EEN)
> *Refer to* **Terbutaline Sulfate.**

Brigance Diagnostic Inventory of Early Development
A *criterion-referenced test* used to evaluate the *psychomotor, self-help*, speech and language, *cognition*, and early academic skills of infants and children from birth to 6 years of age. The results of the Brigance are expressed as the child's *developmental age.* The Brigance is also a curriculum tool. Both professionals and *paraprofessionals* may administer the Brigance.

Broca's Aphasia (BROE-kuhz)
A type of *aphasia* affecting *expressive language*, consisting of nonfluent speech in which the child primarily uses nouns and verbs, but is deficient in *syntax.*
> *Refer to* **Aphasia.**

Broca's Area
An area of the *brain* involved in speech production.

Bronchi (BRONG-kie)
The main tubes that lead from the *trachea* to the *bronchioles*. Air travels in and out of the lungs through the main and the smaller bronchi.
*Refer to **Bronchial Tubes.***

Bronchial Asthma (BRONG-kee-uhl AZ-muh)
*Refer to **Asthma.***

Bronchial Tubes (BRONG-kee-uhl)
The smaller *bronchi* that lead from the *trachea* to the *bronchioles*. Air travels in and out of the lungs through the main and the smaller bronchi.
*Refer to **Bronchi.***

Bronchioles (BRONG-kee-oelz)
Small tubes that branch off from the *bronchial tubes* (the smaller *bronchi*). The bronchioles lead to the *alveoli* within the lungs, which is where the exchange of *oxygen* and *carbon dioxide* takes place.

Bronchitis (brong-KIE-tis)
An *inflammation* or infection of the *mucous membranes* of the *bronchial tubes*. Bronchitis is usually caused by a *viral* (and sometimes *bacterial*) infection, and is characterized by a persistent cough that produces sputum.
*Refer to **Albuterol.***

Bronchodilator Drug (brong-koe-DIE-lay-tuhr)
A drug that widens the airways by relaxing *contractions* of the smooth muscles of the *bronchioles*. This makes breathing easier. Bronchodilators are most commonly used in the treatment of *asthma*.

Bronchopulmonary Dysplasia (BPD)
(brong-koe-PUL-moe-ner-ee dis-PLAY-zee-uh or dis-PLAY-zhuh)
A condition in which *tissue* of the lungs and *bronchioles* become damaged due to *respiratory distress syndrome* (common with *premature infants*) and/or use of the *ventilator*. Breathing problems develop when the damaged tissue dies and is replaced with scar tissue that narrows the airways. Babies recover from BPD (their lungs heal), but are likely to be vulnerable to respiratory illness as infants and preschoolers. BPD is one form of *chronic lung disease*.

Bronchoscopy (brong-KOS-kuh-pee)
An examination of the *bronchi* in which a narrow, lighted tube is inserted through the nose or mouth and into the bronchi to view the tracheobronchial tree (the *trachea*, bronchi, and *bronchial tubes*).

Bronchospasm (BRONG-koe-spazm)
Abnormal contraction of the *bronchi* resulting in temporarily narrowed airways, which causes *wheezing* or coughing. The most common causes of bronchospasm include *asthma* (which is the number one cause), *respiratory* infection, and *chronic lung disease*.

Bronchus (BRONG-kuhs)
Singular of *bronchi*.

Broviac Catheter™
A type of *catheter* that is used as a long-term *central line*.

Brow Presentation
Birth (delivery) of a baby in which the face, specifically the eyebrow/forehead area of the head, is the first part to appear in the mother's *pelvis*.
    Refer to **Fetal Presentation.**

Bruit (BROO-ee or brwee or broo-EE)
An *abnormal* sound or *murmur* in an organ, *vessel*, or *gland* that can be heard through a stethoscope.

Brushfield Spots
Pinpoint speckled pigmented spots on the *iris* of the eye, often seen on the eyes of children with *Down syndrome*. Occasionally, Brushfield spots are seen in children who do not have Down syndrome. Brushfield spots do not affect vision.

Brushing
    Refer to **Wilbarger Deep Pressure and Proprioceptive Technique (DPPT).**

Bruxism (BRUK-sizm)
Unconscious, repetitive grinding or clenching of the teeth.

Bucca (BUK-uh)
The cheek, or fleshy part of the side of the face.

Buccae
Plural of *bucca* (cheek).

Bulbar (BUL-bur)
Pertaining to the *medulla oblongata* of the *brain* and the *cranial nerves*.

BUN
The abbreviation for blood urea nitrogen.

Bunny Hopping
A means of *abnormal locomotion* in which the child with *hypertonia* sits on the floor with her legs in the "W" position and then moves forward by placing her arms in front of her body on the floor and swinging her trunk and legs up to the hand placement.

Bupropion Hydrochloride (byoo-PROE-pee-ahn hie-droe-KLOR-ied)
An *antidepressant drug* sometimes used in the treatment of certain *behaviors* associated with *autism spectrum disorders* and *attention-deficit/hyperactivity disorder.*

BuSpar™ (BYOO-spar)
Refer to **Buspirone Hydrochloride.**

Buspirone Hydrochloride (byoo-SPIE-roen hie-droe-KLOR-ied)
An oral a*nxiolytic drug.* BuSpar™ is the brand name for this drug.

Button
Refer to **Gastrostomy Button.**

Butyrophenone (byoo-ti-roe-FEE-noen)
An *antipsychotic drug* that affects neurochemicals in the *brain* and is used to treat *psychosis* and to suppress *behaviors* such as *tics* associated with *Tourette syndrome.*

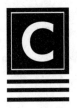

c
The abbreviation for with.

C
The symbol for carbon.
The abbreviation for Celsius.

Ca
The symbol for calcium.

CA
The abbreviation for cancer or carcinoma.

Café au Lait Spots (kaf-ay-oe-LAY)
Light coffee-colored marks on the skin. Café au lait spots may occur without an associated *disorder*, but they are also characteristic of certain *diseases*, such as *neurofibromatosis*.

calc-
A prefix meaning heel.

Calcaneal Tendon (kal-KAY-nee-uhl)
    Refer to **Achilles Tendon.**

Calcaneovalgus (kal-kay-nee-oe-VAL-gus)
A foot deformity in which the foot is turned outward, the ankle upward.

Calcaneus (Kal KAY-nee-uhs)
The heel bone.

Calciferol (kal-SIF-uhr-ol)
    Refer to **Ergocalciferol.**

Calcification
A deposit of *calcium* in body *tissues*.

Calcium (Ca) (KAL-see-uhm)
A chemical necessary for the normal functioning of the *nerves* and *heart,* for muscle *contraction,* for blood clotting, for working with *enzymes,* and for the growth of bones and teeth.

Calcium Gluconate (KAL-see-uhm GLOO-kuh-nayt)
A *calcium* salt that is sometimes given to a child with insufficient calcium.

Calcium Phosphate (KAL-see-um FOS-fayt)
A white powder used to treat excessive stomach acidity and as a *calcium* supplement.

Calvarium (kal-VER-ee-um)
The bones that form the top of the *cranium.*

Camptodactylia (kamp-toe-dak-TIL-ee-uh)
    Refer to **Camptodactyly.**

Camptodactyly (kamp-tuh-DAK-ti-lee)
Permanent *flexion* of the fingers or toes. It most commonly affects the fifth, fourth, and third *digits,* in decreasing order of frequency. Most likely, this *congenital* malformation is caused by the relative shortness of the length of the *flexor tendons* with respect to the growth of the hand.
    Also known as **Camptodactylia.**

Cancer/Cancerous (CA) (KAN-sur/KAN-sur-uhs)
A general term used to indicate any of various types of *malignant* growths (growths that worsen and resist treatment). Cancer is often a fatal *disease* if it spreads uncontrollably to normal *tissue* or to sites within the body that are distant from the original site of *abnormal cell* growth.

Candida Albicans (KAN-di-duh AL-buh-kanz)
A common *fungus* that grows in areas of *mucous membrane* (such as the mouth and vagina) or on the skin and causes *candidiasis* (such as *thrush* or diaper *rash*) and other "*yeast*" infections. Candida growth is encouraged by a warm, moist environment and by drugs that kill the *bacteria* that would normally keep the fungus from growing.
    Also known as **Monilia.**

Candidiasis (kan-di-DIE-uh-sis)
    Refer to **Candida Albicans.**

Cannula (KAN-yoo-luh)
A small tube for insertion into a *vessel* or cavity of the body. A cannula can be used to give or withdraw fluids.

Canthi (KAN-thie)
Plural of *canthus.*

Canthus (KAN-thuhs)
The angle at either end of the opening between the upper and lower eyelids.

CAPD
The abbreviation for *Central Auditory Processing Disorder.*

Capillary
A tiny *blood vessel* that connects the *arteries* and *veins,* thereby nourishing body *tissues* and removing waste products.

Capillary Hemangioma
> *Refer to* **Hemangioma.**

Capitate Bone
The largest bone in the wrist.

Carbamazepine (CBZ) (kar-bam-AZ-uh-peen)
An *antiepileptic drug.* Tegretol™ is the brand name of this drug.

Carbohydrate (kar-boe-HIE-drayt)
A category of foods that includes sugars and starches and is the main source of energy for all body functions.

Carbon (C)
A nonmetallic element that is essential to body chemistry.

Carbon Dioxide (CO$_2$)
A clear, odorless by-product of body *metabolism* that is carried by the blood to the lungs, where it is exhaled.

Carbon Monoxide (CO)
A clear, odorless gas that is formed when there is not enough *oxygen* for proper burning. Carbon monoxide is highly poisonous and can cause *asphyxiation,* which may lead to *central nervous system* damage and death if enough of the gas is inhaled.

carcin-
A prefix meaning *cancer.*

Carcinogen (kar-SIN-oe-jen or KAR-si-noe-jen)
Anything that is capable of causing or accelerating the development of *cancer,* such as tobacco smoke or asbestos.

Carcinoma (CA) (kar-si-NOE-muh)
Any *cancerous (malignant) tumor* that arises from inner or outer body surfaces such as the skin or lungs.

cardi-
A prefix meaning *heart.*

Cardiac
Referring to the *heart*.

Cardiac Arrest
A sudden stop in the pumping of the *heart*. Cardiac arrest in children is most often caused by *respiratory failure*, but other causes include heart attack (which is the common cause in adults), *shock*, blood loss, drug overdose, or *hypothermia*. A person who has suffered cardiac arrest will stop breathing and become unconscious. *Cardiopulmonary resuscitation* is necessary to avoid *brain damage* and death.

Cardiac Catheter
*Refer to **Cardiac Catheterization** and **Catheter**.*

Cardiac Catheterization
A surgical procedure to *diagnose* and assess a *heart* condition. A small incision is made in the arm or leg and a *catheter* is threaded through a large *blood vessel* and into the heart. *Blood pressure* and blood *oxygen* levels are measured, and *x-rays* may be taken to show the inside of the heart as it pumps. If x-rays are taken, a contrast material will first be injected into the heart.

Cardiac Massage
An emergency procedure done during surgery and *cardiopulmonary resuscitation* involving a repeated, rhythmic compression of the *heart*. The procedure is done when the heart stops beating. Cardiac massage forces the heart to pump blood and may stimulate the heart to beat normally on its own.
*Also known as **Heart Massage** or **Chest Compressions**.*

Cardiologist (kar-dee-OL-oe-jist)
A medical doctor who specializes in the evaluation and treatment of *diseases* of the *heart*.

Cardiology
The branch of medicine dealing with the *heart* and blood *circulation*.

Cardiomyopathy (kar-dee-oe-mie-OP-uh-thee)
Any *disease* of the *heart* muscle that causes it to enlarge and that causes a decrease in the force of the heart's *contractions*. This leads to an inability of the heart to efficiently circulate blood through the lungs and the rest of the body. The cause of cardiomyopathy is usually unknown, but it may be an *inherited* condition, or be caused by a *virus*, a *toxin*, scarring of the lining of the heart, an *abnormality* in the chemical activity of the heart muscle *cells* (the cause of the abnormality is unknown), or a *vitamin* or *mineral* deficiency. Drugs may be used to treat the *symptoms* of cardiomyopathy, but often the heart continues to deteriorate.
*Also known as **Myocardiopathy**.*

Cardiopulmonary/Cardiorespiratory
(kar-dee-oe-PUL-muh-ner-ee/kar-dee-oe-RES-pur-uh-tor-ee)
Pertaining to the *heart* and lungs.

Cardiopulmonary Resuscitation (CPR) (kar-dee-oe-PUL-muh-ner-ee)

A method of reviving a person who is not breathing and whose heartbeat is not strong enough to be effective or has stopped. CPR consists of *cardiac massage* (*chest compressions*) and *mouth-to-mouth* (or mouth-to-nose/mouth, in infants) *resuscitation* (rescue breathing).

Cardiovascular System (kar-dee-oe-VAS-kyuh-luhr)

The *heart* and *blood vessels*.
  Refer to **Circulation/Circulatory System.**

Caries (KAYR-eez)

  Refer to **Dental Caries.**

Carnitine (KAR-ni-tin)

A chemical important to the process of *metabolism*. It is sometimes used to treat *myopathy* caused by carnitine deficiency.

Carolina Curriculum for Handicapped Infants and Infants At-Risk

  Refer to **Carolina Curriculum for Infants and Toddlers with Special Needs.**

Carolina Curriculum for Infants and Toddlers with Special Needs (CCITSN)

A *criterion-referenced evaluation* tool used to assess the *cognitive, communication*/language, *fine motor, gross motor, self-help/adaptive,* and *social/emotional* development of the birth to 24-month-old. The Carolina also provides suggested activities for program planning and implementation. The Carolina may be administered by professionals and *paraprofessionals*.
  Formerly known as the **Carolina Curriculum for Handicapped Infants and Infants At-Risk.**

Carotid Arteries (kuh-ROT-id)

The principal *arteries* that carry blood to the neck and head. The carotid arteries can be felt on either side of the neck and are called the left and right common carotid arteries. These arteries each divide into two arteries, the internal and external carotid arteries.

Carpal (KAR-puhl)

Pertaining to the *carpus*, or wrist.

Carpenter Syndrome (KAHR-puhn-tuhr)

An *autosomal recessive disorder* characterized by a *congenital* malformation of the skull caused by premature closure of certain *sutures* (resulting in a head that appears pointed at the top), webbed or fused fingers and/or toes, extra fingers and/or toes, shortened fingers and/or toes, and *mental retardation*.
  Also known as **Acrocephalopolysyndactyly, Type II.**

Carpus (KAR-pus)

The eight small bones of the wrist.

Carrier
1. A person who carries a specific *pathogen* (a *microorganism* capable of producing *disease*) and who is capable of spreading disease, even though he does not show signs of the disease or become ill.
2. A person who carries one *recessive gene* for a particular trait or condition, but shows no signs of the trait or condition himself because he also has a *dominant gene* that overrides the recessive gene. A carrier can, however, pass the recessive trait or condition on if he has a child with someone who also carries the recessive gene and the child inherits the recessive gene from both parents. This is how *autosomal recessive disorders* such as *Tay-Sachs* disease occur.

CARS
The abbreviation for Childhood Autism Rating Scale.

Cartilage
Connective tissue that provides support to body structures. Cartilage also functions to allow smooth motion and decreased friction of *joints*.

Casein (KAY-seen or KAY-see-in)
A *protein* that occurs naturally in dairy products. Some people are sensitive to casein. (It irritates their intestines.) It has been theorized, although not proven by well-controlled scientific research, that casein can irritate or damage the *brain*, causing certain *behaviors* associated with *autism spectrum disorder*.

Case Manager
*Refer to **Service Coordinator**.*

cata-
A prefix meaning down.

Catapres™ (KAT-uh-pres)
*Refer to **Clonidine Hydrochloride**.*

Cataract (KAT-uh-rakt)
An eye *disease* in which the *lens* loses its transparency (becomes opaque), causing partial *blindness*. Cataract may be caused by an infection during the first *trimester* of pregnancy, *prenatal exposure to drugs*, certain *genetic disorders*, injury to the eye, or contact with certain poisons or medications. Cataract occurs most commonly during old age. Cataracts can often be removed to restore vision.

Catastrophic Health Insurance
Health insurance plans against the costs of catastrophic (severe or lengthy) illness or injury. Information on state-offered protection plans can be obtained through public health and welfare departments.

Categorical Placement
Placement of a child with *special needs* in a class setting where all the other children have the same *disability*. For example, placing a child with *visual impairments* in a preschool class of only children with visual impairments.
*Compare **Noncategorical Placement**.*

Catheter (KATH-uh-ter)
A flexible tube used to administer fluids to or drain fluids from the body. There are several sites where catheters are used. Examples of types of catheters (based on location) include the *arterial catheter* (a catheter placed in an *artery* to provide continuous access for withdrawing arterial blood for monitoring *arterial blood gases* and *blood pressure*); *venous catheter* (a catheter placed in a *vein* to give nutrients, medication, or blood, or to withdraw blood); *cardiac catheter* (a catheter that is threaded into the *heart* via a *blood vessel* to diagnose and assess *heart disease*); and *urinary catheter* (a catheter that is inserted into the *bladder* to drain urine). A catheter is sometimes referred to as a "line," such as a *central line*. When a catheter must be left in place for an extended period of time it is called an *indwelling catheter*.

Catheterization
> Refer to **Cardiac Catheterization, Catheter,** and **Urinary Catheterization.**

CAT Scanning
> Refer to **CT Scanning.**

Cattell Infant Intelligence Scale
An *evaluation* tool used to assess the mental development (*sensory, motor,* perceptual, language, and *cognitive* functioning) and *intelligence* of infants and young children between 3 and 30 months of age. The Cattell is typically administered by a professional who holds a doctorate in psychology or education.

Cause-and-Effect
The concept that actions will produce certain responses to those actions. Pushing a button on a toy to make a bunny pop up is an example of a cause-and-effect activity.

Cava (KAY-vuh)
A body cavity such as the *vena cava*.

Cavus (KAY-vus)
A condition in which the height of the arch of the foot is exaggerated.

CBC
The abbreviation for complete blood count.

CBZ
The abbreviation for carbamazepine.

CCITSN
The abbreviation for Carolina Curriculum for Infants and Toddlers with Special Needs.

CCS
The abbreviation for Crippled Children's Services.

CD
The abbreviation for Celiac Disease.

CDD
The abbreviation for Childhood disintegrative disorder.

CDH
The abbreviation for congenital dislocation of the hip.

CE
The abbreviation for conductive education.

Cecum (SEE-kum)
A chamber or blind pouch that forms the first and widest portion of the *large intestine*. At its base is the *appendix*.

Ceiling
The upper limits of a range. On an *evaluation* tool, ceiling refers to the highest test item the child passes.
> *Compare* Basal.

Celestone™ (suh-LES-toen)
> *Refer to* **Betamethasone.**

Celiac (SEE-lee-ak)
Related to the *abdominal* area.

Celiac Disease (CD)
A *malabsorption syndrome* associated with *gluten* (wheat) sensitivity. This *disease* causes diarrhea, *dehydration*, *vitamin* and *mineral* deficiencies, and loss of weight or failure to gain weight. Children usually respond favorably to a *gluten-free* diet. Celiac Disease is an *inborn error of metabolism*.
> *Also known as* **Celiac Sprue, Gluten-Induced Enteropathy,** *and* **Nontropical Sprue.**

Celiac Sprue
> *Refer to* **Celiac Disease.**

Cell
The smallest fundamental unit of living *organisms* capable of independent functioning.

Cellulitis (sel-yoo-LIE-tis)
Inflammation of the skin and the *tissues* beneath it. It is caused by an infection from *bacteria* that has entered a wound. Cellulitis is treated with *antibiotic drugs*.

Celontin™ (suh-LON-tin)
> *Refer to* **Methsuximide.**

-centesis
A suffix meaning puncture.

Central Auditory Processing Disorder (CAPD)
A *disorder* that causes difficulty in processing and interpreting sounds, even though there is no *hearing impairment*. A central auditory processing disorder is caused by a problem that affects the *brain*, such as variations in brain development, an *inherited* condition, a head *trauma*, or *lead poisoning*. CAPD sometimes results in or co-exists with other *learning disabilities*, as well. Children with a CAPD may be easily distracted, have difficulty following directions or conversations, become excessively upset by loud or unexpected noises or by noisy environments, and behave in more appropriate ways when in a quieter or more organized setting.
>*Also known as* **Auditory Processing Disorder.**
>*Compare* **Peripheral Auditory Disorder.**

Central Line
An *intravenous catheter* that is surgically placed into a large *blood vessel* to deliver nutrients or medications, to measure venous pressure (the pressure of circulating blood on the walls of the *veins*), and to withdraw blood samples. A central line is one type of *indwelling catheter*.
>*Refer to* **Catheter.**

Central Nervous System (CNS)
The *brain* and *spinal cord*. The central *nervous system* functions to receive *sensory* information and to initiate the appropriate *motor* response. It works in conjunction with the *peripheral nervous system*.
>*Compare* **Autonomic Nervous System** *and* **Peripheral Nervous System.**

Central Venous Nutrition (CVN)
>*Refer to* **Total Parenteral Nutrition (TPN).**

Central Visual Field
The area seen without moving the head or eyes.

Centromere (SEN-truh-mir)
The constricted region of a *chromosome*. This pinched section separates the smaller segment above the constricted area (the chromosome's "p" arm) from the larger segment below the constricted area (the chromosome's "q" arm).

Centronuclear Myopathy (sen-troe-NOO-klee-ur mie-OP-uh-thee)
>*Refer to* **Myotubular Myopathy.**

cephal-, cephalo-
Prefixes meaning head.

Cephalexin (sef-uh-LEK-sin)
An *antibiotic drug* used to treat some infections. Keflex™ is it the brand name of this drug.

Cephalhematoma (sef-uhl-hee-muh-TOE-muh)

A birth *trauma* characterized by a blood-filled swelling on the newborn's head. This is a *benign* condition that occurs due to pressure on the infant's skull as it passes through the pelvic bones during vaginal delivery. The skull remolds as the infant's head grows during the first year, and the lump (swelling) becomes less noticeable or not noticeable at all. (The blood is usually *reabsorbed* and treatment is not usually necessary.) Cephalhematoma can develop on one or both sides of the head (*bilateral* cephalhematoma), and can be quite dramatic with a vacuum delivery.

Cephalocaudal Sequence of Development (sef-uh-loe-KAH-duhl)

Referring to the progression of human *development*, in that skills develop from the head downward (i.e., *head control* is achieved before control of the legs).

Cephalopelvic Disproportion (CPD) (sef-uh-loe-PEL-vik)

A condition in which the mother's *pelvis* is relatively too small for the baby's head to pass through during vaginal delivery.

Cerebellum (ser-uh-BEL-um)

The part of the *brain* responsible for maintaining *balance* and for coordinating voluntary movements. The cerebellum is located behind the *brainstem* at the base of the skull.

> *Refer to* **Brain.**

Cerebral (suh-REE-bruhl or SER-uh-bruhl)

Of, or pertaining to, the *cerebrum.*

Cerebral Acqueduct (suh-REE-bruhl AW-Kwuh-dukt)

The narrow canal in the *midbrain* through which *cerebrospinal fluid* passes.

> *Also known as* **Aqueduct of Sylvius.**

Cerebral Angiography (suh-REE-bruhl an-jee-OG-ruh-fee)

Angiography (an *x-ray* study of the *blood vessels*) of the *brain.*

Cerebral Cortex

The surface *gray matter* (nervous *tissue*) of the *cerebral hemispheres* (*cerebrum*) of the *brain.* The cerebral cortex is considered responsible for receiving and analyzing *sensory* information, for conscious thought, and for movement.

> *Compare* **Motor Cortex.**

Cerebral Gigantism

> *Refer to* **Sotos Syndrome.**

Cerebral Hemisphere

One half of the paired portions of the *brain.* The two cerebral hemispheres make up the largest part of the brain (the *cerebrum*). Within each cerebral hemisphere is a ventricle that contains *cerebrospinal fluid.* The ventricles are surrounded by the *nerve cells* called the *basal ganglia.* The next layer consists

of nerve fibers, or *white matter*. The outer layer is called the *cerebral cortex*, which is made up of nerve cells, or *gray matter* (nervous *tissue*). Each hemisphere is comprised of four lobes: the *frontal* lobe, which occupies the front third of each hemisphere; the *occipital* lobe, which occupies the back fourth of each hemisphere; the *parietal* lobe, which is located in the middle-upper area of each hemisphere; and the *temporal lobe*, which is located in the lower-middle area of each hemisphere. The two cerebral hemispheres are connected by the *corpus callosum*. The left hemisphere is dominant for speech in most people. Also, the dominant hemisphere determines *hand preference*. For example, if the left hemisphere is dominant, the child will usually be right-handed.
Refer to **Cerebrum.**

Cerebral Palsy (CP) (suh-REE-bruhl or SER-uh-bruhl POL-zee)
A *disorder* of movement and *posture* control resulting from nonprogressive damage to the *brain* during *fetal* life, the newborn period, or early childhood. Both *genetic* and *acquired* factors may be involved. Cerebral palsy may be caused by a lack of normal fetal brain development or by injury to the brain. There are several ways a baby's brain can be injured, including: drug or alcohol exposure, an inadequate supply of *oxygen* to the brain either *prenatally* or during delivery, *maternal* infection that is present during pregnancy, an excess of *bilirubin* during the *neonatal period*, infection of the infant's or young child's brain (such as with *meningitis* or *encephalitis*), or head injury. The extent and location of *brain damage* determine the type of cerebral palsy and the associated *symptoms* (such as *abnormal muscle tone*, *involuntary movements*, or lack of *balance* and coordination). The three main classifications of cerebral palsy are *Pyramidal Cerebral Palsy*, *Extrapyramidal Cerebral Palsy*, and *Mixed-Type Cerebral Palsy*. Most children with cerebral palsy have normal or high *intelligence*, but *mental retardation*, *learning disabilities*, and *seizures* may be included in the *diagnosis* of cerebral palsy.
Refer to **Atonic Cerebral Palsy, Choreoathetoid Cerebral Palsy, Extrapyramidal Cerebral Palsy, Mixed-Type Cerebral Palsy, Pyramidal Cerebral Palsy,** *and* **Rigid Cerebral Palsy.**

Cerebral Visual Impairment
Refer to **Cortical Visual Impairment.**

cerebro-
A prefix meaning *brain*.

Cerebrohepatorenal Syndrome (ser-uh-broe-hep-uh-toe-REE-nuh)
Refer to **Zellweger Syndrome.**

Cerebrospinal Fluid (CSF)
(suh-REE-broe-spie-nuhl or ser-uh-broe-SPIE-nuhl)
Fluid produced in the *brain's* ventricles which circulates around the brain and *spinal column*. The fluid acts as a buffer and also supplies the *central nervous system nutritionally*.
Refer to **Hydrocephalus.**

Cerebrovascular (ser-ee-broe-VAS-kyuh-ler or ser-uh-broe-VAS-kyuh-ler)
Pertaining to the *blood vessels* of the *brain*.

Cerebrovascular Accident (CVA)
>*Refer to* **Stroke**.

Cerebrum (ser-EE-brum or SER-uh-brum)
The largest part of the *brain*. It contains the two *cerebral hemispheres*, which
are joined together by the *corpus callosum*. The cerebrum has *sensory* and
motor functions and is the area where most voluntary thought and activity
is initiated.
>*Refer to* **Brain** *and* **Cerebral Hemisphere**.

Cerumen (se-ROO-men)
Earwax.

Cervical
1. Relating to the neck.
2. Relating to the *cervix*.

Cervical Incompetence
A weakness in the *cervix* which may lead to *miscarriage* or premature delivery.
>*Also known as* **Incompetent Cervix**.

cervico-
A prefix meaning neck.

Cervix
The lowest part of the *uterus* through which the infant passes when born
vaginally.

Cesarean Section (C-Section) (see-SER-ee-uhn or suh-SER-ee-uhn)
The surgical delivery of a baby through incisions in the mother's *abdominal*
and uterine walls.

CF
The abbreviation for cystic fibrosis.

Chaining
>*Refer to* **Backward Chaining** *and* **Forward Chaining**.

Chairs (Adaptive)
Chairs that are used to position a child appropriately to promote a specific
function. Examples of uses include to improve head and trunk control, to increase muscular expansion and *contraction* of the chest for better breathing,
or to assist with maintaining appropriate *posture* to encourage learning, such
as a corner chair that allows the infant or toddler to sit upright on the floor.

Chalasia (kuh-LAY-zhuh or kuh-LAY-zee-uh)
The *abnormal* relaxation of the *sphincter* muscle between the *esophagus* and stomach. This results in *gastroesophageal reflux* (the contents of the stomach come back up into the esophagus).
> *Refer to* **Gastroesophageal Reflux.**

Charcot-Marie-Tooth Disease *(CMT)* (shar-KOE muh-REE tooth)
An *inherited disorder* in which the child progressively develops weakness and wasting of foot and calf muscles and, later, hand and forearm muscles as a result of *peripheral nerve degeneration*. Rarely, progressive *sensorineural hearing impairment* also results. The *disease* usually begins between middle childhood and age 30 and usually progresses slowly. Although the quality of the child's movements will be affected, the resulting *disability* is usually not completely debilitating (frequently the *disease* becomes stationary) and the patient usually lives a normal life span.
> *Also known as* **Peroneal Muscular Atrophy** *and* **Hereditary Motor and Sensory Neuropathy.**

CHARGE Association
A *genetic syndrome* characterized by *Coloboma* (a *cleft*, or area of incomplete fusion of part of the eyeball that results in an area with loss of vision), *Heart disease*, *Atresia choanae* (also called *choanal atresia*, which is blockage of the nasal passage), Retarded growth and *development* (occasional *mental retardation* ranging from mild to profound and growth deficiency), Genital *anomalies*, and Ear anomalies and/or *deafness*.
> *Also known as* **CHARGE Syndrome.**

CHARGE Syndrome
> *Refer to* **CHARGE Association.**

CHAT
The abbreviation for Checklist for Autism in Toddlers.

CHD
The abbreviation for congenital heart disease.

Checklist for Autism in Toddlers (CHAT)
A short questionnaire designed to identify children *at-risk* for social-communication *disorders*. It is completed by the parent and the primary healthcare provider. The CHAT was developed in the U.K. A modified, expanded version (M-CHAT) was developed in the U.S. by Diana L. Robins, Deborah Fein, Marianne L. Barton, and James A. Green.
> *Compare* **Modified Checklist for Autism in Toddlers.**

cheilo-
A prefix meaning lip or edge.

Chelation (kee-LAY-shuhn)
A procedure that uses certain drugs to bind (combine with) an ingested poisonous substance (such as lead or another metal) so the body can *excrete* it through the urine more quickly.

Chemical Dependency
A physical and/or psychological need for a substance such as cocaine.

Chemically Exposed
Referring to the child who has been *prenatally exposed to drugs* or alcohol.
   *Refer to **Prenatally Exposed to Drugs** and **Fetal Alcohol Syndrome**.*

Chemotherapy (kee-muh-THER-uh-pee)
The treatment of *disease* with chemicals (drugs), usually referring to using anticancer drugs that impair the ability of *cancer cells* to multiply.

Chest Compressions
   *Refer to **Cardiac Massage**.*

Chest Percussion
A method of decreasing a child's *respiratory* congestion by "pounding" on his chest with a cupped hand to help him loosen and cough up *mucus* so he can breathe easier. Chest percussion is often accompanied by *postural drainage* and may be used in the treatment of *cystic fibrosis*.
   *Compare **Percussion**.*
   *Refer to **Postural Drainage**.*

Chest Tube (ct)
A tube that is surgically placed to drain fluid or air, and to enable a collapsed lung to re-expand.

Chewing
1. Biting and grinding with the *gums* or teeth. A munching pattern (up and down biting action) is used for chewing food initially (beginning around 6 to 8 months of age), until approximately 18 to 24 months of age, when *rotary chewing* (rotary jaw movement) emerges.
2. An activity to increase arousal in a child who is *hyporesponsive* to *sensory stimulation*. Chewing on a toy or a crunchy food may be part of a child's *sensory diet* designed by his *occupational therapist*.
   *Refer to **Rotary Chewing**.*

CHF
The abbreviation for congestive heart failure.

Chicken Pox
A common, *contagious*, childhood *viral* illness in which a *generalized*, itchy, red *rash* with blisters appears on many parts of the body. Chicken pox is conta-

gious until all *lesions* become crusted with scabs. Young children can be given a *vaccine* by injection to *immunize* them against the *disease*.

>Also known as **Varicella**.
>Refer to **Varicella-Zoster Virus**.

Chicken Pox Vaccine
>Refer to **Varicella-Zoster Virus Vaccine**.

Child Abuse and Neglect
As defined by the Child Abuse Prevention and Treatment Act, Public Law 93-247: "The physical or mental injury, sexual abuse or exploitation, negligent treatment or maltreatment of a child under the age of 18...by a person who is responsible for the child's welfare..."

>Compare **Emotional Abuse** and **Sexual Abuse**.
>Refer to **Mandated Reporter**.

Child-Directed Instruction
Instruction based on the individual interests of the child. Child-directed instruction allows the infant or young child to choose from available and teacher-planned activities designed to stimulate learning and promote the learning objective. The skillful teacher must be able to adjust and adapt so that the child's interests can be used to create new challenges and learning. The teacher must constantly evaluate and add to the activity at the appropriate time so that the child is challenged but not frustrated. A greater emphasis on child-directed instruction over *adult-directed instruction* is appropriate with the infant or young child.

>Compare **Adult-Directed Instruction**.

Child Find
A federal program which requires states to actively locate young children with *disabilities* who are not receiving any or adequate *early intervention* services. This state-wide system is responsible for identifying and making timely referrals of infants and toddlers to service providers, such as for case management, infant *development*, or *physical therapy* services. The Child Find system should provide for the participation by primary referral sources, including hospitals, *physicians*, and child care facilities.

Childhood Autism Rating Scale (CARS)
A brief rating scale that professionals (special educators, *school psychologists*, *physicians*, *speech-language pathologists*, etc.) can be trained to use to recognize and classify children with an *autism spectrum disorder*. It can be used with children over 2 years of age.

Childhood Disintegrative Disorder (CDD)
A very rare *autism spectrum disorder* (*pervasive developmental disorder*), occurring at a rate of approximately 5 in every 10,000 births, affecting boys more than girls. CDD is characterized by loss of skills after typical *development* for at least the first 2 years of life. The *regression* usually occurs when the child is between the ages of 2 and 4, however the "disintegration" can occur up un-

til age 10. The developmental deterioration can occur over a period of weeks or months, but does not continue indefinitely. A *diagnosis* is made based upon 1) lost skills in at least 2 of the following areas: language, social, *adaptive*, play, *motor*, *bowel* or *bladder* control, and 2) frequently observed *abnormalities* of functioning in at least 2 of the following areas: qualitative impairment in social interaction; qualitative impairment in *communication*; and restricted, repetitive, and *stereotyped* patterns of *behavior*, interests, and activities, including motor stereotypies and mannerisms. The child with CDD usually functions at a severely *mentally retarded* level, although new skills may be attained after the period of regression ends.

> Also known as **Disintegrative Psychosis, Heller** or **Heller's Syndrome,** and **Late Onset Autistic Disorder.**
> Formerly known as **Dementia Infantilis.**
> Refer to **Autism Spectrum Disorder.**

Child Protective Agency

An agency that receives and investigates reports of child abuse or *neglect*. The *Department of Children and Family Services* and the police department are examples of child protective agencies.

Chin Presentation

Birth (delivery) of a baby with the face, specifically the chin, appearing first in the mother's *pelvis*.

> Refer to **Fetal Presentation.**

Chloral Hydrate (KLOE-ruhl HIE-drayt)

A drug that can be used to sedate a child such as for an *EEG* (*electroencephalogram*) or *CT scanning*, or for dental work. It is also prescribed to help children with sleeping problems.

Chlorothiazide (kloe-roe-THIE-uh-zied)

A *diuretic* (a drug that helps remove excess water from the body). Diuril™ is the brand name of this drug.

Chlorpromazine (klor-PROE-muh-zeen)

An *antipsychotic drug*. Thorazine™ is the brand name of this drug.

Choanal Atresia (KOE-uh-nuhl uh-TREE-zee-uh)

A *congenital defect* in which one or both of the nasal passages is blocked.

> Also known as **Atresia Choanae.**

chole-

A prefix meaning *bile*.

Cholestasis (koe-lee-STAY-sis)

An interruption in the flow of *bile* as it moves from the *liver* to the *duodenum*. It can be caused by many conditions including *hepatitis*, a *tumor*, or a *genetic disorder*. It is essential that the organ affected (between the liver and the duodenum) be pinpointed so proper treatment can be given.

Cholesteatoma (koe-lee-stee-uh-TOE-muh)
A condition in which skin *cells* from the *auditory canal* grow inward toward the *middle ear*, forming a *cyst* that causes damage to the bones of the middle ear and to the mastoid bone. The growth of the skin cells is usually the result of chronic *otitis media* (*middle ear infection*) that has caused the *tympanic membrane, or eardrum* to burst, but cholesteatoma may be a *congenital* condition. The cyst must be removed surgically. *Auditory impairment* may result.

Choline (KOE-leen or KOE-lin)
A factor found in the *vitamin* B-complex.

chondr-, chondro-
Prefixes meaning *cartilage*.

Chondrodysplasia (kon-droe-dis-PLAY-zee-uh)
An *inherited disease* characterized by *abnormal* growth at the ends of bones. The long bones of the arms and legs are primarily affected (resulting in *short stature*), but the bones of the hands and feet may be affected as well.

Chondrodystrophy (kon-droe-DIS-troe-fee)
A group of *disorders* characterized by disturbance in the early development of the *cartilage* of the long bones of the *extremities*. Chondrodystrophy results in a form of *short stature* in which the arms and legs are *abnormally* short, but the head and trunk are normal-sized. *Achondroplasia* is a type of chondrodystrophy.

Chondroectodermal Dysplasia
(kon-droe-ek-toe-DUR-muhl dis-PLAY-zhuh)
An *autosomal recessive disorder* characterized by short *limbs* and stature, extra fingers and occasionally toes, mouth and teeth *anomalies*, occasional *mental retardation*, and often, a *cardiac* defect that can result in death in infancy.
    Also known as **Ellis-van Creveld Syndrome.**

Chordee (KOR-dee)
Abnormal curving of the penis.

Chorea (koe-REE-uh)
Purposeless, jerking movements. Chorea is caused by damage to the *basal ganglia* of the *brain*.

Choreoathetoid Cerebral Palsy
(koe-ree-oe-ATH-e-toid suh-REE-bruhl POL-zee)
A form of *extrapyramidal cerebral palsy* characterized by *involuntary movements* (relatively slow writhing movements with a jerky component), and by *muscle tone* that fluctuates between low and normal or between low and *spastic*. Choreoathetoid cerebral palsy results from damage to the *nerve* pathways that transmit impulses for controlling movement and maintaining *posture* from the *brain* to the *spinal cord*.
    Refer to **Extrapyramidal Cerebral Palsy.**

Choreoathetoid Movements
Refer to **Choreoathetosis** *and* **Choreoathetoid Cerebral Palsy**.

Choreoathetosis (koe-ree-oe-ath-e-TOE-sis)
Irregular, *involuntary movements* (relatively slow writhing movements with a jerky component) that may involve the face, neck, trunk, *extremities*, or *respiratory* muscles. Choreoathetosis may be present in a child with *cerebral palsy* and is associated with the drug levodopa.
> *Also known as* **Choreoathetoid Movements**.
> *Refer to* **Choreoathetoid Cerebral Palsy**.

Chorionic Villus Sampling (CVS) (koe-ree-ON-ik VIL-us)
A *prenatal* technique for *diagnosing fetal abnormalities* in which a small sample of the chorionic villus (a part of the *placenta*) is removed so the *chromosomes* can be analyzed.

Chorioretinitis (kor-ee-oe-ret-uh-NIE-tis)
An *inflammation* of the *retina* and *choroid* of the eye that can produce visual loss. Chorioretinitis is usually the result of infection. Chorioretinitis can be so minor that, if treated early, the patient may not even be aware that he has it. If the central area of the eye is involved, more eye damage may result.

Choroid (KOR-oid)
The middle layer of the eyeball between the *sclera* and the *retina*. The choroid lines the white of the eyeball and supplies blood to the retina.

chrom-, chromo-
Prefixes meaning color.

Chromosomal Abnormality (kroe-muh-SOE-muhl)
A *genetic disorder* caused by either too few or too many *chromosomes*, or by chromosomes with extra pieces, missing pieces, or pieces attached to another chromosome. An example of a chromosomal abnormality is *Down syndrome* (an extra chromosome 21 is present).
> *Refer to* **Cytogenetic Syndrome**.

Chromosomal Deletion
A condition in which a piece of a *chromosome* is missing. The resulting loss of *genetic* material is microscopically visible. An example of a *disorder* caused by chromosomal deletion is *cri du chat syndrome*.
> *Compare* **Microdeletion**.

Chromosomal Nondisjunction
Failure of a *chromosome* pair to separate during *cell* division (prior to conception), resulting in both chromosomes being carried to one *daughter cell* and none to the other daughter cell. For example, *Down syndrome* may result due to nondisjunction of chromosome pair 21.

Chromosomal Translocation
The transfer of part of a *chromosome* to another chromosome, resulting in a change in the *genetic* material within the body's *cells*. Translocation is a type of *mutation* and can be *inherited* or *acquired* as the result of a new mutation. Often the translocation causes no *abnormality*, but a parent who is a *carrier* of a translocation can have children who are affected. *Down syndrome* is an example of a *disorder* that can occur due to chromosomal translocation.

Chromosome (KROE-muh-soem)
The microscopic rod-shaped structures within *cells* that contain the *genetic* information that determines or influences the individual traits of a child. (Every cell in an individual's body—except for the *sperm* or egg cells—normally carries the exact same chromosomal material.) Normally, human beings have 46 chromosomes (23 pairs) in each cell.

Chromosome Analysis
A procedure to *diagnose chromosome disorders* in which chromosomal materials (from blood, skin, *amniotic fluid*, and other *tissues*) are analyzed by number and structure.
> *Refer to* **Karyotyping.**

Chronic Illness
A sickness that develops slowly and lasts for a long time. Some chronic illnesses persist throughout a person's life.
> *Compare* **Acute Illness.**

Chronic Lung Disease (CLD)
A condition in which there is persistent disruption of the passage of air in and out of the lungs. *Bronchopulmonary dysplasia* is a form of chronic lung disease.

Chronological Age
An infant or child's age stated in hours, days, weeks, months, or years and months since birth.
> *Compare* **Corrected Age** and **Mental Age.**

Cicatrix (SIK-uh-triks or sik-AY-triks)
Scar *tissue*.

CID
The abbreviation for cytomegalic inclusion disease.

Cilia (SIL-ee-uh)
1. Microscopic hairlike projections on some *cells* that sway, causing movement of the fluid that surrounds them. An example of cilia are those found on the *nerve cells* of the *cochlea* of the *inner ear*.

Cimetidine (si-MET-i-deen)
A drug used to decrease stomach acidity and to reduce *inflammation* of the *esophagus*. It is sometimes given to children who experience *gastroesophageal reflux*.

Circle of Communication

A back and forth interaction (one completed cycle of communicating and responding between 2 people) in which the *behavior* and ideas of one person (conveyed by verbalizations, *gestures*, or overtures) are connected to those of the other person. For example, if a parent says to her hidden son, "Where is my little guy hiding?" and the child reappears, or says "Boo!" or "Here I am!", the parent has opened and the child has closed a circle of communication.

Circular Reactions

> *Refer to **Primary Circular Reactions** and **Secondary Circular Reactions**.*

Circulation/Circulatory System

The flow of blood throughout the *heart* and *blood vessels*. Blood circulates in this manner: the left *atrium* (upper chamber) of the heart pumps *oxygenated* blood to the left *ventricle* (lower chamber), where the blood is then forced through the *aorta* to many other *arteries* and even smaller arteries called *arterioles* to get the blood to the rest of the body. The body organs receive blood from the arterioles, which branch off into the *capillaries* of body *tissues*, where oxygen and nutrients are exchanged with *carbon dioxide* and other waste products. From here the blood, which is now *deoxygenated*, flows through the tiny *veins* called venules, the veins, and the *venae cavae*, and on to the right atrium (upper chamber) of the heart. The blood continues on to the right ventricle (lower chamber), which pumps it through the *pulmonary artery* to the lungs. Within the lungs the exchange of carbon dioxide and oxygen is again made, only now the carbon dioxide leaves the blood and the blood is re-oxygenated. Finally, the newly oxygenated blood returns to the left atrium of the heart via the *pulmonary veins* and the cycle continues.

> *Also known as **Cardiovascular System**.*
> *Compare **Fetal Circulation** and **Persistent Fetal Circulation**.*

circum-

A prefix meaning around.

Circumduction Movement

The motion of the head of a bone in its socket, such as a shoulder *joint* when the *distal* end of the arm moves so as to outline an arc. Circumduction is one of the four basic kinds of movement by the joints of the body.

> *Compare **Angular Movement, Gliding Movement**, and **Rotation Movement**.*

Cisapride (SIS-uh-pride)

A drug sometimes used to treat *gastroesophageal reflux*. Propulsid™ is the brand name of this drug.

Citrullinemia (si-truhl-uh-NEE-mee-uh)

An *autosomal recessive disease* in which the *amino acid* citrulline is not metabolized properly due to an *enzyme* deficiency. It can cause vomiting, *seizures*, *coma*, accumulation of ammonia (a gas the body produces, converts to *urea*, then *excretes*), and *mental retardation* beginning in infancy. It is treated with a specialized diet.

CK
The abbreviation for creatine kinase.

CL
The abbreviation for Cutis laxa syndrome.

-clasia
A suffix meaning breaking.

Clavicle
The collarbone. It forms joints with the *sternum* (breast bone) and the *scapula* (shoulder blade).

Clawfoot
> *Refer to* **Pes Cavus.**

Clawing
The action of an infant's toes pressing against the floor while standing, trying to maintain *balance*.

CLD
The abbreviation for chronic lung disease.

-cle
A suffix meaning small.

Clean Intermittent Catheterization
A procedure to drain urine from the *bladder*. A *catheter* is periodically passed through the *urethra*, then into the bladder, not left in place permanently.

Cleft
A split, *fissure*, or elongated opening. For example, a cleft can occur in the lip, *palate*, or skull.

Cleft Lip
A *congenital anomaly* that occurs between the third and tenth weeks of *fetal* life when the upper lip doesn't fuse together, leaving one or more vertical openings that may extend up to the nose. Some babies born with a cleft lip also have a *cleft palate*. Cleft lip is a *multifactorial genetic disorder* (interaction between *genetic* and environmental factors is the cause.) Cleft lip can be repaired surgically.
> *Previously known as* **Harelip.**

Cleft Palate
A *congenital anomaly* that occurs between the third and tenth weeks of *fetal* life when the palatal *tissues* don't fuse together. There is an open space in the roof

of the mouth, either extending through both the *hard* and *soft palates*, or only part way through. Some babies born with a cleft palate also have a *cleft lip.* Cleft palate is a *multifactorial genetic disorder.* (Interaction between *genetic* and environmental factors is the cause.) Cleft palate can be repaired surgically.

Cleocin™ (KLEE-oe-sin)
Refer to **Clindamycin Hydrochloride.**

Click
A brief, sharp sound. A click can be heard during *systole (heart contraction),* and be indicative of various heart conditions. Also, a click may be felt in a child with *congenital* hip *dislocation* when the leg is moved into certain positions.

clin-, clino-
Prefixes meaning slant.

Clindamycin Hydrochloride (klin-duh-MIE-sin hie-droe-KLOR-ied)
An *antibiotic drug* used to treat certain serious *bacterial* infections. Cleocin™ is the brand name of this drug.

Clinical Psychologist
Refer to **Psychologist.**

Clinical Type
Any type of *disability* (especially one that causes *mental retardation*) that can be readily identified by the physical characteristics of individuals who have that disability. *Microcephaly, Down syndrome,* and *fetal alcohol syndrome* are examples.

Clinodactyly (klie-noe-DAK-ti-lee)
A *congenital* condition in which a baby is born with one or more incurved fingers or toes.

Clomipramine Hydrochloride (kloe-MI-pruh-men hie-droe-KLOR-ied)
An *antidepressant drug.* It is sometimes used to treat *obsessive-compulsive disorder* and to reduce *ritualistic behaviors* demonstrated by some children with *autism spectrum disorders.* Anafranil™ is the brand name of this drug.

Clonazepam (kloe-NAZ-uh-pam)
An *antiepileptic drug.* Klonopin™ and Rivotril™ are brand names for this drug.

Clonic Seizures (KLON-ik)
Seizures characterized by fast, jerky movements (repeated muscle *contraction* and relaxation) in part or all of the body.

Clonidine Hydrochloride (KLOE-ni-deen hie-droe-KLOR-ied)
A *drug* used to treat *hypertension* and sometimes used in the treatment of certain *behaviors* associated with *autism spectrum disorders.* Catapres™ is the brand name of this drug.

Clonus (KLOE-nuhs)
The *abnormal* repeated muscle *contraction* and relaxation that occurs when a muscle is stretched (for example, when the foot is bent upward at the ankle). Clonus is an indication of damage to the *nerves* that transmit impulses from the *brain* to a muscle.

Clorazepate (kloe-RAZ-uh-payt)
A *tranquilizer drug* that is also used as an *antiepileptic drug*. Tranxene™ is the brand name of this drug.

Clubbing
Broadening and thickening of the *soft tissues* of the ends of the fingers or toes.

Clubfoot
A *congenital anomaly* in which the foot is twisted in an *abnormal* position. It is believed that clubfoot has a *multifactorial* pattern of *inheritance*. The most common form of clubfoot is *talipes equinovarus*.
    Also known as **Talipes.**

CMT
The abbreviation for Charcot-Marie-Tooth Disease.

CMV
The abbreviation for cytomegalovirus.

CNS
The abbreviation for central nervous system.

CO
The abbreviation for carbon monoxide.

CO_2
The abbreviation for carbon dioxide.

Coarctation of the Aorta (koe-ark-TAY-shuhn)
A narrowing of the *aorta* that causes the *heart* to work harder to get blood to the lower half of the body (the body parts supplied by the aorta past the constricted section). Because the heart has to pump harder, the *blood pressure* above the narrowed part of the aorta is raised. (The blood pressure below the narrowed part is lowered or normal.) This *congenital heart defect* must be repaired surgically. The cause of coarctation of the aorta is unknown, although it is often associated with other heart conditions.
    Also known as **Aortic Coarctation.**

Coarse Facial Features/Coarse Facies
Describing a facial appearance that includes a thickened look to the layer of soft *tissue* just beneath the skin (affecting the lips, the area around the nose, the lower cheeks, and the forehead); a broad nose and forehead; and a prominence of the bone structure above the eyes.
    Refer to **Facies.**

Coccyx (KOK-siks)
The tailbone. The last *vertebra* of the *spine*.

Cochlea (KOK-lee-uh)
The spiral-shaped cavity of the *inner ear* that makes *hearing* possible. The co-chlea functions by transforming sound vibrations into signals that are trans-mitted to the *brain* along the *auditory nerves*.
> *Refer to Ear.*

Cochlear Implant (KOK-lee-ar)
A device to treat severe *sensorineural hearing impairment* in which one or more *electrodes* are surgically implanted in the *inner ear* to electronically stim-ulate any undamaged inner ear *nerves*.

Cockayne Syndrome (kok-AYN)
An *autosomal recessive disorder* characterized by poor growth *(short stature)* with long *extremities* and large hands and feet, *mental retardation, sensorineu-ral hearing impairment, visual impairment*, skin that is sensitive to sunlight, and premature aging. Cockayne syndrome usually results in death by adoles-cence or early adulthood.

Coexisting Condition
> *Refer to Comorbidity.*

Coffin-Lowry Syndrome (KOF-in LOU-ree)
An *X-linked disorder* characterized by deficient growth, downslanting eyes, *coarse facial features, hypotonia* (decreased *muscle tone*), tapering fingers, and *severe mental retardation*. The *gene* that causes this *disorder* is located on *chro-mosome* Xp22.2.

Cognition
Thinking skills, including the ability to receive, process, analyze, and under-stand information.

Cognitive
Referring to the *developmental* area that involves thinking skills, including the ability to receive, process, analyze, and understand information. Match-ing red circles and pushing the button on a mechanical toy to activate it are examples of cognitive skills.

Colace™ (KOE-lays)
> *Refer to Docusate.*

Cold
The common cold is usually a *viral* infection caused by one of many viruses. (A cold can also be a mixed infection or an *allergic* reaction.) It is usually spread by airborne droplets that are inhaled or land on surfaces which are touched (then transferred to the eyes, nose, or mouth by the hand). *Symptoms* include a runny

nose, congestion, a sore throat, a cough, muscle ache, and headache. There is no cure for the common cold, and treatment centers on alleviating discomfort.

Cold Sore
Refer to Herpes Simplex Virus 1 (HSV1).

Colic (KOL-ik)
Sharp *abdominal* pain that some infants experience during the first 3 months of life. (It may last longer than 3 months.) The cause of colic is unclear, but some doctors attribute it to intestinal *spasms* possibly caused by swallowed air, excessive gas in the intestines, or an *allergic* reaction to the baby's formula. Babies who have colic cry excessively and are difficult to console, but are otherwise healthy.

Collagen (KOL-uh-juhn)
A fibrous *protein* that helps hold together the body's *cells* and *tissues* such as the *ligaments* and *tendons*. Collagen is the most common protein in the body.

colo-
A prefix meaning *large intestine.*

Coloboma (kol-uh-BOE-muh)
Most often, a coloboma is a *congenital anomaly* that occurs in early *fetal* development when incomplete fusion of the eyeball results in a space, or *cleft*, in part of the eyeball. (Sometimes the eyelid is also involved.) It can also be caused by eye *disease*. A coloboma results in an area of lost vision within the *visual field,* surrounded by an area of vision.

Colon (KOE-luhn)
The *large intestine*. The colon moves *fecal matter* to the *anus* to be evacuated.

Colonoscopy (koe-lon-OS-koe-pee)
A procedure to examine and *diagnose* problems of the *colon* in which a long, flexible, lighted tube is inserted into the *rectum* so the inside of the colon can be viewed.

Color Vision
The ability to perceive and recognize colors. Color vision is possible when light waves are focused on the light-sensitive cone *cells* in the *retina*, which emit electrical impulses that are transmitted to the *brain* via the *optic nerve.*
Refer to Vision.

Colostomy (koe-LOS-toe-mee)
A surgically created opening to allow the *colon* to pass *feces* directly through the *abdominal* wall, bypassing part of the *digestive tract*. To collect the waste, a colostomy bag is attached to the skin at the point where the colon is brought through the abdominal incision.

Coma (KOE-muh)

A *state* of unconsciousness caused by damage to the *brain* regions responsible for maintaining consciousness. Coma may be due to brain *disease*, drugs, *hypoxia* (a lack of sufficient *oxygen* in the body *cells* or blood), *metabolic disorders, trauma*, or disturbances of the *respiratory* or *circulatory systems*.

Combat Crawl

> *Refer to* **Crawl.**
> *Compare* **Creep.**

Commando Crawl

> *Refer to* **Crawl.**
> *Compare* **Creep.**

Commissurotomy (kom-i-shyoor-OT-oe-mee)

A surgical procedure that divides (by cutting) any fibrous ring of *tissue* connecting parts of a body structure, especially that which surrounds a *heart valve*. This relieves excessive tightness of the *valve* and allows for a more normal flow of blood.

Common Cold

> *Refer to* **Cold.**

Communicable Illness (kuh-MYOO-nuh-kuh-buhl)

Disease that is transmitted person to person via *microorganism* or *parasite*.

Communication

The *developmental* area that involves skills that enable people to understand (*receptive language*) and share (*expressive language*) thoughts and feelings. Communication can be in the form of speech, facial expressions, body language, *gestures*, and written language or print. Waving "bye-bye," using spontaneous single-word utterances, and repeating five-word sentences are all examples of communication skills.

Communication Aid

A nonverbal form of *communication* such as *gesture, sign language, communication boards*, and electronic devices (for example, computers and voice synthesizers).

> *Refer to* **Assistive Technology, Augmentative and Alternative Communication,** *and* **Electronic Communication Aids**.

Communication Board/Book

A board or book with objects or pictures that a child can point to for expression of his needs.

Communication Disorder

Difficulty with understanding and/or expressing messages. Communication disorders include problems with *articulation, voice disorders, stuttering, language disorders*, and some *learning disabilities*.

Comorbidity (koe-mor-BID-i-tee)
The coexistence of 2 or more medical conditions or unrelated *disorders*. This can make *diagnosis* and treatment more difficult.
>   *Also known as* **Coexisting Condition** *and* **Dual Diagnosis.**

Compensatory Movements (kuhm-PEN-suh-tor-ee)
Actions carried out to make up for physical difficulties or inabilities. For example, if a child cannot raise his arm all the way up over his head, he may tilt his body in order to extend his reach.

Complete Blood Count (CBC)
Tests to measure the number and types of *cells* in the blood. Both *red* and *white blood cells* are counted. *Platelet* count is also determined, as well as *hemoglobin* concentration.

Complex Partial Seizure
A seizure similar to a *simple partial seizure*, except that the seizure also spreads into the *brain* areas responsible for maintaining consciousness, which usually results in the child losing consciousness. If the seizure spreads to involve the whole brain, it is called a secondarily *generalized* seizure.
>   *Formerly knows as a* **Psychomotor Seizure** *or* **Temporal Lobe Seizure.**
>   *Refer to* **Partial Seizure** *and* **Epilepsy.**
>   *Compare* **Simple Partial Seizure.**

Compound Presentation
Birth (delivery) of a baby in which more than one of the baby's body parts (most commonly a hand next to the head) are the first to appear in the mother's *pelvis*.
>   *Refer to* **Fetal Presentation.**

Compression
1. Approximation (bringing together) of the components/parts of a *joint*, while they are in *extension*, to promote stability of that joint. Compression encourages *contraction* of the muscles that support the joint and increases *proprioception* in the joint. Compression is a technique commonly used by a *physical* or *occupational therapist*.
2. Approximation (bringing together) of the components/parts of a joint to increase feedback provided to that joint thereby sending *sensory* information to the *brain* in an organized manner. Compression is a technique commonly used by an occupational therapist when treating a child with *sensory integration dysfunction*.
>   *Also known as* **Joint Compression.**

Compulsion (kumh-PUL-shuhn)
An irrational urge to repetitively perform an act in spite of understanding that the repetition is not necessary. Repeating the act does, however, decrease *anxiety*, which usually results from an *obsession*. For example, a child may repeatedly wash his hands even though he knows they were clean after the first washing. The repeated hand-washing relieves anxiety about germs (an obsession.)
>   *Refer to* **Obsession, Obsessive-Compulsive Behavior,** *and*
>   **Obsessive-Compulsive Disorder.**

Computed Tomography
Refer to CT Scanning.

Computerized Axial Tomography
Refer to CT Scanning.

con-
A prefix meaning with or together.

Concerta™
Refer to Methylphenidate Hydrochloride.

Concha (KONG-kuh)
1. A small shell-shaped bone found along the outer side of the nasal cavity.
Also known as Turbinate Bone.
2. The cavity in the *external ear* that surrounds the *external auditory canal*.

Concomitant Symptom (kon-KOM-i-tuhnt)
Any *symptom* that accompanies a primary symptom.

Conditioned Orientation Reflex (COR)
Refer to Visual Response Audiometry.

Conductive Education (CE)
A method of education designed to enable children with *motor* dysfunction to become more independent in *activities of daily living*. A professional trained in education and rehabilitation (the Conductor) helps the student find individualized ways to gain *motor control* through the use of music and/or repetitive rhythmic phrases. Conductive education is delivered in a positive, encouraging, goal-oriented group setting, with the Conductor creating a caring environment in which the child can feel motivated, attempt self-initiated activities, and experience success. No *wheelchairs* are used in the classroom. Students are asked to walk or move with appropriate assistance from one activity to another. Basic wood furniture is used, ideal for *grasping*, pushing, and pulling. The primary goal of conductive education is the development of the child's whole personality. Conductive education was developed by Dr. Andras Peto, a *neurologist*, in Hungary in the early 1940s.
Also known as Peto.

Conductive Hearing Impairment
Auditory impairment caused by problems transmitting sound vibrations to the *brain*, either because of obstruction in the *auditory canal* or because of *disorders* of the *tympanic membrane* or *middle ear*, such as *otitis media* (infection in the middle ear) or an *eardrum perforation*. This type of *hearing loss* can usually be resolved with medicine or surgery, and thus may not be permanent. Conductive hearing impairment can occur *congenitally* or be *acquired*.
Compare Mixed Hearing Impairment and Sensorineural Hearing Impairment.
Refer to Auditory Impairment.

Congenital (kuhn-JEN-i-tuhl)
Referring to a condition present at birth that may be *hereditary* (a *genetic disorder*), may be the result of a problem during pregnancy (such as a *maternal* infection), or may occur due to injury to the *fetus* prior to or at the time of birth.
Compare **Acquired** *and* **Inherited.**

Congenital Anomaly
A problem present at birth, such as *congenital heart disease* or *cleft palate*. A congenital anomaly can be *inherited* (*genetic*), occur due to a factor of the pregnancy (such as *maternal* illness, drug use, *x-ray* exposure, or physical factors in the *uterus*), result from a *chromosomal abnormality*, or occur during childbirth.
Formerly known as **Birth Defect.**

Congenital CMV
Refer to **Cytomegalovirus (CMV).**

Congenital Dislocation of the Hip (CDH)
Refer to **Developmental Dysplasia of the Hip.**

Congenital Facial Diplegia (die-PLEE-jee-uh)
Refer to **Mobius Syndrome.**

Congenital Heart Disease (CHD)
Heart disease that is present at birth. Examples of congenital heart disease include defects such as *patent ductus arteriosus* and *tetralogy of Fallot*.

Congenital Herpes
Refer to **Herpes Simplex Virus 2.**

Congenital Hypothyroidism
A *disorder* present at birth that occurs due to *congenital* lack of thyroid *secretion*. The baby with untreated congenital hypothyroidism may have retarded growth, *mental retardation*, a large tongue, and *floppy muscle tone*. Thyroid *hormone* can be replaced by taking a daily supplement; thus these consequences can be avoided.
Also known as **Cretinism.**

Congenital Infections
Diseases that occur either before birth or when passing through the birth canal by exposure to *viral*, *bacterial*, or other *microorganisms*. Examples of infections acquired before birth include *rubella* and *cytomegalovirus*. Examples of infection obtained during birth include *conjunctivitis*, *herpes*, and possibly *meningitis*.

Congenital Megacolon
Refer to **Hirschsprung Disease.**

Congenital Oculofacial Paralysis
Refer to **Mobius Syndrome.**

Congenital Rocker-Bottom Foot

A *congenital anomaly* in which the bones of the foot are positioned in such a way that the bottom side is rounded like a rocker on a rocking chair. The foot is rigid with a "reversed" arch. This condition is common in *Trisomy 18* and other *disorders*.

> *Also known as* **Congenital Vertical Talus** *and* **Vertical Talus.**

Congenital Rubella

A *viral* infection that produces only mild *symptoms* (slight fever or other signs of *upper respiratory infection*) and *rash* in a child, but can cause severe *congenital anomalies* in the *fetus* of a woman who is infected during the first 4 months of pregnancy. The earlier in pregnancy that a woman is infected, the more likely she will either miscarry or have a baby with serious *congenital* problems such as *deafness*, *heart disease*, *mental retardation*, eye *disorders*, and *cerebral palsy*.

> *Also known as* **German Measles** (however, *rubella* is not all that similar to *measles*).

Congenital Scoliosis

A progressive *congenital anomaly* caused by specific malformations of ribs and *vertebrae*. The *spine* has a C-shaped or S-shaped *lateral* curve that requires treatment (either surgical or nonsurgical, such as use of a *brace*) if it is severe or as it worsens.

Congenital Syphilis

A sexually transmitted infection that may be passed to the *fetus*, possibly causing *jaundice*, *anemia*, damage to the bones, *blindness*, *deafness*, and *mental retardation*. Congenital syphilis can be fatal to a fetus or newborn. Good *prenatal* care should include *maternal* screening for syphilis.

Congenital Toxoplasmosis

> *Refer to* **Toxoplasmosis.**

Congenital Vertical Talus

> *Refer to* **Congenital Rocker-Bottom Foot.**

Congestive Heart Failure (CHF)

The inability of the *heart* to pump enough blood to the lungs and the rest of the body. CHF is treated by determining its cause and treating that condition. Many conditions can cause congestive heart failure, including *congenital* malformations, infection, *hypertension*, a *heart arrhythmia*, *cardiomyopathy*, or *pulmonary hypertension*.

Conjugate Gaze

The eyes working in unison.

Conjugation

The act of joining together.

Conjunctiva (kon-jungk-TIE-vuh)
The *membranes* lining the eyelid and covering the eyeball.

Conjunctivitis (kuhn-jungk-ti-VIE-tis)
Inflammation of the *conjunctiva*. It can be caused by *bacteria*, a *virus*, or an *allergic* response, or be *acquired* from the mother during birth. Conjunctivitis may be infectious and *contagious*, and cause redness, an itch, and discharge.
    Also known as **Pinkeye**.

Connective Tissue
Body *tissue* that supports and holds together various structures within the body. *Tendons* and *cartilage* are made of connective tissue, and connective tissue is found in other structures such as bones.

Consanguinity (kon-san-GWIN-i-tee)
Referring to a blood relationship, especially the mating of close blood relatives, such as cousins.

Consolidation
The process by which dysfunctional or *disorganized behaviors* are replaced with *developmentally* appropriate skills.

Consonant
One of the 21 letters of the alphabet other than the five *vowels* (a, e, i, o, u). Consonants are produced when air flow that passes over the vocal cords is obstructed (mostly by the teeth and tongue) as it moves through the mouth.
    Compare **Vowel**.

Constipation
Hard, rocklike stools from *bowel movements* that may be infrequent and painful.
    Refer to **Glycerin Suppository**.

Constriction (kuhn-STRIK-shuhn)
An *abnormal* reduction in the size of an opening or passage of the body. Sometimes a constriction results in the closure of an opening. Examples include constriction of *sphincter* muscles or *blood vessels*.

Contagious (kuhn-TAY-juhs)
Communicable. Referring to a *disease* that can be passed to another person.

Contiguous Gene Deletion Syndrome
One of many different *syndromes* caused by *chromosomal deletion* that involves several different *genes* lying next to each other (contiguously) on the *chromosome*. For example, *Miller-Dieker syndrome* is a contiguous gene deletion syndrome.
    Refer to **Chromosomal Deletion and Chromosome**.

Continuant
A speech sound produced while the speech organs are held in a relatively constant position, such as the /s/, /m/, /f/, and *vowel* sounds.

Continuous Positive Airway Pressure (CPAP)
A continuous flow of pressurized air (with or without additional *oxygen*), that assists a baby in keeping his lungs expanded as he inhales and exhales.
Refer to **Nasal CPAP.**

contra-
A prefix meaning opposed or against.

Contraction (kuhn-TRAK-shuhn)
1. The brief tightening of a muscle, reducing it in size while it is tightened.
2. A rhythmic tightening of muscles of the *uterus* during *labor*.
Refer to **Uterine Contraction.**

Contracture (kuhn-TRAK-chuhr)
A shortening of muscles, *tendons*, and *fascia* that causes decreased *joint* mobility. The joint is bent and does not have a full *range of motion*. Contractures may be caused by fibrosis (*abnormal* formation of *fibrous tissue*) of the tissues supporting the muscle or joint, by *disorders* of the muscle fibers themselves, injury, or arthritis. Contractures can sometimes be prevented by range of motion exercise and by adequate support of the joints.

Convergence
The coordinated turning of both eyes inward to focus on a near point.

Convergent Strabismus (struh-BIZ-muhs)
Refer to **Esotropia.**

Convolution (kon-voe-LOO-shun)
Refer to **Gyrus.**

Convulsion
An outdated term for a *generalized tonic-clonic seizure*. It is characterized by involuntary muscle *contractions*.
Refer to **Seizure.**

Cooing
Vowel sounds produced by the infant in vocal play. The vowel sounds that are made at the back of the mouth with a more open mouth (such as "ahh") are the first sounds a baby creates because they are the easiest. The next sounds that emerge are made with a more closed mouth (such as "ee"). Cooing typically begins around 2 months of age.
Compare **Babbling, Jabbering,** *and* **Jargon.**

Cookie Insert™
An arch support pad worn inside a child's shoe.

Cooley's Anemia
Refer to **Thalassemia.**

Coombs Test (KOOMZ)
A test that detects *antibodies* to *red blood cells*. It is performed on patients suspected of having *hemolytic disease* (breakdown of red blood cells). In the newborn, hemolytic disease may be caused by *maternal* antibodies, such as when an Rh-positive baby is born to an Rh-negative mother who produced antibodies to Rh-positive blood. A Coombs test is also run in crossmatching blood (testing to establish blood compatibility before transfusion).
> *Refer to **Rh Incompatibility.***

Coprolalia (kop-roe-LAY-lee-uh)
A form of *tic* in which the child involuntarily uses obscene or vulgar words or *gestures*. Many children can learn to suppress coprolalia (and other *tics*). Some children with *Tourette syndrome* exhibit this *behavior*.

Copy
To draw a design (such as a cross or a circle), with an example to imitate, but without a demonstration of it being drawn.

COR
The abbreviation for conditioned orientation reflex.

cordi-
A prefix meaning *heart*.

Cornea (KOR-nee-uh)
The transparent, domelike shell covering the front part of the eye.
> *Refer to **Eye.***

Cornelia de Lange Syndrome (kor-NAY-lee-ah day LAHNG)
A *sporadically* occurring *congenital disorder* characterized by *short stature*, continuous eyebrows, small jaw, *microcephaly*, small or malformed hands and feet, coarse hair growing low on the forehead and on the neck, thin downturned lips, congenital *heart defects*, speech and language *deficits*, and *mental retardation*.
> *Also known as **de Lange Syndrome.***

Corner Chairs
> *Refer to **Chairs (Adaptive).***

Cor Pulmonale (kor pool-muh-NAY-lee)
A condition in which the right ventricle of the *heart* becomes enlarged and strained, which may eventually lead to *heart failure* (a condition in which the *heart* fails to maintain adequate *circulation* of blood). It is caused by *chronic lung disease*.

Corpus Callosum (KOR-pus ka-LOE-sum)
A mass of *white matter* (*nerve* fibers) that joins the *cerebral hemispheres* of the *brain*, allowing them to "communicate" with each other.

Corpus Callosum Agenesis
Refer to **Agenesis of Corpus Callosum.**

Corrected Age
The age a *premature infant* would be if he had been born on his due date. For example, a baby born 2 months prematurely has a corrected age of 6 months when he is actually (chronologically) 8 months old. This is an important consideration when measuring the premature infant's *development,* because the time missed in the *uterus* should be a factor in determining appropriate expectations for the baby.
Also known as **Adjusted Age.**
Compare **Chronological Age.**

Correlation
The relationship between variables, such as the relationship between a premature birth and the presence of *respiratory distress syndrome.*

Cortex
The outer layer of an organ or body structure.
Refer to **Cerebral Cortex.**

Cortical (KOR-ti-kuhl)
Referring to the *cortex,* or outer layer of an organ or body structure.

Cortical Atrophy (AT-roe-fee)
Wasting away of the *gray matter* (nervous *tissue*) of the *brain.*

Cortical Blindness
Refer to **Cortical Visual Impairment.**

Cortical Thumbing
Refer to **Indwelling Thumb.**

Cortical Visual Impairment (CVI)
Visual impairment resulting from an inability of the *occipital lobe* of the *brain* to process visual *stimuli.* (The eye itself is normal.) Cortical blindness can result from an *abnormality* of the brain, head injury, or infection. Depending on the cause of the damage (for example, an infection of the brain), visual impairment may improve.
Also known as **Cerebral Visual Impairment** *and* **Cortical Blindness.**

Corticosteroid (kor-ti-koe-STEER-oid)
One of the *hormones* produced by the *adrenal glands.* Corticosteroids (a type of *steroid* drug) are also made synthetically and are used to replace natural hormones and to reduce *inflammation.*

Corticotropin (kor-ti-koe-TROE-pin)
Refer to **Adrenocorticotropic Hormone.**

Costa (KOS-tuh)
A rib.

Costal (KOS-tuhl)
Pertaining to the ribs. There are 12 ribs on each side of the rib cage.
> Refer to **Intercostal**.

costo-
A prefix meaning rib.

Counterrotation (koun-tuhr-roe-TAY-shuhn)
Rotating in opposite directions, such as when the left shoulder rotates backward and the left hip rotates forward.

Coxa (KOK-suh)
The hipbone and hip *joint*.

Coxae (KOK-say)
Plural of *coxa*.

Coxa Valga (KOK-suh VAL-guh)
A hip deformity in which the angle created by the head and shaft of the *femur* (thigh bone) is increased, angling the femur toward the side of the body.

Coxa Vara (KOK-suh VAY-ruh)
A hip deformity in which the angle created by the head and shaft of the *femur* (thigh bone) is decreased, angling the femur in toward the *midline* of the body. This causes one leg to be shorter, which makes a child limp.

Coxsackievirus (kok-SAK-ee-vie-rus)
An *enterovirus* (a *virus* that thrives mainly in the intestinal tract) that may cause *congenital heart lesions* in the newborn of a woman infected during the first *trimester* of pregnancy. This type of infection can range from mild to serious when contracted by children.

CP
The abbreviation for cerebral palsy.

CPAP
The abbreviation for continuous positive airway pressure.

CPD
The abbreviation for cephalopelvic disproportion.

CPK, C-PK
The abbreviation for creatine phosphokinase.

CPR
The abbreviation for cardiopulmonary resuscitation.

cps
The abbreviation for cycle per second.
> *Refer to* **Hertz.**

CPS
The abbreviation for Child Protective Services.
> *Refer to* **Child Protective Agency.**

Cradle Cap
> *Refer to* **Seborrheic Dermatitis.**

cranio-
A prefix meaning skull.

Craniofacial (kray-nee-oe-FAY-shuhl)
Relating to the skull and bones of the face.

Craniostenosis (kray-nee-oe-stee-NOE-sis)
A *congenital* condition in which the bone *sutures* of the *cranium* close prematurely. *Brain damage* may occur, depending on which bones close prematurely and how early they close. An *abnormally* shaped skull can result when some sutures fuse prematurely and other sutures remain open and allow for expansion of the cranium as the *brain* grows. Surgery may be needed to relieve *cerebral* pressure or for cosmetic reasons.
> *Refer to* **Acrocephalopolysyndactyly** *and* **Acrocephalosyndactyly.**

Craniostosis (krae-nee-os-TOE-sis)
> *Refer to* **Craniosynostosis.**

Craniosynostosis (kray-nee-oe-sin-os-TOE-sis)
Premature formation of the bone substance that forms the skull (with premature closure of the *sutures* of the skull). This results in an *atypically* long and narrow shaped head. Typically with craniosynostosis, the sutures close too early in development because the *brain* has stopped growing.
> *Also known as* **Craniostosis.**

Cranium (KRAY-nee-um)
The part of the skull that encloses the *brain*.

Crawl
To move by using the arms and legs to propel the body forward or backward with the *abdomen* resting on the floor.
> *Also known as* **Belly Crawl, Combat Crawl,** *and* **Commando Crawl.**
> *Compare* **Creep.**

Crawling Aid
A device that supports the child's trunk to enable him to bear weight on his hands and knees.

Creatine Kinase (CK) (KREE-uh-teen KIE-nays)
Refer to **Creatine Phosphokinase**.

Creatine Phosphokinase (CPK, C-PK) (KREE-uh-teen fos-foe-KIE-nays)
An *enzyme* released by damaged *brain tissue, heart* muscle, and skeletal muscle *cells*. There is a high level of CPK in the blood of children with *muscular dystrophy*.
Also known as **Creatine Kinase**.

Creep
To move forward or backward on the hands and knees with the *abdomen* off the floor.
Compare **Crawl**.

Cretinism (KREE-tin-izm)
Refer to **Congenital Hypothyroidism**.

Crib Death
Refer to **Sudden Infant Death Syndrome (SIDS)**.

Crib-O-Gram
A test that detects *deafness* in infants.

Cri du Chat Syndrome (kree-dyoo-shah)
Refer to **5p- Syndrome**.

Crigler-Najjar Syndrome (KREEG-ler NA-hayr)
A *disorder* caused by a lack of glucuronyl transferase, an *enzyme* needed to cause a chemical reaction in the *liver*. Type I Crigler-Najjar syndrome, an *autosomal recessive disorder,* is characterized by *kernicterus* and *brain damage*, and is usually fatal in infancy. Type II Crigler-Najjar syndrome, which can be *inherited* as an *autosomal dominant* or autosomal recessive disorder, is milder and rarely involves neurologic complications.

Crippled Children's Services (CCS)
A state administered program that was established as part of the Social Security Act of 1935 to provide services to children with handicapping conditions. Individual states receive funding under the Maternal and Child Health block grant, as well as from state and local sources. Financial and *diagnostic* eligibility and services vary from state to state. Services often include medical and therapy *intervention*, as well as supplies (such as a *walker*). Most states now use a name other than "Crippled Children's Services" for the agency that offers the services described above. For example, in California the agency is called "California Children's Services" and in Nebraska the agency is called "Medically Handicapped Children's Program." More information on how to receive assistance a child with *disabilities* can be obtained by contacting the local office of the state health agency.

Criterion-Referenced Test

A test that compares a child's performance to specific criteria, thus determining the skills the child possesses. (The child is not measured against norms set by the performance of other children.)

*Compare **Norm-Referenced Test** and **Screening Test.***

Cromolyn Sodium (KROEM-uh-lin)

A drug used to prevent *asthma* attacks in children. It is also used to treat *allergic* conditions.

Cross-Eye

*Refer to **Esotropia.***

"Cross the Midline"

Movement of a *limb* that goes past the center of the body.

Croup (kroop)

Inflammation and swelling of the *trachea* and *bronchi*, characterized by a barking cough and hoarseness. Croup is typically a *viral* infection and affects children up to approximately 4 years of age. *Laryngotracheobronchitis* (inflammation of the *larynx*, trachea, and bronchi) is sometimes used interchangeably with viral croup.

Crouzon Syndrome (kroo-ZON)

An *autosomal dominant disorder* characterized by *craniosynostosis* (a condition in which the *sutures* between the bones of the *cranium* close prematurely), resulting in *brachycephaly* (a short broad shape to the head); shallow, wide-spaced *orbits* (the bony sockets in the skull that contain the eyes) that make the eyes bulge; moderate *auditory impairment*; underdevelopment of the upper jaw bone; and progressive loss of vision (although vision is not always severely affected).

Cruising

Moving (stepping) sideways while holding on to a support (for example, walking while holding on to furniture).

Cryptorchidism (kript-OR-kid-izm)

*Refer to **Undescended Testes.***

Crystalline Lens (KRIS-tuh-lin LENZ)

*Refer to **Lens.***

C-Section

The abbreviation for Cesarean Section.

CSF

The abbreviation for cerebrospinal fluid.

ct
The abbreviation for chest tube.

CT Scanning
Computed Tomography. This is a *diagnostic* procedure in which a computerized machine creates pictures of cross sections of the body. These images of *tissues* are produced by passing *x-ray* beams at various angles through the area of the body to be studied.
Formerly known as **CAT Scanning** *and* **Computerized Axial Tomography.**

Cubitus (KYOO-bi-tus)
The bend of the arm, or the elbow *joint*.

Cuboid (KYOO-boid)
The small bone of the foot that is shaped like a cube. It is between the heel bone and the fourth and fifth *metatarsals* (the bones of the foot to which the toe bones are attached).

Cue (KYOO)
Refer to **Prompt.**

Cued Speech (KYOOD)
A method of *communication* for people with *auditory impairment*. Cued speech supplements the visual aspects of speech (*speechreading*) with *gestures* that make it easier to distinguish between similar-appearing speech sounds (such as /b/ and /p/). There are eight handshapes which symbolize groups of *consonant* sounds and four hand placements around the face which represent groups of *vowel* sounds.

Cultural Competence
The ability to work sensitively and respectfully with children and their families, honoring the diversity of their cultures, spoken languages, and racial and ethnic groups.

Culture
A laboratory test in which *cells*, *tissues*, or *microorganisms* are grown and studied to determine a *diagnosis*. Samples of body tissues or fluids are placed in a growth medium that encourages cultivation of the cells, tissue, or microorganisms.

Cuneiform Bones (kyoo-NEE-i-form)
Any of the small bones of the wrist or foot.

Curvature of the Spine
An *abnormal* condition in which the *spine* is not in alignment.
Refer to **Scoliosis, Kyphosis,** *and* **Lordosis.**

Cutaneous (kyoo-TAY-nee-us)
Referring to the skin.

Cutaneous Papilloma (kyoo-TAY-nee-us pap-i-LOE-muh)
Refer to **Skin Tag**.

Cutaneous Vesicostomy (kyoo-TAY-nee-us ves-uh-KOS-tuh-mee)
Refer to **Vesicostomy**.

Cut-away Cup
Refer to **Cut-out Cup**.

cuti-
A prefix meaning skin.

Cutis (KYOO-tis)
The skin.

Cutis Laxa Syndrome (CL) (KYOO-tuhs LAX-uh)
A very rare *connective tissue disorder* characterized by skin that loses its elasticity, making it loose, and other complications depending on the form of the disorder. *Inherited* forms are more common than the *acquired* form. The exact cause of CL is unknown, but is possibly due to *abnormal elastin metabolism*, resulting in decreased elastin in the skin. Inherited forms include an *autosomal dominant* form that only involves the skin; an *autosomal recessive* form that causes severe internal organ problems, including *genitourinary*, *gastrointestinal*, and lung *disease*, and a *heart* condition (*cor pulmonale*) that can cause death in the very young child; and an *x-linked* form that causes genitourinary and skeletal concerns. Children with cutis laxa syndrome may also have *mental retardation*.

Cutis Marmorata
A brief blue or purple *mottling* (coloring) of the skin, such as sometimes occurs when the skin is exposed to the cold.

Cut-out Cup
A flexible plastic cup that has a semi-circular piece cut out of the rim. Since the cup has a cut-out portion, the adult can monitor the child's intake of fluid and adjust the flow rate while holding the cup in a position that allows the child to drink without overextending his neck. The flexibility of the cup enables the adult to bend it enough to fit the child's mouth.
Also known as **Cut-away Cup**.

CVA
The abbreviation for cerebrovascular accident.

C-V Combination
Combining a *consonant* and *vowel* sound, such as "ba."

CVI
The abbreviation for cortical visual impairment.

CVN
The abbreviation for central venous nutrition.

CVS
The abbreviation for chorionic villus sampling.

Cyanosis (sie-uh-NOE-sis)
A blue or "dusky" color to the skin and *mucous membranes* (most notably the lips, tongue, and beds of the fingernails or toenails) caused by a lack of *oxygen* in the bloodstream. Cyanosis can be a *sign* of *congenital heart disease* in the newborn, other *heart* or lung *disorders*, *disease* of the *central nervous system*, or *hypothermia*.

Cyanotic (sie-uh-NOT-ik)
Refer to **Cyanosis.**

Cylert™ (SIE-lert)
Refer to **Pemoline.**

cyst-
A prefix meaning *bladder*.

Cyst (SIST)
A closed sac in any organ or *tissue* that contains fluid or semisolid material and forms a lump. Cysts are generally harmless, but can disturb the functioning of the organ or tissue where they are growing.

Cystic Fibrosis (CF) (SIS-tik fie-BROE-sis)
An *autosomal recessive disorder* characterized by *abnormally* thick *mucus secretions*, which contribute to chronic lung damage, and a lack of the *enzymes* needed to breakdown and absorb *fats*, which causes *malnutrition*. Cystic fibrosis is a serious illness that nearly always shortens a child's life expectancy.

Cystic Hygroma (hie-GROE-muh)
A quickly growing sac made of *lymphatic tissue* that contains *serous* fluid. It is usually found in the neck and sometimes in the chest. Cystic hygroma is often associated with *Turner syndrome*.
Refer to **Hygroma.**

Cystine Storage Disease
Refer to **Cystinosis.**

Cystinosis (sis-ti-NOE-sis)
An *autosomal recessive metabolic disease* characterized by the *abnormal* presence of *glucose* and excessively large quantities of *protein* and *phosphates* in the urine; *amino acid* compound (cystine) deposits in the *kidneys, liver, corneas, spleen,* muscles, *bone marrow, brain, pancreas,* and *white blood cells*; and growth retardation. It can result in *renal failure*, muscle wasting, *rickets*, diffi-

culty swallowing, *diabetes*, and *hypothyroidism*. A *gene* on *chromosome* 17p13 has been identified as the cystinosis gene. Medication is available to treat cystinosis and, if started early in infancy, can improve a child's *prognosis*.

Also known as **Cystine Storage Disease.**

cysto-
A prefix meaning *bladder.*

Cystourethrography (sis-toe-yoo-ree-THROG-ruh-fee)
A procedure to detect *reflux* of urine, performed by inserting a tube through the *urethra* and into the *bladder*, injecting contrast material into the tube, and taking *x-rays*. The picture, or cystourethrogram, will also reveal any *abnormalities* within the bladder. This procedure is known as *voiding cystourethrography* if x-rays are taken as the patient voids.

cyt-, cyto-
Prefixes meaning *cell.*

-cyte
A suffix meaning *cell.*

Cytogenetics (sie-toe-juh-NET-iks)
The study of the formation, structure, and function of *cells* in relation to *genetics*. Cytogenetic techniques make it possible to *diagnose fetal abnormalities* as early as 11 to 14 weeks of *gestation* (after *amniotic fluid* or *placental* samples are obtained via *amniocentesis* or *chorionic villus sampling*).

Cytogenetic Syndrome (sie-toe-juh-NET-ik)
A *chromosomal disorder* caused by a lack or an excess of genes and their corresponding *proteins*. Thus, the number of *chromosomes* or the structure of the chromosomes may not be normal. For example, *Down syndrome* results when an extra (third) chromosome 21 is present in the body's *cells*, and *Williams syndrome* results when there is a *microdeletion* on the long arm of one of the chromosome 7s.

Compare **Single Gene Disorder.**
Refer to **Gene** and **Chromosome.**

Cytomegalic Inclusion Disease (CID) (sie-tuh-muh-GAL-ik)
A *congenital* infection caused by *cytomegalovirus* (CMV). Although CMV is a common *virus* that causes no significant damage to healthy children and adults, it can cause severe damage to the *fetus* of an infected pregnant woman. CID can result in *low birth weight, microcephaly, jaundice, anemia, liver* and *spleen* damage, *auditory impairment*, and *mental retardation.*

Cytomegalovirus (CMV) (sie-tuh-MEG-uh-loe-VIE-ruhs)
A common herpes-type *virus* that causes no significant damage to healthy children and adults but can infect an unborn baby (known as congenital CMV), causing severe illness and *congenital anomalies*. CMV can persist in an individual for long periods, possibly indefinitely.

Refer to **Cytomegalic Inclusion Disease.**

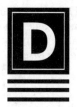

DA
1. The abbreviation for Developmental Age.
2. The abbreviation for Dextroamphetamine.
3. The abbreviation for Dopamine.

DAA
The abbreviation for Digital Auditory Aerobics.

dactyl-
A prefix meaning finger or toe.

Dantrium™ (DAN-tree-uhm)
*Refer to **Dantrolene Sodium.***

Dantrolene Sodium (DAN-troe-leen)
An *antispastic drug* that works directly on the muscle, relaxing *spasms* caused by injury to the *spinal cord* or *brain*. Dantrium™ is the brand name of this drug.

DAT1
The abbreviation for Dopamine Transporter Gene.

Daughter Cell
Any *cell* resulting from the division of a mother, or parent, cell (a cell that divides and gives rise to two or more cells).

dB
The abbreviation for decibel.

dc
The abbreviation for discontinue.

DC:0-3R
The abbreviation for the Diagnostic Classification of Mental Health and Developmental Disorders of Infancy and Early Childhood-Revised.

DCFS
The abbreviation for Department of Children and Family Services.

DD
The abbreviation for developmental disability.

DDST
The abbreviation for Denver Developmental Screening Test (Denver II).

de-
A prefix meaning remove or decrease.

Deaf
Refer to **Auditory Impairment** *and* **Deafness**.

Deaf-Blindness
A condition involving both *auditory* and visual *disability*. A child with the two disabilities usually has such a high degree of *communication* and other *developmental* and educational problems that she cannot be effectively served in a *special education* class solely for children with *auditory* or *visual impairments*. Deaf-blindness may be caused by *genetic* factors (such as *Usher syndrome*), *maternal* illness during pregnancy (such as *rubella*), injury (such as a *brain hemorrhage* associated with prolonged *labor*), or illness (such as *spinal meningitis*, which may lead to *optic* and *auditory nerve* damage if not treated promptly and effectively).

Deafness
A lack of the sense of *hearing* or profound *auditory impairment*.
Refer to **Auditory Impairment** *and* **Prelingual Deafness**.

Decadron™ (DEK-uh-dron)
Refer to Dexamethasone.

Decibel (dB)
A unit for measure of sound intensity, or loudness. The child with normal *hearing* can hear sounds at 20 decibels or less.

Deciduous (dee-SID-yoo-us)
Not permanent. For example, the *primary teeth* (*baby teeth*) are also known as deciduous teeth.

Deciduous Teeth
Refer to **Primary Teeth**.

Decoding
The process of analyzing and making sense of sounds, symbols, *gestures*, or other types of *communication*. Decoding is a part of understanding the meaning of language.

Decongestant
A drug that relieves nasal congestion by reducing the swelling and *inflammation* of the *membranes* of the nose.

Decubitus Ulcer (de-KYOO-bi-tus)
A pressure sore or bedsore.
> *Refer to* **Ulcer.**

Deep Pressure
A type of *sensory* input used to calm, arouse, or organize a child with *sensory processing* difficulties. Deep pressure can be applied by the child or a parent or therapist through firm hugging, *joint compressions*, and or "squishing" the child into or between pillows (with face exposed).

Deep Tendon Reflex (DTR)
An automatic muscle *contraction* in response to a tapping (stretching) of the muscle's *tendon*. Deep tendon reflexes are indicators of the condition of the *nervous system*. An example of a DTR is the *patellar* ("knee jerk") *reflex*.

Defecation
A *bowel movement*. The evacuation of *feces* from the *digestive tract* through the *rectum*.

Deficit
An area of weakness.

Degeneration (di-jen-uh-RAY-shuhn)
The gradual deterioration of normal *cells* and body functions resulting in a lower or dysfunctional form.

Deglutition (dee-gloo-TISH-un)
The act of swallowing.

Dehydration
The loss of excessive amounts of body water. *Symptoms* include extreme thirst; decreased and concentrated (dark) urine output; difficulty in forming tears and saliva; sunken eyes; and dry lips, tongue, and skin. Dehydration is caused by not taking in enough water or by losing body water and not replenishing it (as with perspiration, vomiting or diarrhea, or *disease* such as *diabetes*).

de Lange Syndrome (day LAHNG)
> *Refer to* **Cornelia de Lange Syndrome.**

Deletion
> *Refer to* **Chromosomal Deletion.**

Delta Wave (DEL-tuh)
One of the 4 types of *brain waves* creating the rhythm of electrical activity as

seen on an *EEG*. Delta waves are seen during deep-sleep when a child is not easily aroused. Delta waves are characterized by relatively high voltage and a *frequency* of 4 Hz.

> *Compare* **Alpha Wave, Beta Wave,** *and* **Theta Wave.**
> *Refer to* **Brain Wave.**

Dementia (di-MEN-shuh)
A deterioration of *cognitive* (mental) function caused by *organic* impairment, such as *disease, subdural hematoma,* or drug intoxication.

Dementia Infantilis
> *Refer to* **Childhood Disintegrative Disorder.**

Demyelinating (dee-MIE-uh-luh-nayt-ing)
A condition in which the *myelin sheath* of a *nerve* or nerve fiber is destroyed by *disease*.
> *Refer to* **Myelin Sheath.**

Denis-Browne Splint™
A bar-type *splint* in which the child's shoes are attached at varying degrees of separation and angle. This type of splint is often used as part of the treatment of *clubfoot*.

Dental Caries
Cavities or decay of the teeth.

Dentin
The hard substance that surrounds the tooth pulp and is covered by the enamel.

Dentition
The characteristics (type, number, and arrangement) of teeth. Dentition also refers to the eruption of teeth.

Denver Developmental Screening Test (Denver II) (DDST)
A *screening test* used to evaluate the language, *gross motor, fine motor,* and personal/social *development* of the 6-week to 6-year-old and to identify possible areas of delay. Typically, training on how to administer the test is by a certified master trainer or by a training video.

Deoxygenate (dee-OK-si-juh-nayt)
To remove *oxygen* from a substance.
> *Compare* **Oxygenate.**

Deoxyribonucleic Acid (DNA) (dee-ok-see-rie-boe-noo-KLEE-ik)
The principal component of living *tissue* that contains the *genetic code* responsible for the *inheritance* and transmission of *chromosomes* and *genes*. DNA is made up of molecules called *nucleotides* and its structure is a double-stranded chemical string of sequences of nucleotides. The sequence of nucleotides that form the

2 strands do not match, but rather complement each other, much like the two halves of a zipper. The 2 strands can be separated and the DNA can be analyzed to determine if there are any genetic changes that cause *inherited disorders*.

 Refer to **Gene.**

Deoxyribonucleic Acid (DNA) Analysis
A *diagnostic* procedure done to obtain *genetic* information about a *fetus*. It is used to diagnose conditions such as *fragile X syndrome prenatally*.

Depakene™ (DEP-uh-kayn)
 Refer to **Valproic Acid.**

Depakote™ (DEP-uh-koet)
 Refer to **Valproic Acid.**

Department of Children and Family Services (DCFS)
A protective services agency that investigates, evaluates, and monitors cases of reported *child abuse and neglect*.

 Refer to **Child Abuse and Neglect** *and* **Mandated Reporter.**

Department of Public Social Services (DPSS)
An agency that provides public assistance, such as financial help, food, or shelter, to individuals who qualify.

Also known as **Welfare.**

de Pezzer Catheter™
A type of *urinary catheter*.

 Also known as **Pezzer Catheter.**

Depression
As defined in the *DC:0-3*, "A pattern of depressed or irritable mood lasting at least two weeks, with diminished interest and/or pleasure in developmentally appropriate activities, diminished capacity to protest, excessive whining, and diminished social interactions and initiative." Research has shown that infants can experience depression as early as 4 months of age.

 Refer to **Anaclitic Depression.**

Depth Perception
The ability to blend slightly dissimilar images from the two eyes to judge depth and *spatial relationships*.

derm-
A prefix meaning skin.

Dermatoglyphics (der-muh-toe-GLIF-iks)
The study of the skin ridge patterns (also known as prints, as in fingerprints) on the fingers, toes, palms of the hands, and the soles of the feet. Examining skin ridge patterns is useful in *diagnosing* some *chromosomal abnormalities*.

Derotation Femoral Osteotomy
(dee-roe-TAY-shuhn FEM-or-uhl os-tee-OT-oe-mee)
A surgical procedure in which the shaft of the *femur* (the thigh bone) is cut to change the alignment of the head and neck of the femur with the *acetabulum* (the hip socket).
Refer to **Osteotomy.**

DES
The abbreviation for diethylstilbestrol.

Desat
Refer to **Desaturation.**

Desaturation (dee-sa-chur-AY-shuhn)
A drop in the *oxygen* levels in the baby's blood. The term is sometimes shortened to "desat."

Development
The lifelong process of growth to maturity through which an individual acquires increasingly complex abilities.

Developmental Age (DA)
The age at which a child is functioning (demonstrating specific abilities), based on *assessment* of the child's skills and comparison of those skills to the age at which they are considered typical. For example, at the *chronological age* of 36 months, a child might demonstrate the skills of a 30-month-old, and thus be said to have a developmental age of 30 months.
Also known as **Functional Age.**
Compare **Mental Age.**

Developmental Coordination Disorder
Refer to **Dyspraxia.**

Developmental Delay
The term used to describe the condition of an infant or toddler who is not achieving new skills in the typical time frame and/or is exhibiting *behaviors* that are not appropriate for her age. Some children who are developmentally delayed will be *diagnosed* with a particular *developmental disability*, while other children with delays eventually catch up to their *typically developing* peers. An infant or toddler whose *assessment* scores place her in the developmentally delayed range is eligible to receive *early intervention* services.
Refer to **Global Developmental Delay.**

Developmental Disability (DD)
Any physical or mental condition (such as *mental retardation, cerebral palsy, epilepsy*, an *autism spectrum disorder*, or a *neurological disorder*) that begins before the age of 22 years, causes the child to acquire skills at a slower rate than her peers, is expected to continue indefinitely, and impairs the child's

ability to function in 3 or more *developmental* areas, such as *communication*, learning, and mobility.

Developmental Dysplasia of the Hip (DDH)
(dis-PLAY-zee-uh or dis-PLAY-zhuh)
A condition present at birth in which the head of the thigh bone may be totally out of the hip socket or it may move in and out of the socket. This condition is most correctable when it is discovered very early.
Formally known as **Congenital Dislocation of the Hip.**

Developmental Dyspraxia (dis-PRAK-see-uh)
Refer to **Dyspraxia.**

Developmental, Individual-Difference, Relationship-Based (DIR®) Model
A *developmental* approach created by Drs. Stanley I. Greenspan and Serena Weider that guides the parent and *early interventionist* in addressing a child's developmental challenges through relationship and *affect*, focusing on the child's individual differences and developmental levels:

D—The mastery of the child's 6 <u>D</u>evelopmental milestones (1. *self-regulation* and interest in the world, 2. intimacy, 3. two-way communication, 4. complex communication, 5. emotional, 6. emotional thinking);

I —The child's <u>I</u>ndividual-Differences, such as the child's unique way of experiencing the sights and sounds of her world, as well as her biological challenges;

R—The child's <u>R</u>elationship-Based experiences, in terms of building relationships with *primary caregivers* as a critical element in helping a child to return to a healthy developmental path and achieve *cognitive* growth. These relationship-based experiences in early learning are essential for gaining higher level thinking and problem-solving skills.

Refer to **Floortime.**

Developmental Language Disorder (DLD)
A *disorder* that may occur when a child has difficulty in processing *sensory* information that is received by the *central nervous system* in rapid succession. Examples include *lexical syntactic syndrome* and *verbal auditory agnosia*.

Developmental Milestone
A skill that is recognized as a measurement of a child's functioning, or *development*, and that is typically achieved by a certain age. Taking steps independently is an example of a developmental milestone.

Developmental Profile II (DP-II)
A *developmental* scale used to assess the physical, *self-help*, social, academic, and *communication* development of children between birth and 9½ years of age. An interview format is used. Typically, the DP-II is administered by a *physical* or *occupational therapist* or an MD.
Formerly known as the **Alpern-Boll Developmental Profile.**

Developmental Programming for Infants and Young Children
An *evaluation* tool used to assess the perceptual/*fine motor, gross motor, so-cial/emotional*, self-care, language, and *cognitive development* of infants and young children between birth and 36 months of age. The Developmental Programming for Infants and Young Children is also a curriculum tool. Typically, this test is administered by a professional with a minimum of a college degree or by a *physical* or *occupational therapist*.

Developmental Psychologist
Refer to **Psychologist**.

Developmental Quotient (DQ)
A score similar to an *IQ* that describes an infant's *developmental* level.

Deviation
A moving away from the normal standard or course.

Dexamethasone (dek-suh-METH-uh-soen)
A *steroid* drug that may be used to help reduce *inflammation* and swelling. Decadron™ is the brand name of this drug.

Dexedrine™ (DEKS-uh-dreen)
Refer to **Dextroamphetamine**.

Dextroamphetamine (DA) (deks-troe-am-FET-uh-meen)
A *psychostimulant drug* that may be used to treat a*ttention deficit disorders* and *hyperactivity*. Dexedrine™ is the brand name of this drug.

Dextrostix™ (DEK-stroe-stiks)
A test that measures sugar levels in the blood, performed by placing a drop of blood on a chemically treated plastic strip (also known as a Dextrostix). It is used in the *diagnosis* of *hyperglycemia*.

di-
A prefix meaning two.

dia-
A prefix meaning through or between.

Diabetes Insipidus (die-uh-BEE-teez in-SIP-i-duhs)
A *disease* characterized by excessive urination and excessive thirst. Diabetes insipidus is caused by damage to part of the *pituitary gland* (possibly from a head *trauma*), which results in inadequate *secretion* of antidiuretic *hormone*. Treatment is by healing the injury to the pituitary gland when possible, or by replacing the antidiuretic hormone to control the disease. Diabetes insipidus is more common in the young.

Diabetes Mellitus (die-uh-BEE-teez muh-LIE-tuhs)
A chronic *disorder* of *carbohydrate metabolism* characterized by *abnormally* high
sugar levels in the blood and sugar in the urine, excessive urination and thirst,
and sometimes by abnormally large intake of food, weight loss, and excessive
acidity of body fluids. Diabetes mellitus results from inadequate production or
utilization of *insulin* (a *hormone* that regulates the metabolism of *blood sugar*).
Some patients with diabetes mellitus are insulin-dependent (because the body
produces little or no insulin) and therefore require insulin therapy. (This is referred to as Type I.) Others are non-insulin dependent (the body produces some
insulin) and the *disease* can usually be controlled by diet and medication, although insulin therapy is sometimes needed. (This is referred to as Type II.)

Diagnosis (Dx)
Determination of the nature of a *disease* or *disorder*.
> *Compare* **Misdiagnosis.**
> *Refer to* **Prenatal Diagnosis.**

Diagnostic (die-ag-NOS-tik)
Pertaining to a *diagnosis*.

**Diagnostic and Statistical Manual of Mental Disorders—Text Revision
(DSM-IV-TR)**
A reference book published by the *American Psychiatric Association* that lists
the criteria for classifying *brain*-based *disorders* including mental and emotional disorders and certain *developmental disabilities*, such as *mental retardation, schizophrenia,* and *autism spectrum disorders*. The fourth edition of
the DSM was released in 1994, and the DSM-IV-TR (Text Revision) was published in 2000.

**Diagnostic Classification of Mental Health and Developmental
Disorders of Infancy and Early Childhood-Revised (DC:0-3R)**
A classification system developed by *Zero to Three: National Center for Infants,
Toddlers, and Families*. It guides professionals who diagnose and/or treat infants
and young children in recognizing individual differences (such as abilities, challenges, and coping skills) and it considers the impact the child's interaction with
her primary caregiver(s) and the environment has on her *development*.

Diagnostic Manual for Infancy and Early Childhood (DMIC)
The Interdisciplinary Council on Developmental and Learning Disorder's classification system of infant and early childhood *disorders*. It provides classification of mental health, and *developmental* and learning *disorders* using an approach that is interdisciplinary, developmental (versus *symptom*-based), and
multidimensional (with classification based on the *DIR®*, the *Developmental,
Individual-Difference, Relationship-Based model*). The DMIC's 5 main categories of disorder classification include: *Interactive Disorders, Regulatory-Sensory Processing Disorders, Neurodevelopmental Disorders of Relating and Communicating, Language Disorders,* and Learning Challenges. Using the criteria of
these *diagnoses*, as well as considering other contributing factors (such as the

child's functional and emotional developmental capacities; *regulatory-sensory processing* capacities; language capacities; *visuospatial capacities*; child-caregiver and -family patterns; stress; and other medical and neurological diagnoses), provides a comprehensive description of the child's unique qualities and guides the clinician toward *identification* of the child's primary diagnosis and development of an *intervention* plan.

Refer to **Developmental, Individual-Difference, Relationship-Based (DIR®) Model.**

Diamox™ (DIE-uh-moks)
Refer to **Acetazolamide.**

Diaphoretic (die-uh-foe-RET-ik)
1. Relating to, or causing perspiration.
2. An agent that increases perspiration.
3. Referring to a child who is sweating profusely.

Diaphragm (DIE-uh-fram)
A muscle that assists with *respiration*. It separates the chest cavity from the *abdominal* cavity, and is located above the *liver*.

Diaphysis (die-AF-i-sis)
The shaft of a long bone.

Diastasis (die-AS-tuh-sis)
A separation of two parts of the body that normally are joined together or are in contact.

Diastasis Recti Abdominis
The separation of the 2 rectus muscles that extend from the lower ribs down the length of the *abdomen*. This condition can occur as a *congenital anomaly* due to incomplete development or be the result of injury. It is also occasionally seen in women during or following pregnancy.

Diastole (die-AS-toe-lee)
The period of relaxation when the *heart* chamber dilates and fills with blood to be pumped to the rest of the body. (The time between heart *contractions*.) Diastole coincides with the interval between the second and first heart sound.

Compare **Systole.**
Refer to **Blood Pressure.**

Diazepam (die-AZ-uh-pam)
A drug that works as a *muscle relaxant* by acting on the *central nervous system*. It is usually prescribed for its calming effects. Diazepam can be administered *rectally*, in which case *absorption* is much faster than by *intramuscular injection* or by mouth. It is often administered rectally to stop *status epilepticus*. Valium™ is the brand name of this drug.

DIC
The abbreviation for disseminated intravascular coagulation.

Didactic Materials
Educational tools intended for teaching a specific skill or group of skills. Examples of didactic materials include animal picture cards and a shape sorter.

Diencephalic Syndrome of Infancy (die-en-sef-AL-ik)
A *disorder* that causes *failure to thrive* after initial normal growth in the infant. Babies with this condition usually have a *brain tumor* that affects the appetite center of the brain (the *hypothalamus*).

Diencephalon (die-en-SEF-uh-lon)
The part of the *brain* that contains the *hypothalamus* and *thalamus*.

Diethylstilbestrol (DES) (die-eth-il-stil-BES-trol)
A synthetic estrogen (female sex *hormone*). DES was formerly prescribed to prevent *miscarriage*; however its use with pregnant women was stopped when it was linked to *cancer* and reproductive problems in daughters of women who were given DES during pregnancy.

Differential Diagnosis
The distinguishing of 2 or more *diseases* or *disorders* with similar *symptoms* in which the conditions are systematically compared by signs and symptoms in order to make an accurate *diagnosis*.

Di George Syndrome
A *congenital disorder* characterized by *immune system* deficiencies (caused by failure of the *thymus gland* to develop fully) and *cardiac* defects. Infants typically have a poor *prognosis* and may experience *failure to thrive*, cardiac difficulties, *respiratory* infections, and seizures (caused by low *calcium* that results from lack of development of the *parathyroid glands*, which regulate blood calcium). Children with Di George syndrome usually do not survive beyond 2 years of age. Most infants born with Di George syndrome also have characteristic facial features including uneven placement of the eyes, *palpebral fissures* that are slanted toward the nose, an upturned nose, a short *philtrum*, a cupid-bow shape to the lips, and low-set or rotated ears. Di George syndrome is most often caused by a *deletion* in the upper part of the long arm of *chromosome* 22. Also, Di George features have been associated with *maternal* use of alcohol and *Accutane*™ during pregnancy.
Also known **Thymic Parathyroid Aplasia**.

Digestion
The bodily process by which food is changed into substances that can be absorbed and assimilated. Digestion takes place in the stomach and the intestines.
Refer to **Alimentary** *and* **Nutrition**.

Digestive Tract (die-JES-tiv)
The tube that extends from the mouth to the *anus* and is involved in the process of *digestion*. The digestive tract is lined with *mucous membrane* and includes the mouth, *pharynx, esophagus,* stomach, *small* and *large intestines.*
Also known as **Gastrointestinal Tract (GI Tract).**

Digit
A finger or toe.

Digital Auditory Aerobics (DAA)
A form of *auditory integration training (AIT).* The music therapy equipment used with DAA differs from the equipment originally used for AIT, but the method is the same.
Refer to **Auditory Integration Training/Therapy.**

Digitalis (dij-i-TAL-is)
A drug that is used to treat *heart failure* and other *heart* conditions.

Dilantin™ (die-LAN-tin)
Refer to **Phenytoin.**

Dimetapp™ (DIE-muh-tap)
An over-the-counter *antihistamine* and *decongestant* combination.

Diphenhydramine Hydrochloride
(die-fen-HIE-druh-meen hie-droe-KLOR-ied)
An *antihistamine drug* used to treat *allergic disorders* and motion sickness. Benadryl™ is the brand name of this drug.

Diphtheria (dif-THIR-ee-uh)
An acute, infectious *bacterial disease* that can cause fever, pain, sore throat, and sometimes airway obstruction. Diphtheria can cause *inflammation* of the *heart* muscle and certain *nerves,* and can lead to death. Diphtheria is uncommon now due to the routine administration of the *Diphtheria and Tetanus Toxoids and Acellular Pertussis Vaccine (DTaP).*

Diphtheria and Tetanus Toxoids and Acellular Pertussis Vaccine (DTaP)
An *immunization* against *diphtheria, tetanus,* and *pertussis.* The primary series for the DTaP immunization consists of injections at 2, 4, and 6 months. Two *booster injections* are given, one at 15 -18 months of age, and another prior to beginning school (4½ -5 years of age). Research suggests that consideration should be given as to whether or not the *pertussis vaccine* should be administered to some children, specifically infants with a non-stable *neurological disorder,* such as seizures, or infants who have had a serious reaction to a prior DTaP shot.

Diphthong
A *vowel* sound that is produced when moving from one vowel sound to another within the same syllable, such as the "oy" sound in "boy."

Diplegia (die-PLEE-jee-uh)
Weakness or *paralysis* in the legs and arms caused by *disease* or injury to the *nerves* of the *brain* or *spinal cord* that stimulate the muscles, or by disease to the muscles themselves. Sometimes the word diplegia is used to describe *cerebral palsy* in which the legs are most affected (although the arms, trunk, and face may be slightly affected).
Refer to **Paralysis** and **Pyramidal Cerebral Palsy.**

diplo-
A prefix meaning double.

Diploid (DIP-loid)
Having two of each kind of *chromosome*. Human *cells* are normally diploid (except for the *sex chromosomes* in a male).
Compare **Haploid** and **Triploid.**

Diplopia (dip-LOE-pee-uh)
Double vision.

Diptheria
Refer to *Diphtheria.*

Direct DNA Analysis
A method for detecting the presence of a *mutation* in a *gene* known to be affected in a child's *DNA*. The DNA sample can be obtained from blood, *amniotic fluid,* or other body *tissues*. Direct DNA analysis is available for many *genetic disorders* including *cystic fibrosis* and *fragile X syndrome*.

DIR® Model
The abbreviation for the Developmental, Individual-Difference, Relationship-Based model.

dis-
A prefix meaning apart.

Disability
As described in the *Americans with Disabilities Act* (*ADA*) of 1990, a disability is a substantially limiting physical or mental impairment which affects basic life activities such as *hearing*, seeing, speaking, walking, caring for oneself, learning, or working.
Refer to **Developmental Disability** and **Learning Disability.**

Disassociation
Refer to **Dissociation.**

Discrete Trial Instruction (DTI)
An instructional technique that is part of *Applied Behavior Analysis* (*ABA*). This technique involves 4 steps: 1) presenting a *cue* or *stimulus* to the learner;

2) obtaining the learner's response; 3) providing a positive consequence (*reinforcer*) or correction; and 4) a brief, 3-5 second break until the next teaching trial is provided.

> *Also known as* **Discrete Trial Instruction.**
> *Refer to* **Applied Behavior Analysis** *and* **Lovaas Method.**

Discrete Trial Teaching (DTT)
> *Refer to* **Discrete Trial Instruction.**

Discrimination
1. Showing favor toward one person, race, or group, and prejudice toward another.
2. The act of distinguishing or differentiating between similar *sensory stimuli*, such as two sounds or two written letters of the alphabet.

Disease
Any change or interruption of the normal structure or function of a body part, organ, or system. Disease is indicated by characteristic signs and *symptoms*. The cause and *prognosis* of a disease is not always known.

Disintegrative Psychosis (dis-IN-tuh-gray-tiv sie-KOE-sis)
Another term for *Childhood disintegrative disorder*.
> *Refer to* **Childhood Disintegrative Disorder.**

Dislocated Hip
A condition in which the *femur* (thigh bone) has slipped out of its hip socket. A dislocated hip can be a *congenital* condition, or it can be caused by injury or the unequal pressure of *spastic* muscles at the *joint*.

Dislocation
The separation of two body parts, usually two bones of a *joint*, so that they are no longer in contact.
> *Compare* **Subluxation.**

Disorder
An *abnormality* or disturbance of normal function, such as a *speech disorder*.

Disorganized Behavior
Referring to the infant's decreased ability to make smooth transitions through various *states* of alertness. As the infant approaches toddlerhood, disorganized behavior refers to a decreased ability to organize and tolerate certain types and amounts of *sensory stimulation*.

Displacement
The removal of an organ or structure from its normal position.

Disseminated Intravascular Coagulation (DIC)
(dis-SEM-i-nay-tid in-truh-VAS-kyuh-luhr koe-ag-yuh-LAY-shuhn)
A condition in which too much of the blood's *platelets* and clotting factors is used due to infection, injury, or *disease*. There is uncontrolled activation of

clotting pathways and overproduction of anticlotting substances, which leave the child vulnerable to excessive bleeding.

Dissociation
1. The process of separating into parts.
2. The ability to use selected (smaller) movement patterns rather than gross (large) movement patterns. This allows for independent movement of one body part without movement of another body part. For example, the child is able to move her head in all directions without the rest of her body moving.
    *Also known as **Disassociation**.*

Distal (DIS-tuhl)
Farther from the point of attachment or origin. For example, the fingers are distal to the shoulder, while the elbow is *proximal* to the shoulder.
    *Compare **Proximal**.*

Distance Vision
Distinct vision of objects at a distance, usually 20 feet.

Distractability
A *behavioral* characteristic in which a child has difficulty focusing her attention on what is important because her attention is easily diverted by inconsequential occurrences.

Disuse Syndrome
Problems that result from lack of use of a part of the body. A *contracture* is an example of a physical problem that results from lack of use of a body part, and memory disturbance is an example of a mental problem that results from lack of mental activity.

Diuretic (die-yoo-RET-ik)
A drug that promotes *excretion* of urine from the body.

Diuril™ (DIE-yoo-ril)
    *Refer to **Chlorothiazide**.*

Divergent Strabismus (di-VUR-juhnt struh-BIZ-muhs)
    *Refer to **Exotropia**.*

Division for Early Childhood (DEC)
One of 17 divisions of the Council for Exceptional Children, DEC is an international organization which promotes policies and advances evidence-based practices that support families and enhance the development of young children with disabilities, birth through age eight.

Dizygotic Twins (die-zie-GOT-ik)
Two infants born of the same pregnancy, produced from two eggs and *sperm*. Dizygotic twins each have their own *placentas*, may be the same or opposite sex,

and differ *genetically*. Their similarities are the same as those of any siblings.
>*Also known as* **Fraternal Twins.**
>*Compare* **Monozygotic Twins.**

DLD
The abbreviation for Developmental Language Disorder.

DMIC
The abbreviation for Diagnostic Manual for Infancy and Early Childhood.

DNA
The abbreviation for deoxyribonucleic acid.

DO
The abbreviation for Doctor of Osteopathy.

Doctor of Medicine (MD)
A fully licensed physician trained to practice medicine.

Doctor of Osteopathy (DO)
A fully licensed *physician* trained to practice *osteopathic medicine*.
>*Refer to* **Osteopathic Medicine.**

Docusate (DOK-yoo-sayt)
A stool softener. Colace™ is the brand name of this drug.

dolicho-
A prefix meaning long.

Dolichocephalic (dol-i-koe-si-FAL-ik)
Referring to having a long head.

Dolichocephaly (dol-i-koe-SEF-uh-lee)
A condition in which the skull has a long front-to-back diameter.

Domain
A *developmental* area. The six main developmental areas are the *cognitive*, language (*communication*), *gross motor*, *fine motor* (perceptual), *social/emotional*, and *self-help* (*adaptive*) domains.

Dominant Gene
A *gene* that overrides any *recessive gene* it is paired with in determining what characteristic or condition a child inherits from her parents. For example, the gene for brown eyes is dominant over the gene for blue eyes, so a child who inherits one gene for brown eyes and one for blue eyes will have brown eyes.
>*Compare* **Recessive Gene.**
>*Refer to* **Autosomal Dominant Disorder** *and* **Gene.**

Dominant Hand
Refer to **Hand Preference.**

Dopamine (DA) (DOE-puh-min)
An *amino acid* that functions as a *neurotransmitter* in certain areas of the *brain* and *central nervous system,* enabling electrical impulses to travel from one *neuron* to another across a *synapse.* Dopamine also affects the *myocardium* (the middle and thickest layer of the *heart* wall composed of *cardiac* muscle) by increasing cardiac output, and is presumed to play a major role in regulating movement.

Dopamine Transporter Gene (DAT1)
A *gene,* located on the tip of *chromosome* 5, that has been implicated in the study of children with *AD/HD.*
Refer to **Dopamine.**

Doppler Scanning™ (DOP-ler)
An *ultrasound* imaging technique that can monitor movement of a body structure, such as a *fetal* heartbeat.

dors-
A prefix meaning back.

Dorsal (DOR-suhl)
Referring to a position that is to the back. For example, the back is dorsal compared to the *abdomen,* which is ventral.
Also known as **Posterior.**
Compare **Ventral.**

Dorsal Rhizotomy (DOR-suhl rie-ZOT-uh-mee)
A neurosurgical procedure in which certain *nerves* of the *spine* are cut to reduce *spasticity.*
Also known as **Rhizotomy, Selective Dorsal Rhizotomy,** *and* **Selective Posterior Rhizotomy.**

Dorsiflexion (dor-si-FLEK-shuhn)
Bending or flexing backward or upward. For example, bending the foot toward the upper surface of the foot.
Compare **Plantar Flexion.**

Dorsum
The back or upper surface of a body part. In the foot, the dorsum is the top of the foot.

Double Hemiplegia (hem-ee-PLEE-jee-uh)
Weakness or *paralysis* in both the arms, both the legs, the trunk, and the head caused by *disease* or injury to the *nerves* of the *brain* or *spinal cord* that stimulate the muscles, or by disease to the muscles themselves. Double hemiplegia

also describes *cerebral palsy* in which the arms, legs, face, and trunk are affected, with the arms (and often the face) most affected.

Refer to **Cerebral Palsy** *and* **Pyramidal Cerebral Palsy.**

Double Vision

Refer to **Diplopia.**

Down Syndrome (DS)

A *genetic disorder* caused by a *chromosomal abnormality*. Down syndrome results when an extra (a third) *chromosome* 21, or extra part of chromosome 21, is in the body's *cells*. The presence of this extra *genetic* material can occur several ways: by *chromosomal nondisjunction, translocation,* or *mosaicism. Chromosomal* nondisjunction is the failure of the chromosome 21 pair to separate in the *sperm* or *ovum* (egg), prior to conception. If a sperm or ovum in which the chromosome 21 pair has not separated is involved in forming a fertilized egg, the resulting baby will have 3 (a *trisomy*) chromosome number 21s. (She will have *inherited* two chromosome 21s from one parent and the usual one chromosome 21 from the other parent.) This is the most common way Down syndrome occurs. Translocation occurs when an extra (a third) chromosome 21 becomes attached to another numbered chromosome, again prior to conception. Mosaicism is the *abnormal* separation of the chromosome 21 pair, after conception. Because the separation occurs after some cell division has taken place, not all cells will be affected, and thus there may be fewer characteristic features of Down syndrome. Characteristics of Down syndrome may include *hypotonia*, upward slant to the eyes, *congenital heart defect, epicanthal folds*, a small mouth, small stature and facial features, a flattened back of the head, short broad hands with a *simian crease, Brushfield spots, joint* hyperflexibility, and varying degrees of *mental retardation*. Down syndrome was formerly known as *Mongolism* because the characteristic facial features associated with the condition were erroneously considered to look similar to those of Mongolians.

Also known as **Trisomy 21.**

DP-II

The abbreviation for Developmental Profile II.

DPPT

The abbreviation for Wilbarger Deep Pressure and Proprioceptive Technique.

DPSS

The abbreviation for the Department of Public Social Services.

DPT/DTP

The abbreviation for Diphtheria, Pertussis, and Tetanus Vaccine. The formulation is now used when the *Diphtheria and Tetanus Toxoids and Acellular Pertussis Vaccine (DTaP)* is unavailable.

DQ

The abbreviation for developmental quotient.

Drisdol™ (DRIZ-dol)
Refer to **Ergocalciferol.**

Drop Attack
Refer to **Atonic Seizure.**

Drop Foot
An *abnormal neuromuscular* condition in which the foot is bent downward and the toes drag when walking. This condition is usually caused by *nerve* damage.

Drop Seizure
Refer to **Atonic Seizure.**

Drug
Any substance used to treat or prevent a *disease* or condition. Drugs may be taken by mouth; applied topically (placed on the surface of a part of the body); or injected into a muscle, the skin, a *blood vessel*, or a body cavity (any of the spaces that contain organs). Also known as medicine.

Drug Baby
Refer to **Prenatally Exposed to Drugs.**

DS
The abbreviation for Down syndrome.

DSI
The abbreviation for Sensory Integration Dysfunction. "DSI" is used in place of "SID" to distinguish it from *SIDS (Sudden Infant Death Syndrome).*

DSM-IV-TR
The abbreviation for the fourth edition of the Diagnostic and Statistical Manual of Mental Disorders (Text Revision).

DTaP
The abbreviation for Diphtheria and Tetanus Toxoids and Acellular Pertussis Vaccine.

DTI
The abbreviation for Discrete Trial Instruction.

DTP/DPT
The abbreviation for the Diphtheria, Tetanus, and Pertussis Vaccine. The formulation is now used when the *Diphtheria and Tetanus Toxoids and Acellular Pertussis Vaccine (DTaP)* is unavailable.

DTR
The abbreviation for deep tendon reflex.

DTT
The abbreviation for Discrete Trial Teaching.
> *Refer to* **Discrete Trial Instruction.**

Dual Diagnosis
The existence of two *diagnoses* for a child.
> *Refer to* **Comorbidity.**

Dubowitz Neurological Assessment (DOO-buh-wits noo-roe-LOJ-i-kuhl)
An *assessment* in which the doctor moves and positions the baby to determine her neurological and muscular maturity. It is performed to estimate a newborn's *gestational age* and to track the development of *central nervous system* problems. The assessment is named after Victor Dubowitz, a twentieth century *pediatrician.*

Dubowitz Syndrome (DOO-buh-wits)
A rare *autosomal recessive disorder* characterized by low *birth weight*; *microcephaly*; slight build; *short stature*; sometimes *mild mental retardation*; distinct facial features including *abnormalities* of the jaw, sparse hair, a high sloping forehead, *epicanthal folds*, *ptosis*, flattening of the ridges above the eyes, and prominent or low-set ears; and, in affected males, *cryptorchidism* and *hypospadias*. Usually, infants and young children develop *eczema* on the face and *limbs*, have chronic diarrhea, and have a high-pitched voice. Also, sometimes *behavior disorders* develop, particularly *hyperactivity.*

Duchenne Muscular Dystrophy (dyoo-SHEN MUS-kyoo-ler DIS-troe-fee)
The most common form of *muscular dystrophy*, accounting for 50 percent of all muscular dystrophy *diseases*. This *X-linked recessive disease* is characterized by progressive muscle weakness and wasting, *respiratory* problems, and sometimes *heart failure*. Duchenne muscular dystrophy affects mostly boys and appears slowly in early childhood (between 3 and 5 years of age). Most children do not survive beyond 20 years due to *heart* complications.
> *Also known as* **Pseudohypertrophic Muscular Dystrophy.**

Duck Feet
> *Refer to* **Toeing Out.**

Duct
A tube leading from a *gland* to allow the passage of fluids. The tear ducts are an example.

Ductus Arteriosus (DUK-tus ar-tee-ree-OE-sus)
A *blood vessel* present in the *fetus* that connects the *aorta* with the *pulmonary artery* in order to bypass most blood away from the baby's lungs. Before birth, the *placenta* does the job of *oxygenating* the baby's blood. The blood vessel normally closes within a few days after birth so that blood can flow through the lungs to be *oxygenated*. Often the vessel does not close normally in premature babies. (This condition is called a *patent ductus arteriosus*, or *PDA*.)
> *Compare* **Patent Ductus Arteriosus.**
> *Refer to* **Fetal Circulation.**

Ductus Venosus (DUK-tus vee-NOE-sus)
A small channel that develops in the *embryonic liver,* diverting the *fetus's* blood through the liver. (The blood flows through the channel in the liver rather than through liver *tissue.*) Before birth, the *placenta* does the job of cleansing the baby's blood. After birth, the ductus venosus closes so blood can pass through the liver tissue to be cleansed before returning to the *heart.*
> *Refer to* **Fetal Circulation.**

Dulcolax™ (DUL-koe-laks)
> *Refer to* **Bisacodyl.**

Duodenal Atresia (dyoo-oe-DEE-nuhl or dyoo-OD-uh-nuhl uh-TREE-zhuh)
Blockage in the *small intestine* due to failure of the opening to develop or destruction of the opening.

Duodenal Stenosis (sti-NOE-sis)
Narrowing (*constriction*) of a portion of the *small intestine.*

duodeno-
A prefix meaning *duodenum.*

Duodenum (dyoo-oe-DEE-num or dyoo-OD-uh-nuhm)
The first and widest section of the *small intestine.* It is located between the stomach and the *jejunum.* (The jejunum is the middle section and the *ileum* is the third section of the small intestine.)
> *Refer to* **Small Intestine.**

Dura Mater (DYOO-ruh MAY-tur)
The outermost layer of the *meninges* (the *membranes* surrounding the *brain* and *spinal cord*). The innermost layer is the *pia mater* and the middle layer is the *arachnoid.*
> *Refer to* **Meninges.**

Dwarfism
> *Refer to* **Short Stature.**

Dx
The abbreviation for diagnosis.

Dynamic Splint
A device used to properly position a *joint* (such as the wrist) while also assisting other parts of the body (such as the fingers) to engage in purposeful movement.
> *Compare* **Static Splint.**

dys-
A prefix meaning painful, *abnormal,* or difficult.

Dysacusis (dis-uh-KOO-sis)
1. Difficulty in *hearing.*
2. Pain or discomfort in the ear caused by loud noises.

Dysarthria (dis-AR-three-uh)
Speech *articulation* problems due to damage to the vocal structures or the *nerves* that control these structures, resulting in decreased muscle control. Children with dysarthria have language skills (they understand and can formulate language), but have difficulty with spoken expression.

Dysautonomia (dis-o-tuh-NOE-mee-uh)
> *Refer to* **Riley-Day Syndrome.**

Dyschondroplasia (dis-kon-droe-PLAY-zee-uh)
> *Refer to* **Enchondromatosis.**

Dysfluent Speech (dis-FLOO-uhnt)
Speech that includes breaks that interrupt the smooth, meaningful flow of words. Examples of dysfluent speech include *stuttering* and the speech hesitations of the very young child who is learning to speak.

Dysfunction in Sensory Integration (DSI)
> *Refer to* **Sensory Integration Dysfunction.**

Dyskinesia (dis-ki-NEE-see-uh)
Difficulty in performing voluntary movement, usually due to damage to the *basal ganglia* of the *brain*. Examples of dyskinesia include *chorea, athetosis,* and *choreoathetosis*. Dyskinesia is usually characterized by extra (involuntary) movements that may affect a specific muscle group or the whole body.

Dyskinetic
> *Refer to* **Dyskinesia.**

Dyslexia (dis-LEK-see-uh)
A *learning disability* in which the child has difficulty with reading due to difficulty distinguishing written symbols. She may, for example, transpose letters and words (for example, reading "top" as "pot").

Dysmaturative Myopathy (dis-muh-CHOOR-uh-tiv mie-OP-uh-thee)
A rare form of *muscular dystrophy*.

Dysmature
1. Lacking in development, or having faulty development.
2. Referring to a *fetus* or newborn who is *abnormally* small due to a failure to gain weight in the weeks before birth.

Dysmetria (dis-MEE-tree-uh)
Difficulty with voluntary movement in which the child is unable to stop the movement at the desired point (either overreaching or falling short of the desired point).

Dysmorphic (dis-MOR-fik)
Referring to a deformed shape.

Dysmyelinating (dis-MIE-uh-luh-nayt-ing)
A condition in which the *myelin sheath* of a *nerve* or nerve fiber fails to develop.
Refer to **Myelin Sheath.**

Dysostosis (dis-os-TOE-sis)
Defective bone formation.

Dysphagia (dis-FAY-jee-uh)
Swallowing difficulty or the inability to swallow.

Dysphonia (dis-FOE-nee-uh)
Any *disorder* of the voice, such as hoarseness when speaking.

Dysplasia (dis-PLAY-zee-uh or dis-PLAY-zhuh)
A growth *abnormality* of a body structure or an individual *cell*. The size, shape, or number of cells may be a factor.

Dysplastic (dis-PLAS-tic)
Pertaining to *dysplasia*.

Dyspnea (disp-NEE-uh)
Difficult breathing.

Dyspraxia (dis-PRAK-see-uh)
Difficulty with planning and performing coordinated movements, although there is no apparent physical *disorder* or *mental retardation*. For example, a 3-year-old with dyspraxia may have difficulty standing on one foot or stomping her feet on request, even in imitation of someone else.
Also known as **Developmental Coordination Disorder** *and* **Developmental Dyspraxia.**

Dyssemia (dis-EE-mee-uh)
Difficulty using and understanding nonverbal signs and symbols.

Dystocia (dis-TOE-see-uh)
Difficult childbirth due to a large or malpositioned *fetus*; a fetus with an *anomaly* such as *hydrocephalus*; or a mother with a pelvic or uterine condition.

Dystonia (dis-TOE-nee-uh)
1. *Abnormal muscle tone*, either increased or decreased tone.
2. A *genetic disorder* in which the child experiences severe muscle *spasms* and exhibits abnormal movements and *postures*, especially when walking.

Dystopia Canthorum (dis-TOE-pee-uh)
Lateral displacement of the inner angle of the opening between the upper and lower eyelids.

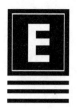

Ear
The organ responsible for the sense of *hearing*. The ear consists of the *outer ear* (*external ear*), the *middle ear*, and the *inner ear*. The outer ear consists of the *pinna* (the part of the ear seen on the outside of the head) and the *auditory canal* (the canal leading from the outside inward to the *tympanic membrane*, or *eardrum*), and the *concha* (the cavity in the external ear that surrounds the *external auditory canal*). The eardrum separates the outer and middle ear. The middle ear consists of the small cavity between the eardrum and the inner ear and the three tiny bones (*auditory ossicles*) of the ear (the *malleus*, the *incus*, and the *stapes*). Also in the middle ear is the opening to the *eustachian tube* which joins the back of the throat to the ear. The inner ear, also called the *labyrinth*, consists of the *cochlea* and the *vestibular apparatus*. It is through the cochlea that the *auditory nerve* passes as it extends to the *brain*.
>*Refer to **Hearing**.*

Ear Canal
>*Refer to **Auditory Canal**.*

Eardrum
>*Refer to **Ear** and **Tympanic Membrane**.*

Eardrum Perforation
A rupture of the *tympanic membrane* that can be caused several ways, including by acute or chronic *otitis media*, a hard blow to the ear, or puncture with a sharp object. *Antibiotic drugs* are used to treat infection, but a perforated eardrum usually heals on its own. Once healed, if there is no damage to the bones of the *middle ear*, normal *hearing* returns.
>*Also known as a **Perforated Eardrum**.*

Ear Infection
>*Refer to **Otitis Media**.*

Early Childhood Special Education (ECSE) Program
An educational program for the child between 3 and 5 years of age who has a *developmental disability* and is eligible for preschool services under the *Individuals with Disabilities Education Improvement Act of 2004*.

Early Educator
*Refer to **Infant Educator.***

Early Head Start
*Refer to **Head Start/Early Head Start.***

Early Infantile Autism
*Refer to **Autistic Disorder.***

Early Intervention
Specialized services provided to infants and toddlers who are *at-risk* for, or are showing signs of, *developmental delay*. Services emphasize the continued development of basic skills through planned interactions that will minimize the effects of the baby's condition. Several types of qualified professionals may plan and implement early intervention services, provided in conformity with an *Individualized Family Service Plan*. These professionals include *service coordinators, infant educators* (who use *developmental* play activities to promote the infant's acquisition of basic skills), *physical* or *occupational therapists, speech-language pathologists, audiologists*, and *social workers*. They may also include other individuals who are trained to help infants and young children with acquiring new skills and *behaviors* or to provide other services such as family training, screening, *assessment*, or health care. Early intervention services are provided under public supervision and at no cost (except where federal or state law provides for a system of payment by families).
*Refer to **Early Interventionist.***

Early Intervention Educator
*Refer to **Infant Educator.***

Early Interventionist
An *infant educator* or other professional who is trained to assess and/or plan and implement a program which addresses the infant or young child's *developmental* needs.
*Refer to **Infant Educator.***

Early Intervention Multidisciplinary Team
*Refer to **Multidisciplinary Team.***

Ear Tube
A small plastic tube that is surgically placed through the *tympanic membrane* into the *middle ear* to treat chronic ear fluid or chronic *ear infections*. The tube is not placed permanently, and usually falls out on its own.
*Also known as **Tympanostomy Tube, Myringotomy Tube, PE Tube, Pressure Equalization Tube**, and **Ventilation Tube**.*
*Refer to **Myringotomy.***

ECG
The abbreviation for electrocardiogram and electrocardiography.

Echocardiography (ek-oe-kar-dee-OG-ruh-fee)
An *ultrasound* imaging technique that creates a picture of the *heart* (*echocardiogram*) produced by the echo of sound waves.

Echolalia (ek-oe-LAY-lee-uh)
Involuntary repetition of another person's words or phrases, including voice *tone*, usually without comprehension. Echolalia is sometimes seen in children with an *autism spectrum disorder, mental retardation, Tourette syndrome,* or *schizophrenia.* (In very young children, imitating or echoing another's speech is normal, and helps in the development of expressive speech and language skills.)

Echovirus (EK-oe-vie-ruhs)
A usually harmless *enterovirus* (a *virus* that thrives mainly in the intestinal tract) associated with many infections.

Eclampsia (e-KLAMP-see-uh)
A serious complication of pregnancy in which the woman who has *pre-eclampsia* also has seizures and sometimes goes into a *coma.* Eclampsia can be fatal to the pregnant woman, and termination of the pregnancy or early delivery may be necessary if the woman's condition cannot be stabilized.
    Compare **Pre-eclampsia.**

ECMO
The abbreviation for extracorporeal membrane oxygenator.

ECSE
The abbreviation for Early Childhood Special Education.

ect-, ecto-
Prefixes meaning outside.

-ectasis
A suffix meaning dilation.

Ectasis (EK-tuh-sis)
Dilation or distention of any tubular *vessel.*

-ectomy
A suffix meaning surgical removal.

Eczema (EK-ze-muh)
Inflammation of the outer layer of skin, resulting in an itchy, weeping *rash* that blisters and scales. The cause of eczema is often unknown; however, it may result from an *allergy.*

ED
The abbreviation for emotionally disordered.

EDC
The abbreviation for estimated date of confinement.

Edema (e-DEE-muh)
Fluid retention in the body *tissues* that often causes swelling.

Edematous (e-DEE-muht-us)
Pertaining to *edema.*

Educable (EJ-uh-kuh-buhl)
An old term for *mild mental retardation.*
>   *Refer to* **Intelligence.**

**Education for All Handicapped Children Act of 1975
(Public Law 94-142)**
A federal law passed in 1975 that mandates that states provide *special educa-tion* services ("a *free appropriate public education* in the *least restrictive environ-ment*") to meet the needs of children with *disabilities* from ages 5 to 21 years.
>   *Refer to* **Individuals with Disabilities Education Improvement Act of 2004.**

**Education of the Handicapped Act Amendments of 1986
(Public Law 99-457)**
A federal law passed in 1986 that amended and became a part of *PL 94-142.*
PL 99-457 mandates that states provide preschool education for children with *special needs* (beginning at age 3 years). Part C (originally known as Part H) focuses on the development of services to infants and toddlers who are *at-risk* or have *disabilities.*
>   *Refer to* **Individuals with Disabilities Education Improvement Act of 2004.**

Edward Syndrome
>   *Refer to* **Trisomy 18.**

EEG
The abbreviation for electroencephalogram and electroencephalography.

EENT
The abbreviation for ears, eyes, nose, and throat.

ef-
A prefix meaning out of or away from.

Efferent (EF-uhr-uhnt)
Directed away from center, such as a *nerve impulse* that travels from the *cen-tral nervous system* to a nerve or muscle.
>   *Compare* **Afferent.**

Effexor™ (e-FEKS-or)
>   *Refer to* **Venlafaxine Hydrochloride.**

Efficacy (EF-uh-kuh-see)
The extent to which a specific *intervention*, procedure, regimen, or service produces a desired effect.

Ehlers-Danlos Syndrome (AY-lerz DAN-los)
A group of *congenital hereditary connective tissue disorders* characterized by deficiency in the quality or quantity of *collagen*, which may result in very stretchy skin with poor wound healing, fragile *tissue*, and *hyperextensible joints* that easily dislocate. *Spine* and *heart* problems may also be present.

Eighth Cranial Nerve
> *Refer to* **Auditory Nerve.**

Eisenmenger Syndrome (IE-suhn-meng-uhr)
A serious *heart* condition that occurs when the *pulmonary blood vessels* become so narrow from thickening (due to *pulmonary hypertension*) that right-to-left (reversed) *shunting* of blood and *cyanosis* results. Eisenmenger syndrome is especially prevalent in children with *Down syndrome*.
> *Refer to* **Occlusive Pulmonary Vascular Disease.**

EKG
The abbreviation for electrocardiogram and electrocardiography.

Elastin (i-LAS-tin)
The main component that forms elastic *tissue* fibers in the body, such as in the *ligaments* of the *spinal column*.

ELBW
The abbreviation for extremely low birth weight infant.

Elective Mutism
> *Refer to* **Selective Mutism.**

Electrocardiogram (EKG, ECG) (ee-lek-troe-KAR-dee-oe-gram)
A recording of the *heart's* electrical impulses.

Electrocardiography (EKG, ECG) (ee-lek-troe-kar-dee-OG-ruh-fee)
A test to study the electrical impulses of the *heart*. *Electrodes* attached to an electrocardiograph machine are applied to the individual's chest, wrist, and ankles. The machine records the heart's electrical impulses (and thus detects any *abnormal* electrical activity), which are displayed on a screen or printout. The procedure causes no discomfort.

Electrode (ee-LEK-troed)
A device attached to an adhesive pad that is placed on the body to record electrical activity such as when obtaining an *electroencephalogram* or *electrocardiogram*.

Electroencephalogram (EEG) (ee-lek-troe-en-SEF-uh-loe-gram)
A recording of the electrical impulses of the *brain*.

Electroencephalography (EEG) (ee-lek-troe-en-sef-uhl-OG-ruh-fee)
A test to study the electrical impulses produced by the activity of the *brain*. *Electrodes* attached to a recording machine are applied to the individual's scalp. The machine measures the brain's electrical impulses, which are displayed on a printout. Electroencephalography is useful in *diagnosing* certain conditions such as *epilepsy* and certain *tumors*.

Electrolyte (ee-LEK-troe-liet)
A substance that, when dissolved or melted, splits into ions that can conduct an electrical current. The body requires adequate, balanced amounts of electrolytes for normal *metabolism* and function. Deficiency or imbalance among them can result in serious conditions such as *hypovolemia* and *shock*.

Electromyogram (EMG) (ee-lek-troe-MIE-oe-gram)
A recording of the electrical activity of muscles.

Electromyography (EMG) (ee-lek-troe-mie-OG-ru-fee)
A test to study the electrical activity of muscles.

Electronic Communication Aids
Computers, voice synthesizers, printers, and other electrical devices that enable a child with speech difficulties to communicate.
>	*Refer to **Assistive Technology** and **Augmentative and Alternative Communication**.*

Elfin Facies Syndrome (EL-fin FAY-shi-eez or FAY-shee-eez)
>	*Refer to **Williams Syndrome**.*

Ellis-van Creveld Syndrome
>	*Refer to **Chondroectodermal Dysplasia**.*

Emaciated (i-MAY-shee-ay-tid)
>	Referring to an extremely lean, wasted condition of the body.

Embryo (EM-bree-oe)
The unborn, developing infant from conception through approximately the eighth week.

Embryonic
Referring to an *embryo*.

Emesis (EM-e-sis)
Vomiting.

EMG
The abbreviation for electromyogram and electromyography.

-emia
A suffix meaning blood.

Emotional Abuse
Continual belittling, threatening, blaming, ignoring, or rejecting of a child that can disable him emotionally and *behaviorally*. The parent or caregiver who verbally abuses, is always negative, or responds in unpredictable ways toward a child in his care is considered to be maltreating him. Although emotional abuse is difficult to prove, the *mandated reporter* should report any observed or suspected abuse.
*Refer to **Child Abuse and Neglect** and **Mandated Reporter.***

Emotionally Disordered (ED)
Having a *learning disability* or *behavioral* disturbance characterized by an inability to learn, and/or maintain normal relationships with peers and teachers. The child who is emotionally disordered may have a *neurodevelopmental disorder* or a *psychiatric* disorder and usually has average or above-average *intelligence*, yet is unable to function in the regular education classroom.

Empirical (em-PIR-i-kuhl)
Derived from or relying upon observation, experimentation, or experience.

Encephalitis (en-sef-uh-LIE-tis)
An *inflammation* of the *brain*, usually caused by an infection. Encephalitis can be mild, but is more commonly serious, and may result in *seizures, paralysis* of one side of the body, *brain damage, coma,* or death.

Encephalocele (en-SEF-uh-loe-seel)
A *congenital anomaly* in which the *brain, meninges* (the *membranes* surrounding the brain and *spinal cord*), or both protrude through an opening in the skull. With this form of *spina bifida*, severe *brain damage* usually results due to the brain *tissue* exposure.
*Refer to **Spina Bifida.***

Encephalofacial Angiomatosis
(en-sef-uh-loe-FAY-shuhl an-jee-oe-muh-TOE-sis)
*Refer to **Sturge-Weber Syndrome.***

Encephalomalacia (en-sef-uh-loe-muh-LAY-shee-uh)
Softening of the *cerebrum* (the largest part of the *brain*, containing the two *cerebral hemispheres*, which are joined together by the *corpus callosum*). Encephalomalacia is often caused by a poor or interrupted supply of blood to the brain. This results in death to the brain *tissue* that did not receive blood. The level of *brain damage* will depend upon the part of the brain tissue that died.

Encephalomeningocele (en-sef-uh-loe-men-IN-goe-seel)
*Refer to **Meningoencephalocele.***

Encephalomyelitis (en-sef-uh-loe-mie-el-IE-tis)
An *inflammation* of the *brain* and *spinal cord*, usually caused by a *virus*. Encephalomyelitis can result in *seizures*, partial *paralysis*, loss of sensation, *mental retardation*, and death.

Encephalomyelopathy (en-sef-uh-loe-mie-el-OP-uh-thee)
Any *disease* or *disorder* of both the *brain* and the *spinal cord*.

Encephalopathy (en-sef-uh-LOP-uh-thee)
Any *disease* or *disorder* of the *brain*. *Kernicterus* and *Reye syndrome* are examples of encephalopathies.

Encephalotrigeminal Angiomatosis
(en-sef-uh-loe-trie-JEM-i-nuhl an-jee-oe-muh-TOE-sis)
    Refer to **Sturge-Weber Syndrome.**

Enchondromatosis (en-kuhn-droe-muh-TOE-sis)
A *congenital disorder* characterized by an increase of *cartilage* within the extremities of the shafts of bones. This may result in shortened or deformed bones and an increased susceptibility to broken bones.
    Also known as **Dyschondroplasia** *and* **Ollier Disease.**

Encoding
1. The stage of memory when information received through the senses is modified and stored.
2. The process of changing ideas into words or written expressions. Encoding is part of expressing language.

Encopresis (en-koe-PREE-sis)
The inability to hold *bowel movements* long enough to eliminate in the toilet. (The term encopresis applies to children who are old enough to have gained bowel control.) There is no specific physical cause and the condition rarely occurs after 10 years of age. Encopresis usually involves a vicious cycle of stool withholding, *constipation* and leakage of stool, and painful passage of stool.

end-, endo-
A prefix meaning inside.

Endocardial Cushion (en-doe-KAR-dee-uhl)
One of a pair of raised areas, or masses, on the *atrioventricular canal* of the *embryonic heart*. These raised areas of *tissue* are concerned with development of the atrioventricular canals and *valves*.
    Refer to **Endocardial Cushion Defect.**

Endocardial Cushion Defect
A complex *heart defect* involving one or more parts of the *endocardial cushion*. Endocardial cushion defects occur frequently in children with *Down syndrome*.

Endocardial Fibroelastosis
(en-doe-KAR-dee-uhl fie-broe-ee-las-TOE-sis)
An *abnormal* condition of the *endocardium* (the lining of the chambers of the *heart*). The lining becomes thick and *fibroelastic* which can make the heart unable to pump enough blood to body *tissues*.

Endocarditis (en-doe-kar-DIE-tis)
Inflammation of the inner lining of the *heart* (the endocardium), including the *heart valves*. Endocarditis is usually caused by infection and can result in heart damage and/or the need for *valve* replacement. If left untreated, endocarditis can be fatal.

Endocardium (en-doe-KAR-dee-uhm)
The lining (comprised of *epithelial tissue* and *connective tissue*) of the chambers of the *heart*.

Endocrine (EN-doe-krin or EN-doe-krien or EN-doe-kreen)
Pertaining to the *glands* of the endocrine system, or glands that *secrete* directly into the bloodstream.

Endocrine Disorders
Disorders of the *glands* that produce *hormones* and regulate body functions. *Diabetes mellitus* is an example.
> *Refer to* **Adrenocorticotropic Hormone** *and* **Endocrine.**

Endocrine Gland
Glands that *secrete* important *hormones* into the bloodstream and influence *metabolism* and other body functions. The endocrine glands include the pituitary, thyroid, parathyroid, and *adrenal glands*, the *pineal body*, and the *gonads*.

Endocrinologist
A medical doctor who specializes in treating problems of the *endocrine* system.

Endoscopy (en-DOS-koe-pee)
A procedure in which a narrow, flexible tube is inserted into a body cavity for visual examination.

Endotracheal (en-doe-TRAY-kee-uhl)
Referring to within the *trachea*.

Endotracheal Tube (ET Tube)
A narrow plastic tube inserted into the *trachea* to improve *respiration*.

Enema (EN-e-muh)
A procedure in which fluid is introduced into the *rectum*. An enema is given to rid the *bowel* of *feces*, to administer medicine, or as part of an *x-ray* study of the intestines.

Engagement
The ability to remain focused and interactive with (or responsive to) a person. Engagement builds intimacy and a rhythm to interactions, and is the foundation for higher level functional, emotional interactions, and for learning.

entero-
A prefix meaning pertaining to the intestines.

Enterobius Vermicularis (en-ter-OE-bee-us ver-mik-yoo-LAR-is)
Pinworms.
> *Refer to* **Worms.**

Enterocolitis (en-ter-oe-koe-LIE-tis)
An *inflammation* of the *small* and *large intestines.*

Enteropathy (en-tuh-ROP-uh-thee)
A *disease* or *disorder* of the intestines.

Enterovirus (EN-tuhr-oe-vie-ruhs)
A *virus* that thrives mainly in the intestinal tract.

ENT Specialist
The abbreviation for Ear, Nose, and Throat Specialist.
> *Also known as an* **Otolaryngologist.**

Enucleation (ee-noo-klee-AY-shuhn)
Surgical removal of the entire eye.

Enunciate (i-NUN-see-ayt)
To pronounce, or speak clearly.

Enuresis (en-yoo-REE-sis)
The inability to control the need to urinate after the age 5, when most children have achieved *bladder* control. *Nocturnal enuresis* (commonly referred to as bedwetting) occurs in approximately 10 percent of healthy children. Causes of enuresis include: immaturity of the *nervous system* functions concerned with bladder control; stress; or a physical *abnormality*, such as an infection, *spinal cord* damage, or an anatomic defect of the *urinary tract*. Usually children no longer wet the bed after about 10 years of age.

Environmental Risk
> *Refer to* **At-Risk.**

Enzyme (EN-ziem)
A *protein* that speeds up a chemical change in the body, such as in the *digestion* of foods.

EOM
1. The abbreviation for extraocular muscles.
2. The abbreviation for equal ocular movements.

Ependyma (e-PEN-di-muh)
The lining of the central canal of the *spinal cord* and of the ventricles of the *brain*.

epi-
A prefix meaning upon, after, or above.

Epicanthal Fold/Epicanthus (ep-i-KAN-thuhl/ep-i-KAN-thuhs)
A vertical skin fold at the inner corner of the eye.

Epidermis (ep-i-DUR-mis)
The outer 5 layers of skin.

Epidural Anesthesia (ep-i-DOOR-uhl an-es-THEE-zee-uh)
A local *anesthetic* injected into the space surrounding the *dura mater* of the *spinal cord*. Epidurals are often administered to mothers during *labor* and delivery. Epidural anesthesia has the potential for causing stress to the *fetus* (most likely an inadequate delivery of oxygen), but this outcome is rare if the epidural is properly managed.
Refer to Anesthesia.

Epiglottis (ep-i-GLOT-is)
The *cartilage* flap that covers the *trachea* when swallowing to prevent food from entering the lungs.

Epilepsy (EP-i-lep-see)
A group of neurologic *disorders* characterized by recurrent *seizures* that are caused by *abnormal* electrical activity in the *brain*. The cause of epilepsy is often unknown, but seizures can occur for many reasons, including damage to the brain due to infection, injury, birth *trauma, tumor, stroke,* drug intoxication, and chemical imbalance. *Seizures* that have a known cause are called *symptomatic* or secondary. Seizures that do not have an identifiable cause are thought to occur due to a *genetic* predisposition (but not as an *inherited genetic disorder*), and are referred to as *idiopathic* or primary seizures. There are several types of seizures, classified according to the area of the brain affected and the associated *behaviors*. Seizures are classified as either *generalized seizures* or *partial seizures*. Generalized seizures affect the whole brain and usually cause a loss of consciousness. The types of generalized seizures include *tonic-clonic (grand mal) seizures, absence (petit mal) seizures, myoclonic seizures,* and *atonic (drop) seizures*. Partial seizures affect specific areas of the brain (although the electrical disturbance may not remain confined to one area and may spread to the whole brain, thus causing a generalized seizure). The child may retain consciousness during a partial seizure. The types of partial seizures include *simple partial seizures* and *complex partial seizures*. Epilepsy is usually treated with *antiepileptic drugs* to control the seizures.

Epiloia (ep-i-LOY-uh)
Refer to **Tuberous Sclerosis.**

Epinephrine (ep-i-NEF-rin)
A *hormone* released by the *adrenal glands*, along with *norepinephrine*, to increase the *heart's* ability to work, especially in response to stressors on the body such as exercise or fear. It also relaxes the smooth muscles of the *bronchioles* and intestines and has other muscular and *metabolic* effects. Epinephrine can also be made synthetically and is used to treat *allergic* reactions.
Also known as **Adrenaline.**
Refer to **Allergy.**

EpiPen™
A device that an individual can use to inject himself with synthetic *epinephrine* if he is exposed to an *allergen* and is at-risk for *anaphylaxis*.
Refer to **Epinephrine.**

Episodic (ep-i-SOD-ik)
An incident, such as a seizure, that occurs at intervals.

Epithelial (ep-i-THEE-lee-uhl)
Pertaining to the outer layer of the skin, or lining of other body structures such as the lungs and intestines.

Epithelium (ep-i-THEE-lee-um)
Tissue that covers the internal or external surfaces of the body, such as the skin and the lining of the lungs.

Epogen™ (EP-oe-jen)
A drug used to signal the *bone marrow* to make *red blood cells.*

EPs
The abbreviation for Evoked Potential Studies.

Epstein-Barr Virus (EP-stien BAR)
A herpes-like *virus* that causes *infectious mononucleosis.*

Equilibrium (ee-kwuh-LIB-ree-uhm)
Balance.

Equilibrium Reactions (ee-kwuh-LIB-ree-uhm)
Any of several *reflexes* that enable the body to restore *balance* when the center of gravity has shifted. Children learn to compensate for a loss of balance by moving in ways to counteract the pull of gravity.
Refer to **Automatic Reflex.**

Equinovalgus (ee-kwi-noe-VAL-gus)
Refer to **Talipes Equinovalgus.**

Equinovarus (ee-kwi-noe-VAY-rus)
*Refer to **Talipes Equinovarus**.*

Equinus (EE-kwi-nuhs)
A condition in which the foot is held in *extension*, which results in *toe walking*. It is caused by a shortening of the calf muscles and *tendons* and is usually associated with *clubfoot*.

ERA
The abbreviation for Evoked Response Audiometry.
*Refer to **Auditory Brainstem Response**.*

Erb's Palsy
A condition in which the *brachial plexus* is injured during delivery, resulting in weakness and *paralysis* of the upper arm on the damaged side. Functional use of the arm usually improves with treatment, including *physical therapy*.

Ergocalciferol (er-goe-kal-SIF-uh-rol)
Vitamin D2. Drisdol™ is the brand name drug of this vitamin.
*Also known as **Calciferol**.*

Errorless Learning
A teaching technique that involves *prompting* the child immediately following a request, which allows the child to always respond correctly. The prompts are faded as soon as possible until the child is responding independently.

Erythema (er-i-THEE-muh)
Inflammation of the skin, resulting in redness. Examples of causes include fever, mild sunburn, or blushing.

Erythema Infectiosum
A mild, *contagious disease* caused by *human parvovirus B-19*. It is transmitted via *respiratory secretions* and results in illness consisting of fever, headache, malaise, and an itchy, red *rash*. The rash appears first on the face (about 10 days after the onset of the other *symptoms*), and consists of red spots that run together on the cheeks giving a "slapped face" appearance. Several days after the facial rash appears, red spots may develop on the trunk, arms, and legs. The rash usually lasts about a week. Erythema infectiosum can be very serious, even fatal, to the *fetus* if a pregnant woman passes it to her baby.
*Also known as **Fifth Disease**.*

erythro-
A prefix meaning red.

Erythroblastosis Fetalis (e-rith-roe-blas-TOE-sis fee-TAY-lis)
A severe type of *hemolytic anemia* of the *fetus* or newborn infant that is typically caused by *Rh incompatibility*. Rh incompatibility occurs when a pregnant woman who has Rh negative blood is carrying a fetus with Rh positive

blood, and the woman was previously exposed to Rh positive blood (either through a pregnancy in which the woman carried a baby with Rh positive blood or through a blood transfusion of Rh positive blood). Due to this prior exposure to the Rh positive blood, the woman produced *antibodies* to Rh positive blood, which react to the Rh positive blood of the fetus she is currently carrying as a foreign substance and destroy the fetus's *red blood cells*. Erythroblastosis fetalis results in serious *fetal disease* (*generalized edema*, enlargement of the *liver* and the *spleen*, hemolytic anemia, and *jaundice* that leads to *kernicterus*) or in death.

> Also known as **Hemolytic Disease of the Newborn** and **Hemolytic Anemia of the Newborn.**
> Refer to **Rh Incompatibility** and **Rh Factor.**

Erythrocyte (e-RITH-roe-siet)
A *red blood cell.*

Erythromycin (e-rith-roe-MIE-sin)
An *antibiotic drug* used to treat infection.

eso-
A prefix meaning inside or inward.

Esophagitis (ee-sof-uh-JIE-tis)
Inflammation of the *esophagus* caused by *reflux* (backflow) of gastric juice from the stomach, infection, or irritation from a tube inserted through the nose to the stomach.

Esophagus (ee-SOF-uh-gus)
The tube that carries food from the throat to the stomach.

Esotropia (es-oe-TROE-pee-uh)
A form of *strabismus* in which one eye turns inward (is convergent) while the other eye focuses straight ahead.

> Also known as **Cross-eye** and **Convergent Strabismus.**
> Compare **Exotropia.**
> Refer to **Strabismus.**

Established Medical Diagnosis
An eligibility designation that may allow a preschooler to receive *special education* services, based on a previous medical condition that was *diagnosed* in infancy.

Established Risk
A *diagnosed* condition that indicates a high probability of eventual *developmental delay.*

esthe-
A prefix meaning perceive or sense.

Estimated Date of Confinement (EDC)
The pregnant woman's estimated date of delivery, or due date.

Ethmoid Bone (ETH-moid)
A small bone of the skull that forms part of the *orbit* (the bony socket that contains the eye) and the nose.

Ethosuximide (eth-oe-SUK-si-mied)
An *antiepileptic drug*. It is used most commonly to treat *absence seizures*. Zarontin™ is the brand name of this drug.

Etiology (ee-tee-OL-oe-jee)
The study of the cause of *disease*.

ET Tube
The abbreviation for endotracheal tube.

eu-
A prefix meaning good, well, or true.

Eustachian Tube (yoo-STAY-shuhn or yoo-STAY-kee-uhn)
A tube lined with *mucous membrane* that joins the *nasopharynx* (the passageway between the nasal area behind the nose and the throat area behind the *soft palate*) with the *middle ear*. The tube regulates air pressure in the ear, such as when it opens during yawning and swallowing. (The air pressure must be equal on each side of the *tympanic membrane* for it to function properly.) The eustachian tube also functions as a passageway through which fluids can drain.
    Refer to Ear.

Evaluation
    Refer to Assessment.

Eversion
Turning a part of the body outward (for example, turning the foot toward the direction of the little toe).
    Compare Inversion.

Evoked Potential/Evoked Response
A refined or specialized *EEG* to assess the condition of the visual, auditory, or *tactile* pathways of the neurological system.
    Refer to Electroencephalogram.

Evoked Potential Studies (EPs)
Tests to evaluate the electrical response in the *brainstem* or the *cerebral cortex* to specific *sensory stimulation*. EP studies are useful in assessing the condition of the visual, auditory, or *tactile* pathways of the neurological system in individuals who are unable to voluntarily respond to *stimulation*, such as a newborn or a person unconscious during surgery. Examples include *visual-evoked*

responses (VERs), *auditory brainstem-evoked potentials* (*ABEPs*), and *somato-sensory-evoked responses* (*SERs*).

>   *Also known as* **Evoked Response Studies.**
>   *Refer to* **Electroencephalogram.**

Evoked Response Audiometry (ERA)

A *hearing* test useful in *diagnosing nerve* defects of the *inner ear* and *brainstem* auditory pathways.

Evoked Response Studies

>   *Refer to* **Evoked Potential Studies.**

ex-

A prefix meaning out or away from.

Exchange Transfusion

A type of blood transfusion in which the infant's blood is withdrawn in small amounts and replaced with equal amounts of donor blood.

Excrete

To eliminate or discharge waste product from the body.

>   *Compare* **Secrete.**
>   *Refer to* **Gland.**

Excretion

The process by which the body (beginning at the *cell* level) gets rid of waste products. Excretion is the final stage of *nutrition*.

>   *Refer to* **Nutrition.**

exo-

A prefix meaning outside.

Exomphalos (eks-OM-fuh-lus)

>   *Refer to* **Omphalocele.**

Exophthalmia (eks-of-THAL-mee-uh)

Exophthalmos caused by a variety of *diseases*. It can result in *visual impairment*. Treatment of the underlying disease is required.

Exophthalmos (eks-of-THAL-moes)

Abnormal protrusion of the eyeball.

Exotropia (eks-oe-TROE-pee-uh)

A form of *strabismus* in which one eye turns outward (is divergent) while the other eye focuses straight ahead. The child may have *visual impairment*.

>   *Also known as* **Wall-Eye** and **Divergent Strabismus.**
>   *Compare* **Esotropia.**
>   *Refer to* **Strabismus.**

Expectorant
A drug given to encourage the coughing up of *mucus*/sputum (material coughed up from the lungs, important in the *diagnosis* of many illnesses).

Expressive Aphasia
*Refer to **Aphasia**.*

Expressive Language
The ability to communicate thoughts and feelings by *gesture, sign language,* verbalization, or written word.
*Compare **Receptive Language**.*

Extension
Straightening of the neck, trunk, or *limbs*. This movement increases the angle between two bones of a *joint*.
*Compare **Flexion**.*
*Refer to **Hyperextension**.*

Extensor
Any muscle whose function is to straighten out a *joint* of the body.
*Compare **Flexor**.*

Extensor Pattern
A pattern of muscle movement that causes a straightening out of a *limb*.

Extensor Thrust
A *reflex*, normally present during the first 2 months of life, in which the infant's flexed leg uncontrollably extends when the sole of the foot is stimulated (i.e., scratched lightly).
*Compare **Flexor Withdrawal**.*

Extensor Thrust Pattern
An *abnormal* pattern of muscle movement (when it persists beyond 4 months of age) in which the child's body becomes rigid and extends (straightens out) while the child is lying on his back.

External Auditory Canal
*Refer to **Auditory Canal**.*

External Ear
The *outer ear*.
*Refer to **Auditory Canal, Concha, Ear,** and **Pinna**.*

External Rotation
A turning outward or away from the *midline* of the body. An example of external rotation is turning a leg outward so that the toes are pointed to the side, away from the body's midline.

Extinction (ik-STINGK-shuhn)
Lessening the frequency or intensity of an inappropriate or otherwise unwanted *behavior* in a child by no longer *reinforcing* a previously reinforced response.

Extracorporeal Membrane Oxygenator (ECMO)
(ek-struh-kor-POR-ee-uhl)
A *heart*-lung bypass machine that *oxygenates* a baby's blood outside his body then returns it to his *circulatory system*. For example, it may be used to treat persistent *pulmonary hypertension* in the newborn.

Extraocular Muscle (EOM) (ek-struh-OK-yoo-luhr)
One of the six sets of muscles attached to each eye that control movements of the eyeball.

Extrapyramidal Cerebral Palsy (eks-truh-pi-RAM-i-duhl)
Cerebral palsy that results from damage to the *nerve* pathways (outside the *pyramidal tract*) that transmit impulses for controlling movement and maintaining *posture* from the *brain* to the *spinal cord*. There are several forms of extrapyramidal cerebral palsy, such as *choreoathetoid cerebral palsy*, *rigid cerebral palsy*, and *atonic cerebral palsy*.
> *Compare* **Pyramidal Cerebral Palsy.**
> *Refer to* **Cerebral Palsy.**

Extrapyramidal Tract
The *nerve* pathways that transmit impulses for controlling movement and maintaining *posture* from the *brain* to the *spinal cord*.
> *Compare* **Pyramidal Tract.**

Extremely Low Birth Weight Infant (ELBW)
A baby who weighs less than 1000 grams (approximately 2 pounds, 4 ounces) at birth.
> *Compare* **Birth Weight, Low Birth Weight Infant, and Very Low Birth Weight Infant.**
> *Refer to* **Premature Infant.**

Extremity
An arm or leg.

Extrusion Reflex
A normal response in infants up to 4 months, in which the baby pushes his tongue out when the tongue is depressed.
> *Refer to* **Primitive Reflex.**

Extubation (eks-too-BAY-shuhn)
The removal of the *endotracheal tube* (plastic tube inserted into the *trachea* to improve *respiration*).
> *Compare* **Intubation.**

Eye

The organ responsible for vision. The eye consists of the *pupil*, which is the opening in the center of the *iris* (the clear *tissue* of the eye under which are pigment *cells* that give the eye its color); the *cornea*, which is the transparent, domelike shell covering the front part of the eye; the *lens* (*crystalline lens*) which is between the iris and the *vitreous humor* (the gel-like substance of the eye); the *retina*, which is the *membrane* lining the back of the inside of the eyeball; and the *optic nerve*, which is the bundle of *nerve* fibers that lead from the retina to the *brain*.

Refer to **Ophthalmologist** and **Vision.**

Eye Dominance

Preferring one eye to assume the major function of seeing, such as when using one eye to look through a microscope or door peephole.

Eye-Hand Coordination

The ability to use visual *input* to assist in manipulation of an object with the hands. For example, seeing a desired object and successfully reaching toward and *grasping* it.

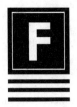

F
1. The abbreviation for female.
2. The abbreviation for frequency.

Face Presentation

Birth (delivery) of a baby in which the face area of the head is the first to appear in the mother's *pelvis*.

Refer to **Fetal Presentation.**

Facies (FAY-shi-eez or FAY-shee-eez)

The face's expression or appearance. For example, the characteristic facies of *fetal alcohol syndrome* includes small eyes, *epicanthal folds* (a vertical skin fold at the inner corner of the eyes), small jaw, flat *midface*, indistinct or long *philtrum* (the grooved area between the upper lip and the nose), thin upper lip, short nose, and short *palpebral fissures* (the opening between the upper and lower eyelids).

Compare **Coarse Facial Features/Coarse Facies.**

Facilitated Communication (FC)

A teaching method originally designed to help children with *motor* difficulties to communicate (such as nonverbal children with *cerebral palsy* whose hands *tremor*). In using this method, a "facilitator" holds the child's hand or forearm, steadies the extended index finger, and helps the child type out letters on a keyboard or spell out words by pointing to letters on a piece of paper. The theory is that the child can then read and type, enabling her to express her feelings. Facilitated communication has also been tried with children with *autism spectrum disorders*. Research indicates, however, that children do not improve their *communication* skills, and that it is the facilitator's thoughts that are being expressed, not the child's.

FACP

The abbreviation for Fellow, American College of Physicians.

FACS

The abbreviation for Fellow, American College of Surgeons.

Fading
Slowly phasing out *prompts* until no prompting is needed, as the child begins to show signs of learning a new skill (i.e., she demonstrates correct responses).
Refer to **Prompt.**

FAE
The abbreviation for fetal alcohol effects.
Refer to **Alcohol-Related Neurodevelopmental Disorder.**

Failure to Thrive (FTT)
A condition of infancy and early childhood characterized by lower weight/slower weight gain than that which is expected by comparison to a standardized growth chart. FTT may occur when the baby does not receive sufficient nutrients. This may be due to physical or psychosocial problems, such as *chromosomal abnormalities, acute illness, malnutrition,* or severe *maternal* deprivation.

False Negative
A test result that fails to show evidence of a substance, condition, or *disease* when it is actually present.
Compare **False Positive.**

False Positive
A test result that shows evidence of a substance, condition, or *disease* when it is not actually present.
Compare **False Negative.**

Familial (fuh-MIL-yuhl)
Pertaining to a *disease* that is common to, or occurs in more members of a family than expected by chance alone.

Familial Autonomic Dysfunction
Refer to **Riley-Day Syndrome.**

Familial Disorder
A condition that occurs in more members of a family than would be expected to occur in the general population. Familial disorders are usually, but not always, *hereditary.*
Compare **Hereditary.**

Familial Dysautonomia (fuh-MIL-yuhl dis-aw-toe-NOE-mee-uh)
Refer to **Riley-Day Syndrome.**

Family Dynamics
The interaction and influence of members of a family on each other.

Fanning
The action of an infant's toes extending and separating while standing and trying to maintain *balance.*

FAPE
The abbreviation for free appropriate public education.

Farsightedness
> *Refer to* **Hyperopia.**

FAS
The abbreviation for fetal alcohol syndrome.

fasc-, fasci-
Prefixes meaning *band.*

Fascia (FASH-ee-uh or FASH-uh)
Fibrous *connective tissue* in the body that surrounds structures and supports organs.

Fasciculation (fa-sik-yoo-LAY-shuhn)
The involuntary twitching of a single muscle group that is innervated by a single *nerve*. It can be a *symptom* of certain *diseases*, result from fever or dietary deficiency, or occur as a *side effect* of some drugs.

Fascioscapulohumeral Muscular Dystrophy (FSH, FSHD)
(fay-shee-oe-skap-yoo-loe-HYOO-mer-uhl)
An *autosomal dominant* form of *muscular dystrophy* that affects the muscles of the face, shoulder, and upper arms (and occasionally the hips and legs), which weaken slowly. This is a relatively *benign* form of muscular dystrophy.
> *Also known as* **Landouzy-Déjérine Muscular Dystrophy.**

FASD
The abbreviation for Fetal Alcohol Spectrum Disorder.

Fats
One of the categories of essential nutrients. Fats are the body's most concentrated source of food energy and the form in which extra energy is stored.

Fatty Acid
Any of several acids found in *fats* (nutrients that provide the body with stored or potential energy). Fatty acids are either saturated or unsaturated. A diet high in saturated fatty acids is linked to a high level of *cholesterol* in the blood and to *heart disease*. An important type of unsaturated fatty acid, the essential fatty acids, cannot be produced by the body and must be added to the diet to maintain proper growth and functioning.

fauci-
A prefix meaning throat.

FBA
The abbreviation for Functional Behavior Analysis.

FC
The abbreviation for facilitated communication.

Fe
The chemical symbol for *iron*.

Feature Matching
Selecting an *assistive technology* device or software that has features that will match (meet) the needs of a child with a *disability*.

Febrile (FEE-bril or FEE-briel or FEB-ril)
Having a fever.
>   Compare **Afebrile.**

Febrile Seizure
A *seizure* that is associated with a rapidly rising high fever. Febrile seizures are the most common type of seizure in children under age 5. They are not considered to be a form of *epilepsy*.

Feces/Fecal Matter (FEE-seez/FEE-kuhl)
Referring to the waste material from the *digestive tract* (*bowel movements*).

Feeding Tube
A tube placed into part of the *digestive tract* to feed babies who cannot take food by mouth. Examples include the NG Tube (*nasogastric tube*) or the *G-Tube* (*gastrostomy tube*).
>   *Refer to* **Gastrostomy, Gastrostomy Tube, Nasogastric Tube, Nasojejunal Tube,** *and* **Oral Gastric Tube.**

Femur (FEE-mur)
The thigh bone.

Fer-In-Sol™
The over-the-counter liquid form of *iron* (*ferrous sulfate*).

Ferrous Sulfate (FER-us SUL-fayt)
Iron.
>   *Refer to* **Fer-In-Sol™.**

Fetal (FEET-l)
Pertaining to the *fetus*.

Fetal Alcohol Effects (FAE)
>   *Refer to* **Alcohol-Related Neurodevelopmental Disorder (ARND).**

Fetal Alcohol Spectrum Disorder (FASD)
An umbrella category that includes *Fetal Alcohol Syndrome (FAS)*, *Partial Fetal Alcohol Syndrome (PFAS)*, and *Alcohol-Related Neurodevelopmental Disorder (ARND)*.

Fetal Alcohol Syndrome (FAS)

A combination of *congenital anomalies* caused by *maternal* consumption of alcohol during pregnancy. Characteristics can include growth retardation; *central nervous system neurodevelopmental abnormalities*; *heart, liver,* and *kidney* problems; abnormalities of the arms, legs, hands, or feet; and a characteristic facial appearance, including small eyes, *epicanthal folds* (a vertical skin fold at the inner corner of the eyes), small jaw, flat *midface*, indistinct or long *philtrum* (the grooved area between the upper lip and the nose), thin upper lip, short nose, ear anomalies, and short *palpebral fissures* (the opening between the upper and lower eyelids). Children with *FAS* typically have significant *developmental delays/mental retardation* and *attention-deficit/hyperactivity disorder*, and often *vision* and *hearing* problems.

> *Refer to* **Fetal Alcohol Spectrum Disorder (FASD)**.

Fetal Circulation

The unique pattern of blood flow in the *fetus* in which blood flows to and from the *placenta* to receive *oxygen* and nutrients, and to discharge wastes. The fetal lungs are (largely) bypassed in the process of *circulation*.

> *Compare* **Circulation** *and* **Persistent Fetal Circulation**.

Fetal Dilantin Syndrome

> *Refer to* **Fetal Hydantoin Syndrome**.

Fetal Face Syndrome

> *Refer to* **Robinow Syndrome**.

Fetal Hydantoin Syndrome (FHS) (FEET-l hie-DAN-toe-in)

A combination of *congenital anomalies* caused by use of *phenytoin* during pregnancy for seizure control, resulting in *microcephaly*, small size, facial/finger/toe *abnormalities*, poor growth, *mild mental retardation*, and *heart defects*.

> *Also known as* **Fetal Dilantin Syndrome**.

Fetal Monitor

An electronic device used for monitoring fetal *heart rate* during pregnancy and *labor*. Fetal *heart* monitoring is done by placing an *ultrasound* transmitter on the mother's *abdomen* or by inserting an *electrode* through the mother's vagina and placing it on the head of the *fetus*.

Fetal Presentation

The body part of the *fetus* that is first seen in the mother's *pelvis* at the time of delivery. Types of fetal presentation include *vertex* (head first, specifically the crown, or top of the head first), *brow* (head first, specifically the eyebrow/forehead area first), *face* (head first, specifically the face first), *chin, shoulder, breech* (feet, knees, or buttocks first), and *compound* (entry of more than one body part, such as the hand next to the head, in the mother's pelvis).

Fetoscopy (fee-TOS-koe-pee)

A *diagnostic* procedure for visualizing a *fetus* while in the *uterus*. Fetoscopy involves placing a fetoscope (stethoscope) into the mother's uterus, through a small *abdominal* incision, to view the fetus (take photographs) or obtain blood or *tissue* samples.

Fetus (FEE-tuhs)
The developing unborn child from the end of the *embryonic* stage (about the eighth week of pregnancy) until birth.

FG Syndrome
An uncommon *X-linked recessive disorder* that affects males. The *disorder* is characterized by *mental retardation*; a large head; facial differences including a prominent forehead, small ears, *hypertelorism*, a *frontal*, upswept cowlick of the hair, short, down-slanting *palpebral fissures*, *epicanthal folds*, prominent lower lip, a narrow *palate*, and large appearing *corneas*; spinal defects; *short stature*; *imperforate anus* (and other *gastrointestinal anomalies*); seizures; con-*stipation*; finger and toe anomalies; *hypotonia* and/or delayed *motor* development; an outgoing, friendly personality, yet *prone* to *tantrums*/outbursts; short *attention span* and *hyperactivity*. Approximately one-third of children born with FG syndrome die prior to 2 years of age, usually due to complications of the *cardiac* defect or imperforate anus.
Also known as **Opitz-Kaveggia Syndrome.**

FHS
The abbreviation for fetal hydantoin syndrome.

Fibroelastic Tissue (fie-broe-ee-LAS-tik)
Refer to **Fibrous Tissue.**

Fibrotic (fie-BROT-ik)
Pertaining to the formation of fibrous, thickened *connective tissue* such as the formation of scar *tissue* as a reparative response to injury.

Fibrous Tissue (FIE-bruhs)
The tightly woven elastic fibers and fluid-filled spaces that form the *connective tissue* of the body.
Also known as **Fibroelastic Tissue.**

Fibula (FIB-yoo-luh)
The outer and smaller of the two bones of the lower leg. (The other bone is the *tibia*.)

Field of Vision
Refer to **Visual Field.**

Fifth Disease
Refer to **Erythema Infectiosum.**

Fine Motor
The *developmental* area that involves skills which require the coordination of the small muscles of the body, including those of the hands and face. Exam-

ples of fine motor skills include stacking small blocks, stringing beads, *tracking* an object with the eyes, and smiling.

Finger Feeding
Independently picking up small bites of food with the fingers and placing them in the mouth.

Finger Opposition
Refer to **Opposition Movement.**

Fingerspelling
A form of *sign language* in which the fingers are used to represent letters of the alphabet. The letters (signs) are strung together to spell words. The American Manual Alphabet is an example of a fingerspelling system.
Refer to **American Sign Language** *and* **Manual Alphabet.**

FISH
The abbreviation for fluorescent in situ hybridization.

Fissure (FISH-uhr)
1. A crack or groove on the surface of an organ. This may be a normal or *abnormal* condition. The division between the lobes of the lungs is a normal fissure. A crack in the skin around the *anus* that may bleed (called an anal fissure) is not a normal condition.
2. One of many deep grooves that separate the *gyri* (*convolutions*) of the surface of the *cerebral hemispheres* of the *brain*.
Compare **Sulcus.**

Fisting
Keeping the hand(s) tightly clenched with the thumb held against the palm and the fingers flexed around the thumb. A baby with *hypertonicity* may keep her hands fisted. Keeping the hands fisted approximately 50 percent of the time is normal in the first 3 months of life.

Fistula (FIS-chuh-luh)
An *abnormal* passage between two hollow organs or between an organ and the surface of the body. An example of a fistula is a *tracheoesophageal fistula* found between the *esophagus* and the *trachea*. Fistulas may be *congenital* or may be *acquired* as a result of infection or damage to *tissue*, such as during *abdominal* surgery.

Fixation
Directing the eye to an object so its image, in the normal eye, centers on the fovea (the part of the *retina* that provides the area of most distinct vision).

Flat Affect
Having no visible emotional reaction. A child whose visible expression of feelings varies little in response to her environment, even in situations that typically induce anger or excitement, would be said to have flat affect.
Compare **Affect.**

Flatfeet
Refer to **Pes Planus.**

Flexion (FLEK-shuhn)
To bend, bringing the body parts that a *joint* connects toward each other. Bending the neck, trunk, and *limbs* are examples of flexion.
Compare **Extension.**

Flexor
A muscle that controls *flexion* of a *joint.*
Compare **Extensor.**

Flexor Tone
Muscle tone that tends to keep the arms and legs close to the body ("folded") and never completely extended. (This is normal in a newborn and typically disappears by 4 months of age as the infant gains voluntary control of her head and body.)

Flexor Withdrawal
A *reflex*, normally present during the first 2 months of life, in which the infant's extended leg forcefully pulls into a flexed position when the sole of her foot is stimulated (i.e., lightly scratched), as she lies on her back.
Compare **Extensor Thrust.**

Floortime
The centerpiece of (and often used as another name for) the *Developmental, Individual-Difference, Relationship-Based (DIR®) model*, describing the teaching approach of literally getting down on the floor with the child and, by following her lead in what interests her, engaging her in activity that mobilizes her communicative, *cognitive*, and emotional capacities. The 4 goals of floortime are to 1) encourage attention and intimacy, 2) engage in *two-way communication*, 3) encourage the expression and use of feelings and ideas, and 4) encourage logical thought.
Refer to **Developmental, Individual-Difference, Relationship-Based (DIR®) Model.**

Floppy Infant
Referring to a baby with *hypotonia.*

Flu
Refer to **Influenza.**

Fluctuating Tone
Muscle tone that fluctuates between *low tone* ("floppiness," or *hypotonicity*) and *high tone* (*spasticity*, or *hypertonicity*).

Fluorescent In Situ Hybridization (FISH)
A process for viewing and analyzing *DNA* at the molecular level in order to detect the presence or absence of *genetic* material along a *chromosome.* A fluo-

rescent substance "tags" (is added to) a specific *molecular probe*, which is then placed with the DNA sample being studied. The fluorescent chemical "labels" the molecular probe and gives it a detectable signal. The laboratory scientist can observe whether the probe finds its complementary sequence of *nucleotides* (the molecules of which DNA is made), in the DNA being analyzed, and what the chromosomal location of the sequence is.

>   *Refer to* **Molecular Probe.**

Fluorescent Treponemal Antibody Absorption Test (FTA-ABS Test)
(floor-ES-uhnt trep-uh-NEE-muhl AN-ti-bod-ee uhb-SORP-shuhn)
A blood test to confirm the *diagnosis* of *syphilis*.

Fluoride
A *mineral* used to prevent tooth decay.

>   *Refer to* **Poly-Vi-Flor™.**

Fluoxetine Hydrochloride (floo-OK-suh-teen hie-droe-KLOR-ied)
An *antidepressant drug* sometimes used in the treatment of certain *behaviors* associated with an *autism spectrum disorder*. Prozac™ is the brand name of this drug.

FMR1 Gene
The abbreviation for the fragile X mental retardation 1 gene.

FO
The abbreviation for foot orthosis.

Focal (FOE-kuhl)
Referring to a limited or *localized* area or part of an organ or of the body.

Focal Seizure
An older term for a *partial seizure*.

>   *Refer to* **Partial Seizure and Epilepsy.**

Focus (FOE-kuhs)
A specific *localized* area/part of an organ or of the body, such as the site of an infection or the area of the *brain* where a *seizure* begins.

Foley Tube/Catheter™ (FOE-lee)
A type of *urinary catheter*.

Folic Acid (FOE-lik or FOL-ik)
A water-soluble *vitamin* essential for *cell* growth and reproduction. The daily requirement for folic acid increases in pregnancy, infancy, and during periods of stress. Adequate daily intake of folic acid prior to conception and during early pregnancy has been found to decrease the risk of *fetal neural tube defects*.

Following the Child's Lead
An interactive play process, important to the development of *engagement* and

to learning, in which the adult plays with the child in such a way that the adult becomes involved with the child's focus of interest. This creates the opportunity to expand on the child's focus of interest by adding a playful, compatible extension to the child's play. For example, if the child is rubbing his face on a pillow for *sensory input*, the adult may begin by also rubbing her face on a pillow, then slowly using her pillow to begin a game of peek-a-boo. Or if the child also has a favorite stuffed toy (Elmo, for example), Elmo could also "rub" his face on a pillow and begin playing peek-a-boo with the child. This expansion of play allows for a natural opportunity for engagement and more meaningful *reciprocity* within the play activity. Following a child's lead is a significant part of Drs. Stanley I. Greenspan and Serena Weider's *Developmental, Individual-Difference, Relationship-Based (DIR®) model.*

> *Refer to* **Floortime.**

Fontan Operation

A surgical procedure done to allow blood to bypass obstruction associated with a *heart defect.*

Fontanel/Fontanelle (fon-tuh-NEL)

One of the two "soft spots" on the top of the infant's head between the bones of the skull before they completely fuse. The *posterior* (rear) fontanelle usually closes by 2 months of age and the *anterior* (front) fontanelle usually closes by 18 months of age.

Foot Orthosis (FO)

A plastic heel, foot support, or *brace* that fits in a shoe or into corrective shoes that are prescribed by an *orthopedist.*

> *Refer to* **Orthosis.**

Foramen Magnum (for-AY-muhn)

An opening in the *occipital bone* of the skull through which the *spinal cord* enters the *spinal column.*

Foramen Ovale (for-AY-muhn oe-VAY-lee or oe-VAH-lay)

An opening in the wall between the right and left *atria* in the *fetal heart*. After the newborn takes her first breath the foramen ovale begins to close, which is necessary for her blood to be able to circulate through her lungs for *oxygenation*. A *heart defect* results if the opening does not close off.

Forefoot

The part of the foot consisting of the *metatarsus* and the toes.

Forelock

A front lock of hair.

Formboard

A flat puzzle-type board with one or more geometric shapes cut out and matching pieces that can be placed in the cut-outs on the board.

Forward Chaining

A method of teaching a skill in which the skill is broken down into steps. The child receives *reinforcement* upon learning step 1, then steps 1 and 2, and so on.

Compare **Backward Chaining.**

Four-Point Position

On the hands and knees.

Fragile X Mental Retardation 1 Gene (FMR1 Gene)

The *gene* responsible for causing *fragile X syndrome*. The discovery of this gene, and *direct DNA analysis*, have made it possible to test unaffected family members to determine if they are *carriers* of fragile X syndrome, to gain information that may help to determine an affected child's *prognosis*, and to obtain a *prenatal diagnosis*.

Fragile X Syndrome (FXS)

An *X-linked developmental disability* that often, but not always, causes *mild* to *moderate mental retardation*. Some children with fragile X syndrome have average *intelligence*, with or without a *learning disability*. Other *symptoms* may include a long, narrow face with prominent forehead, nose, jaw, and ears; *macroorchidism*; *attention-deficit/hyperactivity disorder*; *heart murmurs*; *strabismus*; and occasional *autistic-like behaviors*, including problems relating to others. Boys with fragile X syndrome are usually more *cognitively* affected than girls. The condition is so-called because *chromosomal analysis* often reveals a partially broken (fragile) site on some *X chromosomes*. *Direct DNA analysis* of the fragile X *gene*, *FMR1 gene* (fragile X mental retardation 1), can identify fragile X *carriers* and provide *prenatal diagnosis*. Fragile X syndrome is the most common known *inherited* cause of mental retardation.

Also known as **Martin-Bell Syndrome.**

Fragilitas Ossium

Refer to **Osteogenesis Imperfecta.**

Franceschetti Syndrome (fran-ches-KET-ee)

An *autosomal dominant disorder* characterized by a flattening of the cheek bones; *coloboma* (a space, or *cleft*, of part of the eyeball); downslanting *palpebral fissures*; lower jaw defects; *external ear* malformation; *auditory hearing impairment*; and *respiratory* problems. The child usually has *normal intelligence*, but may have a *learning disability*. Franceschetti syndrome is the complete form of *mandibulofacial dysostosis*. (*Treacher Collins syndrome* is the incomplete form.)

Fraternal Twins

Refer to **Dizygotic Twins.**

Free Appropriate Public Education (FAPE)

The federal requirement (established in 1975 with the passage of *Public Law 94-142*) that states ensure that a "free appropriate public education is available to

all children with *disabilities*, residing in the state," at age 3. The *Individuals with Disabilities Education Improvement Act of 2004* reauthorized this mandate.
Refer to **Education for All Handicapped Children Act of 1975.**

Frejka Pillow Splint™ (FRAY-Kuh)
A *splint* consisting of a pillow that is belted between the baby's legs. It is used to correct *dislocated hips.*

Frenulum (FREN-yoo-lum)
Refer to **Frenum.**

Frenum (FREE-nuhm)
A narrow fold of *tissue* that connects a movable body part to an immovable part, such as the *mucous membrane* that attaches the tongue to the floor of the mouth.
Also known as **Frenulum.**
Refer to **Lingual Frenum.**

Frequency (F)
The number of repetitions of any occurrence or event (such as heartbeats or complete cycles a sound wave makes) within a specified period of time.

Fricative
A *consonant* sound that is produced by closing off most of the air flow as it passes through the mouth, such as /f/, /v/, and /z/.

Friedreich's Ataxia (FREED-riks uh-TAK-see-uh)
A *hereditary disorder* involving *degeneration* of *nerves* in the *spinal cord.* This progressive disorder is characterized by muscle weakness, unsteadiness and loss of coordinated movement (*ataxia*), speech impairment, *scoliosis*, and possible *cardiomyopathy* (*heart* muscle *disease*).
Also known as **Hereditary Spinal Ataxia** *and* **Spinal Cerebellar Degeneration.**

Frontal
Pertaining to the forehead.

Frontal Lobe
Refer to **Cerebral Hemisphere.**

FSC
The abbreviation for Functional Spontaneous Communication.

FSH
The abbreviation for Fascioscapulohumeral Muscular Dystrophy.

FSHD
The abbreviation for Fascioscapulohumeral Muscular Dystrophy.

FT
The abbreviation for full term.

FTA-ABS Test
The abbreviation for fluorescent treponemal antibody absorption test.

FTT
The abbreviation for failure to thrive.

Full Inclusion
    *Refer to **Inclusion**.*

Full Term (FT)
Relating to an infant born between the 38th and 42nd weeks of *gestation*.

Functional Age
    *Refer to **Developmental Age**.*

Functional Behavior Analysis (FBA)
A method of *behavior* management that uses *behavioral assessment* to analyze the function, or purpose, of a child's unacceptable behavior (commonly, the function is the desire to communicate a need or wish), in order to develop strategies to reduce the behavior. For example, a child may scream or hit to express her feelings, or to convey that she needs assistance, or that she wants to escape her current situation. Once the function of the behavior has been determined, it may be possible to prevent the behavior by changing the situation that elicits the behavior, or to teach the child more acceptable ways of communicating. Practicing and rewarding acceptable behaviors and making sure the unacceptable behavior no longer gets the child's needs met are essential steps in functional behavior analysis.
    *Refer to **Positive Behavior Support**.*

Functional Behaviors
Behaviors (basic skills, such as meal-time skills) the child has mastered, or needs to master, in order to get along as independently as possible in society.

Functional Spontaneous Communication (FSC)
Communication that is unprompted and elicits a desired effect. It is a critically important skill for a person with *autism spectrum disorder* and a predictor of high quality of life outcomes.

Fundal Plication (FUN-duhl plie-KAY-shuhn)
    *Refer to **Fundoplication**.*

Fundi
Plural of fundus.

Fundoplication (fun-duh-pli-KAY-shuhn)
A surgical procedure to correct severe *gastroesophageal reflux* in which the opening from the *esophagus* to the stomach is tightened by wrapping the upper end of the stomach around the lower end of the esophagus and sewing it in place.
    *Also known as **Fundal Plication** and **Nissen Fundoplication.***

Fundus
The base of a hollow organ, or the part farthest from the entrance.

Fungal
Referring to a *fungus*.

Fungi
Plural of *fungus*.

Fungus
A simple *parasitic* plant (a plant that takes *nutrition* from a living *organism* of another species) or a saprophytic plant (a plant that takes nutrition from dead *organic* matter), such as a *yeast* or mold, that can produce *infections* in humans.
    *Refer to **Antifungal Drug.***

FUO
The abbreviation for fever of undetermined origin.

Furosemide (fyoo-ROE-suh-mied)
A *diuretic* (a drug that helps remove excess water from the body). Lasix™ is the brand name for this drug.

FXS
The abbreviation for fragile X syndrome.

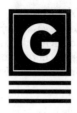

g.
The abbreviation for gram.

Gabatril™
>   *Refer to **Tiagabine Hydrochloride.***

Gag Reflex
A gagging response elicited when the *soft palate* or back of the throat is stimulated. The gag response is a lifetime *reflex*, but it is increased in newborns, usually until the ability to chew food develops. *Oral stimulation* (*mouthing* of safe toys) is important for developing tolerance of various food textures and sensations.

Gait
The manner or style of walking. Walking is normally a progression of *reciprocal movement* in which one foot steps forward and weight is placed on it, then the second foot steps forward (ahead of the placement of the first foot).
>   *Refer to **Non-Reciprocal Gait.***

galact-
A prefix meaning milk.

Galactosemia (guh-lak-toe-SEE-mee-uh)
An *autosomal recessive disorder* characterized by the body's *inborn* inability to metabolize galactose (a sugar substance derived from *lactose*, i.e., milk sugar). This causes high levels of galactose and, if untreated, results in *liver* and *kidney disease, cataracts,* and *mental retardation.*

Gallop Rhythm
An *abnormal heart* rhythm in which 3 or 4 sounds (rather than 2) are heard in each cycle (beat). At certain *heart rates,* the 3 or 4 sounds resemble the sound of a horse gallop.

Gamete (GA-meet)
A sex *cell.* An *ovum* (female sex cell, or egg) and *sperm* (male sex cell) are necessary for reproduction. Each gamete has half the complement of *chromosomes* of a normal cell.

Gamma Globulin (GAM-uh GLOB-yoo-lin)
A class of *immune proteins* formed in the blood.

Gamma Radiation (GAM-uh)
The use of high-*frequency* electromagnetic radiation to *diagnose* and destroy *diseased tissue*, such as a *tumor*.
>Also known as **Gamma Ray.**

Gamma Ray
>*Refer to* **Gamma Radiation.**

Ganglioside (GANG-glee-uh-sied)
A chemical found in the *gray matter* (nervous *tissue*) of the *brain* and other *nervous system* tissues. An *inborn error of metabolism* can cause gangliosides to accumulate, resulting in *disorders* such as *Tay-Sachs disease*.

Gantrisin™ (GAN-tris-in)
>*Refer to* **Sulfisoxazole.**

gastr-, gastro-
Prefixes meaning stomach or *abdomen*.

Gastrocnemius (gas-trok-NEE-mee-us)
A muscle in the back of the calf of the leg.

Gastroenteritis (gas-troe-en-ter-IE-tis)
Inflammation of the stomach and intestines that results in nausea, diarrhea, and vomiting. Gastroenteritis can be caused by many things, including a *virus* or *bacteria* that has contaminated food or water, certain drugs, or ingesting *toxic* substances.

Gastroenterologist (gas-troe-en-ter-OL-oe-jist)
A doctor who specializes in the study and treatment of problems of the stomach and intestinal tract.

Gastroesophageal (GE) (gas-troe-uh-sof-uh-JEE-uhl)
Pertaining to the stomach and the *esophagus*.

Gastroesophageal Reflux (GE Reflux, GER, GERD)
An *abnormal* backflow of stomach acid and other contents into the *esophagus* caused by a weakness in the *sphincter* muscle that closes off the passageway between the esophagus and stomach. GE reflux may cause *esophagitis*. Feeding the infant smaller meals more frequently and in a more upright position may help decrease the vomiting that usually occurs after meals.
>*Also known as* **Gastroesophageal Reflux Disorder.**

Gastrointestinal (GI) (gas-troe-in-TES-ti-nuhl)
Pertaining to the organs of the *gastrointestinal tract*.

Gastrointestinal Disorder
Any illness involving one or more parts of the body related to *digestion* and elimination. *Gastroesophageal reflux* is an example of a *gastrointestinal* disorder.

Gastrointestinal Tract (GI Tract)
> *Refer to* **Digestive Tract.**

Gastroschisis (gas-TROS-ki-sis)
A *congenital anomaly* in which the *abdominal* wall fails to close completely. This results in a hole through which the intestines bulge.

Gastrostomy (gas-TROS-toe-mee)
A surgically created opening in the *abdominal* wall through which a *feeding tube* is inserted directly into the stomach. A gastrostomy tube (*G-tube*), also known as a stomach tube, may be temporarily or permanently placed, depending on the reason for needing tube feeding. G-tube placement may be necessary if the *esophagus* is blocked, if the child is not able to receive adequate *nutrition* orally, or to provide drainage after abdominal surgery.

Gastrostomy Button
A small flexible *gastrostomy tube* with a one-way *valve* used to tube feed.

Gastrostomy Tube (G-Tube)
> *Refer to* **Gastrostomy.**

Gaucher Disease (goe-SHAY)
An *autosomal recessive lipid metabolism disorder* characterized by lack of the *enzyme* necessary for fat processing. This creates an excessive amount of fat in body *tissue*. Gaucher disease can be fatal.

Gavage Feeding (guh-VAZH)
Liquid feedings given via a tube passed through the nose or mouth and into the stomach.

GDS
The abbreviation for Gesell Developmental Schedules.

GE
The abbreviation for gastroesophageal.

Gene (JEEN)
The basic unit of *inheritance* that carries individual traits from parent to child. The gene is capable of reproducing itself at each *cell* division. Each gene is located at a specific point on a particular *chromosome* and consists primarily of *DNA* and *protein*.
> *Refer to* **Dominant Gene** *and* **Recessive Gene.**

General Anesthesia/Anesthetic (an-es-THEE-zee-uh/an-es-THET-ik)
> *Refer to* **Anesthesia.**

Generalization
1. The ability to make inferences about the properties of an object based on awareness of the properties of a similar object.
2. The ability to transfer a skill learned in one environment to new environments.
3. Becoming widespread, as when a local process or *disease* becomes *systemic*.

Generalized Anxiety Disorder
*Refer to **Anxiety Disorder**.*

Generalized Seizure
A *seizure* that affects the whole *brain*, causing loss of consciousness. Types of generalized seizure include *absence seizures, myoclonic seizures, atonic seizures*, and *tonic-clonic seizures*.
*Compare **Partial Seizure**.*
*Refer to **Epilepsy**.*

General Practitioner (GP)
A family *physician*. General practitioners are trained to take care of most non-surgical *diseases*.

-genesis
A suffix meaning origination or production.

Genetic (gen-ET-ik)
Inherited or pertaining to *heredity*.
*Refer to **Gene**.*

Genetic Code
The information carried by *DNA* that is responsible for the *inheritance* and transmission of *chromosomes* and *genes*. A change in the genetic code can cause a *mutation*.
*Refer to **Gene**.*

Genetic Counselor
A specialist who provides information about *hereditary disorders*, including confirming a suspected *genetic diagnosis*, determining which other family members might be affected, and assisting with comprehension of the diagnosis.

Genetic Disorder
An *inherited disorder* caused by defective *genetic* material. Types of genetic disorders include *chromosomal abnormalities, unifactorial* defects, or *multifactorial* defects.

Genetic Evaluation
An evaluation done to determine the presence of a *genetic disorder*. The evaluation usually includes obtaining the family health *history* (covering several generations) and determining the family's racial and ethnic background, the parents' ages, the mother's health during her pregnancy, *labor*, and delivery,

and the baby's health as a newborn. The infant's growth and *development* are also reviewed. Finally, the infant is given a physical examination and tests (such as *chromosome analysis*) may be performed.

Geneticist (juh-NET-i-sist)
A specialist who evaluates individuals for *genetic disorders*.

Genetic Material
> *Refer to* **Gene.**

Genetic Mutation
> *Refer to* **Mutation.**

Genitalia (jen-i-TAYL-ee-uh)
The reproductive organs visible on the outside of the body.

Genitals
> *Refer to* **Genitalia.**

Genitourinary (GU) (jen-i-toe-YOOR-i-nayr-ee)
Pertaining to the *genitalia* and the *urinary* system.

Genotype (JEN-oe-tiep)
The individual's complete set of *inherited* characteristics (as determined by the combination and location of the *genes* on the *chromosomes*).
> *Compare* **Phenotype.**

Gentamicin Sulfate (jen-tuh-MIE-sin SUL-fayt)
An *antibiotic drug* used to treat infections.

Genu Recurvatum (JEE-nyoo ree-kuhr-VAY-tuhm)
Abnormal hyperextension of the knee *joints.*
> *Also known as* **Back Knee** *and* **Knee Joint Hyperextensibility.**

Genu Valgum (JEE-nyoo VAL-guhm)
A deformity in which the legs are curved inward so that the knees are close together.
> *Also known as* **Knock Knees.**

Genu Varum (JEE-nyoo VER-uhm)
A deformity in which one or both of the legs curve outward at the knee.
> *Also known as* **Bowleg.**

GER
The abbreviation for gastroesophageal reflux.

GERD
The abbreviation for gastroesophageal reflux disorder.
> *Refer to* **Gastroesophageal Reflux.**

GE Reflux
The abbreviation for gastroesophageal reflux.

Germ (JURM)
Any *microorganism* that causes *disease*. *Viruses* and *bacteria* are examples of germs.

German Measles
>Compare **Measles.**
>*Refer to* **Congenital Rubella** *and* **Rubella.**

Gesell Developmental Schedules (GDS) (gi-ZEL)
An *evaluation* tool used to measure the *communication, adaptive, gross motor, fine motor,* and personal/social *development* of the birth to 6-year-old.

Gestation (jes-TAY-shuhn)
The length of time between the first day of the mother's last menstrual period before conception and the delivery of the baby. The gestational period is usually approximately 284 days (270 days plus the 14 days prior to conception).
>*Refer to* **Trimester.**

Gestational Age
The age of a *fetus* or infant stated in weeks from the first day of the mother's last menstrual period before conception until the baby reaches term (40 weeks).

Gesture/Gesturing
A form of non-verbal *communication* involving body movements. Examples include waving "hi," motioning with the hand "come here," and patting the seat to invite someone to "sit down."

GF
The abbreviation for gluten-free.

GI
The abbreviation for gastrointestinal.

Gilles de la Tourette Syndrome (ZHIL duh lah too-RET)
>*Refer to* **Tourette Syndrome.**

Gingiva (JIN-ji-vuh)
>*Refer to* **Gum.**

Gingival Hyperplasia (JIN-ji-vuhl hie per-PLAY-zee-uh)
Gingiva (gum) overgrowth, or enlargement. It is usually a plaque-induced or medication-induced (such as by *Dilantin*) *gingivitis.*
>*Refer to* **Hyperplasia.**

Gingivitis (jin-ji-VIE-tis)
Inflammation and swelling of the *gums.*

gingivo-
A prefix meaning *gums*.

GI Tract
The abbreviation for gastrointestinal tract.
> *Refer to* **Digestive Tract.**

Glabella (gluh-BUHL-uh)
The smooth, most forward-projecting, bony area of the forehead above the nose.

Glabella Response
Reflexive (involuntary) eyelid blinking in response to a finger tap on the *glabella*. The glabella response is checked as part of the newborn infant's neurological *assessment*.

Gland
An organ formed by a clumping of *cells* that *secrete* (release cell products for use in the body) or *excrete* (eliminate or discharge waste product from the body) fluid and material. The *pituitary gland* is an example of a gland that secretes *hormones* and a sweat gland is an example of a gland that excretes waste product.

Glaucoma (glaw-KOE-muh)
A condition in which there is increased pressure inside the eye which can damage the *optic nerve* and cause *blindness*. Glaucoma in children is usually the result of a *congenital anomaly* in which there is a structural *abnormality* in the eye.
> *Refer to* **Goniotomy.**

Glide Consonants
The consonant speech sounds /w/ and /y/.
> *Refer to* **Consonant.**

Gliding Movement
A smooth, continuous *joint* movement that allows one bone surface to glide over another. Gliding is one of the four basic kinds of movement by the joints of the body.
> *Compare* **Angular Movement, Circumduction Movement,** *and*
> **Rotation Movement.**

Global Developmental Delay
Delay in the child's acquisition of skills in most areas of *development*. A child with global developmental delay may not have an identified *diagnosis*, but is functioning similarly to a child who has *mental retardation*.
> *Refer to* **Developmental Delay.**

Glossa (GLOS-uh)
The tongue.
> *Also known as* **Lingua.**

glosso-
A prefix meaning tongue.

Glossoptosis (glos-op-TOE-sis)
Downward *displacement* or *retraction* of the tongue.

Glottal Fricative (GLOT-uhl)
The /h/ speech sound.

Glottal Stop
A speech sound made by the closure of the *glottis,* followed by a forceful release. The /k/ speech sound is an example of a glottal stop.

Glottis (GLOT-is)
The two vocal cords and the space between them.

Glucose (GLOO-koes)
A type of sugar that is found in foods and also produced as a product of *digestion.* It circulates in the blood and is used by the body for energy.

Gluteal Muscle/Gluteus (GLOO-tee-uhl or gloo-TEE-uhl/gloo-TEE-uhs)
One of the three muscles on each side of the buttocks.

Gluten (GLOO-tuhn)
A *protein* found in wheat, rye, and barley. Some people are sensitive to gluten. (It irritates their intestines.) It has also been theorized that gluten can irritate or damage the *brain,* causing certain *behaviors* associated with *autism spectrum disorder.* This theory has not yet been proven by well-controlled scientific research.
  Refer to **Celiac Disease.**

Gluten-Free (GF)
Containing no *gluten.*
  Refer to **Celiac Disease** *and* **Gluten.**

Gluten-Induced Enteropathy (GLOO-tuhn en-tuh-ROP-uh-thee)
  Refer to **Celiac Disease.**

Gluten Intolerance
  Refer to **Celiac Disease.**

glyc-
A prefix meaning sugar or sweet.

Glycerin Suppository (GLIS-uh-rin suh-POZ-uh-tor-ee)
A *suppository* used to treat children with *constipation.*
  Refer to **Suppository.**

gm/GM
The abbreviation for gram.

Gnashing (NASH-ing)
Grinding of the teeth.

-gnosis
A suffix meaning knowledge.

Goiter (GOI-tuhr)
An enlarged *thyroid gland*, usually seen as a swelling in the neck. Goiter may be a result of a lack of *iodine* in the diet.

Goldenhar Syndrome (GOLE-duhn-hahr)
A *sporadically* occurring *disorder* characterized by poor development of facial structures (usually including one side of the face appearing smaller than the other); a *cleft*-like extension to the side of the corner of the mouth; *skin tags* in front of the ears; outer and *inner ear* defects, often with *conductive hearing impairment; cleft palate* or other oral defects; a *benign* fatty *tumor* in the outer eye; *visual impairment; spinal column abnormalities; congenital heart defect* and *hydrocephalus* in more severe cases; and, rarely, *mental retardation*.
>   *Also known as* **Oculoauriculovertebral Dysplasia, OAV Syndrome,** *and* **Vertebroauriculofacial Syndrome.**

Gonads
The *ovaries* and the *testes*. The gonads are responsible for producing male or female reproductive *cells*.

Goniometer (goe-nee-OM-uh-ter)
A device that measures the *range of motion* of a *joint*.

Goniotomy (goe-nee-OT-oe-mee)
A surgical procedure for treating *glaucoma* in which an opening is made in the eye so the increased fluid in the eye can drain to relieve the pressure.

Goodman Syndrome
An *autosomal recessive disorder* characterized by a *congenital* malformation of the skull caused by premature closures of certain *sutures* (resulting in a head that appears pointed at the top), webbed or fused fingers and/or toes, extra fingers and/or toes, congenital *heart defects*, sideways *deviation* and *abnormal flexion* (bending) of fingers and/or toes, deviation of the *ulna* bone, and *normal intelligence*.
>   *Also known as* **Acrocephalopolysyndactyly, Type IV.**

Goodness of Fit
A compatibility between a parent and child in relation to each individual's *temperament*. A parent's natural or developed acceptance and appreciation for his child's unique temperament (even if it is extremely different than his

own) creates a goodness of fit between the two. Both emotional fit and behavioral fit contribute to a good parent-child fit.

GP
The abbreviation for general practitioner.

Grade I, II, III, or IV Bleed
Refer to **Intraventricular Hemorrhage.**

Gram (GM, gm, g.)
The basic unit of weight in the metric system. There are 28 grams in 1 ounce.

Grammar
All the rules that govern how a given language is spoken and written, including the rules specifying how words are formed, pronounced, and arranged into meaningful phrases and sentences. An example of a rule of language is the need for the subject and the verb within a sentence to agree in person and number "He is tall" (a singular noun and a singular verb) compared to "They are tall" (a plural noun and a plural verb).

Grand Mal Seizure (grahn-MAHL)
Refer to **Tonic-Clonic Seizure** *and* **Epilepsy.**

Grasp
The manner in which an object is held. There are several types of grasp that an infant uses as his *fine motor* skills develop. A newborn demonstrates a *grasp reflex* that is present for the first 4 months of life. The first voluntary grasp to develop is the *ulnar palmar grasp,* which emerges around 4 months and is grasp of an object with the ring finger and little finger against the palm of the hand. The second grasp to develop is the *palmar grasp,* which emerges around 5 months and is grasp of an object with all 4 fingers pressing the palm of the hand; the thumb is not involved. The third type of grasp to develop is the *radial palmar grasp,* which emerges around 6 months and is grasp of an object with the thumb, index, and middle fingers against the palm of the hand. The fourth type of grasp to develop is the *radial digital grasp,* which emerges between 7 and 9 months and is grasp of an object with the thumb, index, and middle fingers without the involvement of the palm of the hand. The fifth grasp to develop is the *inferior pincer grasp,* which emerges between 8 and 10 months and is grasp of a small object with the index finger and thumb, the thumb to the side of the bent index finger. The final grasp to develop is the *neat pincer grasp,* which emerges between 10 and 12 months and is grasp of a tiny object with precise thumb and index *finger opposition* (i.e., tip to tip).

Grasp Reflex
An involuntary *fisting* of the hand triggered by placement of a cylindrical object (such as an adult's finger) in the middle part of an infant's palm. The grasp reflex is a normal *reflex* in infants up to 4 months of age.
Also known as **Palmar Reflex.**
Refer to **Grasp** *and* **Primitive Reflex.**

Gravida (GRAHV-i-duh)

A Latin word meaning a pregnant woman. She is referred to as gravida 1 during the first pregnancy, gravida 2 during the second, etc. *Primigravida* is used interchangeably with gravida 1.

Compare **Para.**

Gray Matter/Substance

The gray *tissue* of the *central nervous system*. It is responsible for processing *sensory* information.

Compare **White Matter/Substance.**

Greenspan, Dr. Stanley I.

Refer to **Developmental, Individual-Difference, Relationship-Based (DIR®) Model, Following the Child's Lead,** *and* **Interdisciplinary Council on Developmental and Learning Disorders (ICDL).**

Grieving Process

The normal emotional response to a loss. The five stages of grieving, according to Elisabeth Kubler-Ross, *psychiatrist* and authority and counselor on death, include denial, anger, bargaining, depression, and acceptance. Some authorities include shock with denial, and understanding with acceptance.

Gross Motor

The *developmental* area that involves skills which require the coordination of large muscle groups, such as those in the arms, legs, and trunk. Examples of gross motor skills include walking, *jumping*, and throwing a ball.

G Syndrome

A rare (sometimes *autosomal dominant,* sometimes *X-linked) disorder* characterized by *hypertelorism* (widely-spaced eyes); *epicanthal folds;* an upturned nose with a flat bridge; *hypospadias* (a condition in which the *urethra* opens on the undersurface of the penis, before it reaches the tip of the penis); severe swallowing difficulty; and *mental retardation* (in half to two-thirds of affected children). The features of G syndrome can range from mild to severe. Some affected children have no functional impairment and other infants are unable to survive due to the swallowing problems (which can result in *aspiration* of food into the lungs). G syndrome is named after the family in which it was first identified. (The family's last name began with the letter "G.")

Also known as **Opitz Syndrome, Opitz-Frias Syndrome,** *and* **Hypertelorism-Hypospadias Syndrome.**

G-Tube

The abbreviation for gastrostomy tube.

Refer to **Gastrostomy.**

GU

The abbreviation for genitourinary.

Guanfacine Hydrochloride (GWAHN-fuh-seen hie-droe-KLOR-ied)

A medication originally used to lower *blood pressure* that is sometimes used to treat certain *behaviors* associated with *autism spectrum disorder* and *attention-deficit/hyperactivity disorder*. Tenex™ is the brand name of this drug.

Guard

An arm position used to maintain *balance*. When the arms are held low, closer to the body, it is considered low guard. When the arms are held high (as seen in a newly walking toddler), it is considered *high guard*.

Gum

1. The *soft tissue* that surrounds the base of the teeth.
      Also known as **Gingiva.**
2. *Mouthing* objects or food with the gums.
      Refer to **Mouthing.**

Guthrie Test (GUTH-ree)

A blood test to detect *Phenylketonuria (PKU)*.

gyn-

A prefix meaning woman.

Gyri (JIE-rie)

Plural of *gyrus*.

gyro-

A prefix meaning ring, circle.

Gyrus (JIE-ruhs)

One of the *convolutions* or folds of the surface of the *cerebral hemispheres* of the *brain*.

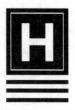

h
The abbreviation for height.

HA
The abbreviation for hyperalimentation.

Habituation
1. A gradual adaptation (and thus decreased response) to a *stimulus* or to the environment, based upon repeated exposure to the stimulus or the environment. This is an indicator of the infant's increasing *cognition*. For example, the infant's interest in and attention to a picture will decrease when she becomes "bored" with it after seeing it many times; she requires a more complex picture to hold her interest. The ability to habituate is observed, too, in the newborn who is able to ignore irritating stimulation (such as noise), and to sleep or remain in a calm, alert *state*.
2. The process of forming a habit.

Haemophilus Influenzae (hee-MOF-i-luhs)
   Refer to **Hemophilus Influenzae Type B.**

Hair Whorl (hwurl)
A spiral or twist of hair.

Haldol™ (HAL-dol)
   Refer to **Haloperidol.**

Half-Kneeling Position
Bearing weight on one knee and the other foot (placed forward of the knee).

Halitosis (hal-i-TOE-sis)
Foul mouth odor.

Hallucal (HAL-yoo-kuhl)
Pertaining to the *hallux*, or the great toe.

Hallux (HAL-uks)
The great toe.

Haloperidol (ha-loe-PER-i-dol)
An *antipsychotic drug* (tranquilizer) sometimes used in the treatment of certain *autistic-like behaviors* and in the treatment of *Tourette syndrome*. Haldol™ is the brand name for this drug.

Hammer
> *Refer to **Malleus.***

Hammock
An *adaptive* device used to encourage proper body alignment and to decrease *abnormal postures*. A hammock can help the child with *hypertonicity* to maintain a more flexed position while on her back, and can keep the child with *hypotonicity* from sleeping with her legs in a frog-like position. Gently swinging the hammock may be used to help the child who is sensitive to movement in space and to help relax the child with tight muscles.

Handedness
> *Refer to **Hand Preference.***

Hand Flapping/Hand Biting
Perseverative behaviors often seen in children with *developmental disabilities*. These behaviors may be motivated by a *sensory* need, or a desire to focus and calm oneself or to escape from a demand.

Handling
Referring to the correct methods for lifting and carrying an infant or child with *special needs*. By properly holding the infant or child who has *muscle tone* problems, the adult can inhibit *abnormal postures* and help the child feel secure while being held.

Hand-Over-Hand Guidance
Physically guiding a child through the movements involved in a *fine motor* task. Helping the child to *grasp* a spoon and bring it to her mouth is an example of hand-over-hand guidance.

Hand Preference
The natural tendency to use the preferred hand (either the right or left hand) for most voluntary *motor* (manipulative) activities. For activities that require two-hand involvement, the preferred hand does the manipulating while the other hand assists. The dominant (preferred) hand may not be apparent until the child is between 3 and 4 years of age, although it frequently appears by age 3. Hand preference is related to which side of the *brain* is dominant. For example, if the left *hemisphere* of the brain is dominant, the child usually will be right handed.
> *Also known as **Dominant Hand, Handedness**, and **Laterality.***

Hands-Feet Position
Bearing weight on the hands and feet with the *abdomen* off the floor.

Hanen Approach (HAN-en)
A model of *early intervention* designed to teach parents and other caregivers strategies to encourage and expand the *communication* skills of young children. The approach teaches parents ways to maximize their child's language abilities using naturally-occurring daily situations as the child passes through the *developmental* stages involved in acquiring communication skills.

Haploid (HAP-loid)
Referring to a single complete set of *chromosomes* (½ of the usual paired set; that is, 23 single chromosomes, rather than 23 pairs of chromosomes). *Sperm* and eggs (ova) are haploid because they only have one chromosome of each kind.
> *Also known as* **Monoploid.**
> *Compare* **Diploid** *and* **Triploid.**

Happy Puppet Syndrome
> *Refer to* **Angelman Syndrome.**

Hard-of-Hearing
Auditory impairment that may be improved by the use of *hearing aids*.

Hard Palate
The bony front part of the roof of the mouth. Certain speech sounds (such as the /t/ and /d/ sounds) are produced when the tongue touches or approximates the ridge of the hard palate (the *alveolar ridge*), which is slightly behind the upper teeth.
> *Compare* **Soft Palate.**
> *Refer to* **Aveolar Ridge** *and* **Palate.**

Harelip
> *Refer to* **Cleft Lip.**

Harrington Rod™
A metal rod that is surgically placed along the *spine* during the *spinal fusion* procedure to maintain proper alignment in children with severe *scoliosis*.

Hashimoto's Disease (hah-shi-MOE-toez)
An *autoimmune* thyroid *disorder* that results in *goiter* and thyroid deficiency. It is more common in females and primarily affects 30- to 50-year-olds, but young children can be affected as well. Thyroid *hormone* replacement therapy may be needed.

HAV
The abbreviation for hepatitis A virus.

Hawaii Early Learning Profile (HELP)
Criterion-referenced tests used to evaluate the *cognitive*, language, *gross motor*, *fine motor*, social, and *self-help development* of the newborn to 36-month-old and the 3- to 6-year-old. The Hawaii may be administered by a professional or *paraprofessional*. It includes an activity guide that can be used for curriculum planning.

Hb
An abbreviation for hemoglobin.

HBV
The abbreviation for hepatitis B virus.

hct
The abbreviation for hematocrit.

HCV
The abbreviation for hepatitis C virus.

Head Banging
A form of *self-stimulation* in which the child repetitively bangs her head on the floor or another surface.
*Refer to **Self-Stimulation** and **Self-Injurious Behavior.***

Head Circumference
An important body measurement that doctors use to estimate the rate at which the infant's *brain* is growing. Head circumference is measured just above the eyebrows and around the *occiput* (the back part of the base of the head).
*Refer to **Body Measurements.***

Head Control
The ability to lift and keep the head up, holding it in line with the body. In a *typically developing* infant, head control is attained around 4 months of age. Head control is required for sitting.

Head Lag
The backward lag of the head when an infant without *head control* is pulled to a sitting position.
*Refer to **Head Control.***

Head Righting Reflex
An automatic response to hold the head in an upright, *midline* position, even if the body is tilted to the side.
*Refer to **Automatic Reflex.***

Head Start/Early Head Start
A federal program aimed at providing a comprehensive program for infants and toddlers (Early Head Start), and preschool-aged children (Head Start)

of low-income families. Planned activities are designed to address individual needs and to help children attain their potential in growth and mental and physical *development* before starting school. Head Start started in 1965. Ten percent or more of enrollment opportunities are for children with *disabilities*.

Hearing

Hearing is a process involving both the ears, the *auditory nerve*, and the *brain*. For hearing to occur, sound waves in the air must pass through the *pinna* (the part of the ear seen on the outside of the head) and enter the *auditory canal* (the *ear canal* leading from outside the ear inward to the *tympanic membrane*, or *eardrum*). The sound waves then hit the eardrum causing the eardrum to vibrate. (For the eardrum to vibrate properly, the air pressure on each side of the eardrum must be equal. Equalizing the air pressure is the job of the *eustachian tube*.) The vibrations then pass through the *middle ear* by moving along a tiny chain of bones (the *malleus*, *incus*, and *stapes*), and into the *inner ear* via the last bone, the stapes, which extends into the *cochlea*, located in the inner ear. As the stapes vibrates, it causes the fluid within the cochlea to ripple, stimulating the cochlea's *nerve cells* and beginning the motion of the *cilia* (the microscopic hairlike projections on the cells). The motion transmits sound impulses along the auditory nerve to the brain. Finally, when the impulses reach the brain, the *cerebral cortex* of the brain receives and analyzes the impulses, recognizing them as meaningful sound.

Refer to **Auditory Impairment** *and* **Ear.**

Hearing Aid

A device for amplifying sound (but not for making the sound clearer). For the child to benefit from hearing aids, she must have some degree of *hearing*.

Compare **Vibrotactile Hearing Aid.**

Hearing Impairment/Loss

Refer to **Auditory Impairment.**

Heart

The organ located in the center of the chest that pumps blood throughout the body. The heart is divided into four chambers. The upper two chambers are the *atria* and the lower two chambers are the *ventricles*. The openings between the atria and the ventricles are the *valves*.

Refer to **Circulation.**

Heart Arrhythmia (uh-RITH-mee-uh)

Refer to *Arrhythmia.*

Heart Defect

Any structural *abnormality* of the *heart* that obstructs or creates abnormal blood flow through the heart. Examples of heart defects include *patent ductus arteriosus*, *atrial septal defects*, and *tetralogy of Fallot*. Heart defects are often treated with drugs or surgery.

Heart Disease

Refer to **Congenital Heart Disease.**

Heart Failure
Refer to **Congestive Heart Failure.**

Heart Massage
Refer to **Cardiac Massage.**

Heart Murmur
A *heart* sound made by blood flow or by the *heart valves* which may be normal or *abnormal* depending on the cause. Many murmurs that occur when the heart contracts are *benign*; murmurs that occur when the heart is at rest are more likely dangerous, possibly indicating that one or more *valves* are not functioning properly.

Heart Rate (HR)
The rate at which the *heart* beats. The heart rate is expressed in beats per minute. There are normal ranges for each age group. Normally, the newborn heart rate is over 100 beats per minute and the heart rate of 1- to 3-year-olds is in the 100 to 160 range.

Heart Valve
One of the 4 structures within the *heart* that prevent a backward flow of blood by opening and closing with each heartbeat.
Refer to **Aortic Valve, Mitral Valve, Pulmonary Valve,** *and* **Tricuspid Valve.**

Heel Cord
Refer to **Achilles Tendon.**

Heel Cord Lengthening
Refer to **Achilles Tendon Lengthening.**

Heel Stick/Puncture
Pricking the baby's heel to obtain a small blood sample.

Heel Strike
The part of walking with a normal heel-toe *gait* pattern when the heel comes in contact with the floor.

HEENT
The abbreviation for head, eyes, ears, nose, and throat.

Heimlich Maneuver (HIEM-lik)
A life-saving procedure used when someone is choking. The rescuer puts pressure on the victim's *diaphragm* by thrusting inward and upward on the *abdomen* between the hips and the lower edge of the ribs. This pressure forces some of the air that was in the lungs upward, expelling the lodged object out of the *trachea*.
Also known as **Abdominal Thrust** *and* **Manual Thrust.**

Helix (HEE-liks)
1. A coiled formation found in *DNA* (*deoxyribonucleic acid*) and other *organic* molecules.
2. The rounded rim portion of the *external ear*.

Heller Syndrome/Heller's Syndrome
　　Refer to **Childhood Disintegrative Disorder.**

HELP
The abbreviation for Hawaii Early Learning Profile.

Helper T Cell
　　Refer to **T Cell.**

hema- (HEE-muh or HEM-uh)
A prefix meaning blood.

Hemangioma (hee-man-jee-OE-muh)
A usually harmless *tumor* caused by an *abnormal* distribution of *blood vessels*. Hemangiomas can occur as birthmarks or develop later in life. They can either be flat, such as a *port wine stain*, or raised, such as a *strawberry mark*. Hemangiomas can occur anywhere in the body but are usually found in the skin.

Hemapoiesis (hem-uh-poi-EE-sis)
The formation of *blood cells*.

Hemapoietic (hem-uh-poi-ET-ik)
Referring to *hemapoiesis*.

hemato-
A prefix meaning blood.

Hematochezia (hem-uh-toe-KEE-zee-uh)
The presence of red blood in passed stools.

Hematocrit (hct) (hee-MAT-oe-krit)
A measure of the number of *red blood cells* found in the blood. It is expressed as a percentage of the total blood volume and it yields an estimate of the amount of *hemoglobin* in the blood.

Hematology (hee-muh-TOL-oe-jee or hem-uh-TOL-oe-jee)
The study of blood and blood *disorders*.

Hematoma (hee-muh-TOE-muh)
A swelling, or collection, of blood (usually clotted) that develops in a *localized* area of an organ, *tissue*, or body space. A hematoma is caused by bleeding from a broken *blood vessel* resulting from *trauma* or surgery. Hematomas range in severity from minor to potentially fatal conditions.

Hematopoiesis (hee-muh-toe-poi-EE-sis)
The formation and development of *blood cells* in the *bone marrow*.

Hematopoietic (hee-muh-toe-poi-ET-ik or hem-uh-toe-poi-ET-ik)
Referring to *hematopoiesis.*

Hematuria (hee-muh-TUR-ee-uh or hem-uh-TUR-ee-uh)
Blood in the urine. This condition can be caused by a variety of *kidney, urinary,* and genital *diseases* or *disorders,* by *trauma,* and by poisoning.

hemi-
A prefix meaning half.

Hemiamblyopia (hem-ee-am-blee-OE-pee-uh)
Blindness or *visual impairment* in one half of the *visual field* in one or both eyes.
    Refer to **Amblyopia.**

Hemianopia/Hemianopsia
(hem-ee-uh-NOE-pee-uh/hem-ee-uh-NOP-see-uh)
    Refer to **Hemiamblyopia.**

Hemiparesis (hem-i-puh-REE-sis)
Muscular weakness of one half of the body.

Hemiplegia (hem-ee-PLEE-jee-uh)
Weakness or *paralysis* of one side of the body caused by *disease* or injury to the *nerves* of the *brain* or *spinal cord* that stimulate the muscles, or by disease to the muscles themselves. Nerve damage to the left *pyramidal tract* of the brain results in hemiplegia on the right side of the body, and nerve damage to the right pyramidal tract of the brain results in hemiplegia on the left side of the body. Sometimes the word hemiplegia is used to describe *cerebral palsy* in which the arm, leg, trunk, or face on one side of the body is affected. The arm is usually more affected than the leg, trunk, or face.
    Refer to **Paralysis** *and* **Pyramidal Cerebral Palsy.**

Hemisphere
    Refer to **Cerebral Hemisphere.**

Hemivertebra (hem-ee-VUR-tuh-bruh)
A *congenital* condition in which half of a *vertebra* is missing. One or more vertebrae may be affected. *Scoliosis* can result. *Spinal fusion* may be required.

hemo-
A prefix meaning blood or *blood vessels*.

Hemoglobin (Hb, Hgb) (hee-moe-GLOE-bin or hem-oe-GLOE-bin)
The *oxygen*-carrying, *iron*-containing pigment in *red blood cells*.

Hemoglobinopathy (hee-moe-gloe-bi-NOP-uh-thee)
Any of a group of *genetic disorders* in which there are changes (errors) in the structure of the *hemoglobin* molecule. An example of a hemoglobinopathy is *sickle cell anemia.*

Hemolysis (hee-MOL-i-sis)
The destruction of *red blood cells*. This is a normal body process, except when the breakdown occurs prematurely or in great amounts, which may cause *anemia* and *jaundice*. *Abnormal* hemolysis in the newborn (*hemolytic disease of the newborn*) is usually caused by *Rh incompatibility* between the mother and *fetus.*

Hemolytic Anemia (hee-moe-LIT-ik uh-NEE-mee-uh)
A blood disorder characterized by chronic premature destruction of *red blood cells*. The condition may be associated with certain *diseases* and *inherited* blood disorders, or it may be a response to drugs or other *toxins.*

Hemolytic Anemia of the Newborn
*Refer to **Erythroblastosis Fetalis.***

Hemolytic Disease of the Newborn
*Refer to **Erythroblastosis Fetalis.***

Hemophilia (hee-moe-FIL-ee-uh or hem-oe-FIL-ee-uh)
A group of *X-linked recessive disorders* caused by deficiency in one of the *proteins* necessary for blood clotting. Children with hemophilia have varying degrees and sites (internal and external) of spontaneous bleeding (most often bleeding is into the muscles and *joints*), and should avoid play activities that pose the risk of injury. Hemophilia is treated by giving infusions (slowly introducing the deficient blood protein into the bloodstream by means of *IV*) either at the time of bleeding or on a regular, preventive basis.

Hemophilus Influenzae Type B (Hib) (hee-MOF-il-us)
A *bacterium* spread by nose and mouth *secretions* that can cause serious illness in infants and young children, including *meningitis, pneumonia, sepsis,* and other infections. Children can carry the *bacteria* without actually having the infection or any of the *diseases* it causes. A *vaccine* is available.
*Also known as **Haemophilus Influenzae** and **H.flu.***

Hemophilus Influenzae Type B Vaccine
*Refer to **Hib-Immune Vaccine.***

Hemopoietic (hee-moe-poe-ET-ik)
Related to the formation and development of various types of *blood cells.*

Hemorrhage (HEM-or-ij)
A large amount of bleeding in a short period of time.
*Refer to **Intracerebral Hemorrhage, Intracranial Hemorrhage, Intraventricular Hemorrhage, Periventricular Hemorrhage,** and **Subarachnoid Hemorrhage.***

HepA
The abbreviation for hepatitis A vaccine.

hepat-
A prefix meaning *liver*.

Hepatitis (hep-uh-TIE-tis)
An *inflammation* of the *liver*, usually due to an infection, and sometimes due to *toxic* agents.

Hepatitis A Vaccine (HepA)
An *immunization* against *hepatitis A virus*. The *vaccination* is recommended between 12-23 months of age. It is administered in 2 doses, separated by 6-12 or 6-18 months, depending on the formulation. HepA is administered by *intramuscular injection*.

Hepatitis A Virus (HAV)
A *virus* transmitted most commonly through exposure to contaminated water or food. The illness is usually mild, but can be severe. Teaching the young child (and care givers) good hygiene, especially adequate hand-washing, can help prevent the spread of this infection.
    Refer to **Hepatitis**.

Hepatitis B Vaccine (HepB)
An *immunization* against *hepatitis B virus*. The child receives her first dose shortly after birth, with a total of three doses by 18 months of age. It is administered by injection.

Hepatitis B Virus (HBV)
A *virus* transmitted most commonly through exposure to the blood or body fluids of an infected person. It can be passed from mother to *fetus* during pregnancy. *Symptoms* include decreased appetite, nausea, and fatigue followed by *jaundice*. Blood for transfusion is screened for HBV infection. A *vaccine* is available to prevent hepatitis B infection.
    Also known as **Serum Hepatitis**.
    Refer to **Hepatitis**.

Hepatitis C Virus (HCV)
A *virus* transmitted most commonly through exposure to the blood or body fluids of an infected person. Acute infections from hepatitis C virus are similar to infections caused by *hepatitis B*. Of patients acutely infected with hepatitis C, 80 percent progress to chronic infection.
    Refer to **Hepatitis**.

hepato-
A prefix meaning *liver*.

Hepatomegaly (hep-uh-toe-MEG-uh-lee)
An enlarged *liver* that can result from many liver *disorders*.

Hepatosplenomegaly (hep-uh-toe-splee-noe-MEG-uh-lee)
An enlarged *liver* and *spleen* that can result from many *disorders*.

HepB
The abbreviation for hepatitis B vaccine.

Hereditary/Heredity
Referring to a trait (such as eye color) or defect or *disease* (such as *cystic fibrosis*) that is *genetically* determined (*inherited*). Not all hereditary *disorders* are apparent at birth and not all *congenital anomalies* are hereditary.
    Also known as **Inherited** *and* **Genetic.**

Hereditary Motor and Sensory Neuropathy (noor-OP-uh-thee)
    Refer to **Charcot-Marie-Tooth Disease.**

Hereditary Spinal Ataxia
    Refer to **Friedreich's Ataxia.**

Hermaphrodism (huhr-MAF-ruh-diz-uhm)
    Refer to **Hermaphroditism.**

Hermaphroditism (huhr-MAF-ruh-die-tiz-uhm)
A rare condition caused by a *chromosomal abnormality* in which a baby is born with both testicular and ovarian *tissue*.
    Also known as **Hermaphrodism.**

Hernia
A protrusion of an organ through an opening in the muscle wall that surrounds it. Hernias can occur *congenitally* or be *acquired* as the result of injury or muscle weakness. Examples include *hiatal hernia* and *inguinal hernia*.

Herniorrhaphy (hur-nee-OR-uh-fee)
The surgical repair of a *hernia*.

Herpes Simplex Virus 1 (HSV1) (HER-peez)
A *virus* typically associated with infectious *lesions* of the mouth and face (but sometimes found in the genital area). The virus is transmitted by direct contact with the lesions (cold sores).

Herpes Simplex Virus 2 (HSV2)
A *virus* typically associated with infectious *lesions* of the genital area (but sometimes found in the mouth). The virus is usually sexually transmitted. Herpes Simplex 2 can be passed on to a baby at the time of birth (*congenital herpes*) and can cause severe illness in the baby. The effects can range from *disease* of the skin and *mucous membranes* to neurological damage and death.

Hertz (Hz) (HURTS)
A unit of measurement of wave *frequency* equal to 1 cycle per second (cps). For example, alpha *brain waves* have a frequency of 8 to 13 Hz.

hetero-
A prefix meaning varied or different.

Heterochromia Iridis (het-uh-roe-KROE-mee-uh IE-ri-dis)
A condition in which there is more than one color of the *iris* of one or both eyes, or each eye is a different color.

Heterotopia (het-er-oe-TOE-pee-uh)
1. Development of a normal *tissue* in a part of the body where that tissue is not normally found.
2. A condition in which a part of the body is in an *abnormal* location.

H.flu
> *Refer to* **Hemophilus Influenzae Type B.**

HFV
The abbreviation for high frequency ventilation.

Hgb
An abbreviation for hemoglobin.

Hiatal Hernia (hie-AY-tuhl)
A condition in which part of the stomach pushes upward through an opening (hiatus) in the *diaphragm*. Hiatal hernia in children is usually a *congenital* condition. The child with hiatal hernia usually suffers from *gastroesophageal reflux*.

Hib
The abbreviation for Hemophilus Influenzae Type B.

Hib-Immune Vaccine
A *vaccine* that protects children against the type of *meningitis* caused by *Hemophilus Influenzae Type B.*

Hickman Catheter™ (HIK-muhn)
A type of *catheter* that is used as a long-term *central line*.
> *Refer to* **Total Parenteral Nutrition.**

High Frequency Ventilation (HFV)
A method for providing a patient with breathing assistance.
> *Refer to* **Ventilation.**

High Guard
An early standing position in which the infant keeps her arms flexed so that the hands are at shoulder level, in order to keep her *balance*.
> *Refer to* **Guard.**

High Risk
> *Refer to* **At-Risk.**

High Tone
Refer to **Hypertonia.**

Hip Adduction Release
A surgical procedure in which the muscles and/or *tendons* that *adduct* the thighs are cut to lengthen them.

Hip-Knee-Ankle-Foot Orthosis (HKAFO)
A long leg *brace* with a *pelvic band* that is used to passively stretch muscles and to stabilize the *joints*.
Refer to **Orthosis.**

Hirschsprung Disease (HIRSH-sprung)
A *congenital disorder* characterized by absence or marked decrease in the number of *nerve* endings that cause the *bowel* to move *feces*. This causes a segment of the intestines to become dilated, resulting in *constipation* and poor appetite. The treatment for Hirschsprung Disease is removal of the *abnormal* section of bowel.
Also known as **Aganglionic Megacolon** *and* **Congenital Megacolon.**

Hirsutism (HUR-syoot-izm)
Excessive body hair. Hirsutism is frequently used to describe coarse hair on females that grows in patterns that are typically male, such as facial hair and hair growth on the trunk of the body. It can be caused by a high level of male *hormones*, be associated with certain *disorders* such as *Scheie syndrome*, or be a normal occurrence in some women.

Histamine
Refer to **Antihistamine Drug.**

histo-
A prefix meaning *tissue*.

History (Hx)
The circumstances preceding an event, which may be relevant to the current condition or status. For example, the factors of a woman's health history while she was pregnant may be relevant to the newborn's health status.

HIV
The abbreviation for human immunodeficiency virus.

Hives
Refer to **Urticaria.**

HKAFO
The abbreviation for hip-knee-ankle-foot orthosis.

HLHS
The abbreviation for hypoplastic left heart syndrome.

HMD
The abbreviation for hyaline membrane disease.

Hole in the Heart
A *septal defect*, or hole in the *septum* (wall) that divides the right and left *atria* or the right and left ventricles of the *heart*.
  Refer to **Atrial Septal Defect** *and* **Ventricular Septal Defect.**

Holoprosencephaly (hol-oe-pros-en-SEF-uh-lee)
A *congenital anomaly* in which the forebrain does not divide into two *cerebral hemispheres* or form lobes. This results in facial differences, including *cleft lip and palate*, ear *anomalies* and *deafness*, and eye anomalies (ranging from an *abnormally* decreased space between the eyes to a single, fused eye); *microcephaly*; *seizures*; *heart defect*; *motor* deficiency; *mental retardation*; and infant mortality.

homeo-
A prefix meaning alike.

Homeostasis (hoe-mee-oe-STAY-sis)
The bodily process of maintaining a balanced internal *state*. Steady breathing and heartbeat are indicators of homeostasis.
  Also known as **Body Homeostasis.**

homo-
A prefix meaning same.

Homocystinuria (hoe-moe-sis-ti-NOOR-ee-uh)
A rare *autosomal recessive disorder* characterized by excess homocystine (an *amino acid*) in the blood and urine; *dislocation* of the *lens* of the eye; tall, lanky stature; *vascular abnormalities* (such that could lead to a *blood vessel* being obstructed by a clot); and *mental retardation*. Homocystinuria is caused by any of several *enzyme* deficiencies.

Homonymous Hemianopia/Hemianopsia
(hoe-MON-i-mus hem-ee-uh-NOE-pee-uh or hem-ee-uh-NOP-see-uh)
A *visual field defect* on the right or left *visual field* of both eyes. The child is *blind* or *visually impaired* in these visual fields and should be taught to turn her head to see. This *disorder* may occur with children affected by *hemiplegia*.

Hormone (HOR-moen)
A chemical substance produced in one part or organ of the body that starts or regulates the activity of an organ or group of *cells* in another part of the body. For example, *epinephrine* released by the *adrenal glands* increases the *heart's* ability to work.

Hospice Care (HOS-pis)
A hospital that provides *palliative* and supportive care for terminally ill patients and their families, either on an out-patient or in-patient basis.

HPI
The abbreviation for history of present illness.

HR
The abbreviation for heart rate.

hs
The abbreviation for the Latin words meaning at bedtime.

HSV1
The abbreviation for herpes simplex virus 1.

HSV2
The abbreviation for herpes simplex virus 2.

Human Immunodeficiency Virus (HIV)
(HYOO-muhn im-yuh-noe-di-FISH-uhn-see VIE-ruhs)
A serious *virus* that damages the *immune system* and attacks the *brain*, resulting in *developmental delay and increased susceptibility* to infection. HIV is transmitted when the virus enters the bloodstream, and can be passed to a *fetus* by her mother. HIV causes *AIDS (Acquired Immune Deficiency Syndrome)*.

Humerus (HYOO-muhr-uhs)
The long bone of the upper arm that extends from the shoulder to the elbow.

Hunter Syndrome
An *X-linked recessive mucopolysaccharidosis* (a *metabolic disease* in which complex sugars or *carbohydrates* accumulate in the urine) characterized by skeletal deformity (partial *contracture* of *joints* and *short stature*), *coarse facial features, macrocephaly,* progressive *hearing loss, hepatosplenomegaly,* and *mild* to *severe mental retardation*. Only males are affected. Death may occur by 20 years of age, but some patients live longer.
Also known as **Mucopolysaccharidosis II or MPS II.**

Hurler Syndrome
An *autosomal recessive mucopolysaccharidosis* (a *metabolic disease* in which complex sugars or *carbohydrates* accumulate in the urine) characterized by *coarse facial features,* clouding of the *cornea, macrocephaly,* short misshapen bones, *short stature,* excessive body hair, *heart disease,* and *severe mental retardation*. Death usually occurs by around 10 years of age when left untreated. Early signs include *hepatosplenomegaly, joint* stiffness, chronic *rhinitis,* and recurrent *otitis media,* as well as the characteristics listed above.
Also known as **Mucopolysaccharidosis I or MPS I.**

Hutchinson-Gelford Syndrome
Refer to **Progeria.**

Hx
The abbreviation for history.

Hyaline Membrane Disease (HMD) (HIE-uh-lien)
*Refer to **Respiratory Distress Syndrome**.*

Hydantoin (hie-DAN-toe-in)
A class of drugs used to treat epileptic *seizures*.

Hydramnios (hie-DRAM-nee-uhs)
Excessive *amniotic fluid* during pregnancy. It is sometimes associated with *fetal abnormality*, *maternal* illness such as *diabetes mellitus*, or with multiple pregnancy. Hydramnios may cause premature *labor*.
*Also known as **Polyhydramnios**.*
*Compare **Oligohydramnios**.*

Hydranencephaly (hie-dran-en-SEF-uh-lee)
A *congenital* condition characterized by the absence of *cerebral hemispheres* (the space is instead filled with fluid). Affected infants rarely survive beyond 1 year of age.

hydro-
A prefix meaning water.

Hydrocephalus (hie-droe-SEF-uh-luhs)
An *abnormal* accumulation of *cerebrospinal fluid* in the ventricles of the *brain*. Hydrocephalus occurs when too much cerebrospinal fluid is produced, when the *circulation* of the fluid is blocked, or when both conditions are present. Hydrocephalus can occur as a *congenital anomaly* (as in *spina bifida*) or as a result of *brain injury*, infection, bleeding, or *tumor*. Children with hydrocephalus are treated by draining away the excess fluid via a *shunt* that channels the fluid to another part of the body, where it is absorbed. The fluid must be removed so that *brain damage* does not occur.
*Formerly known as **Water on the Brain**.*
*Refer to **Shunt**.*

Hydronephrosis (hie-droe-nef-ROE-sis)
Distention of the *kidney*(s) resulting from blockage or narrowing of the *ureter*. *Aspiration* or surgical removal of the cause of the blockage (for example, a kidney stone, a *tumor*, or a narrowing that's present from birth) is necessary to prevent or treat *renal failure*.

Hydrops (HIE-drops)
The *abnormal* accumulation of *serous* fluid (a thin, watery liquid) in body *tissues* or a body cavity, such as the *middle ear*.

Hygroma (hie-GROE-muh)
A sac within the body that contains fluid. It can be caused by an injury or be a *congenital* malformation.

Hyoid (HIE-oid)
The U-shaped bone located in the front of the neck beneath the chin and above the *larynx* (the voice box).

hyper-
A prefix meaning above, elevated, or excessive.
Compare hypo-.

Hyperactivity (hie-puhr-ak-TIV-i-tee)
A nervous system-based difficulty that makes it hard for a child to control *motor* (muscle) *behavior*. It is characterized by frequent movement, rapidly switching from one activity to another, and difficulty with concentrating on one task, sitting still, or controlling restless movements. Due to their overactivity and *impulsivity*, children who are hyperactive often have difficulty with learning, even if they score in the normal range on *IQ* tests. Hyperactivity can occur with *attention deficit disorder, mental retardation, seizure disorder, sensory deficit disorders* (such as *auditory impairment*), or other *central nervous system* damage.
Also known as Hyperkinetic.
Compare Hypoactivity.

Hyperacuity (hie-puhr-a-KYOO-i-tee)
Excessive sensitivity to sounds.

Hyperacusis (hie-puhr-uh-KYOO-sis)
Excessive sensitivity to sounds wherein the child experiences certain sounds as painful and unpleasant.

Hyperalimentation (HA) (hie-puhr-al-i-men-TAY-shuhn)
An *intravenous* solution that is given through an intravenous line to provide *nutrition* to the baby who cannot take any or enough food by mouth.
Also known as Intravenous Feeding or Total Parenteral Nutrition (TPN).

Hyperbilirubinemia (hie-puhr-bil-i-roo-bin-EE-mee-uh)
Excess *bilirubin* in the blood caused by poor functioning of the *liver*. *Jaundice* occurs with increased *bilirubin* levels. Infants with hyperbilirubinemia must be treated to prevent *brain damage*. Often the baby is treated by placing her under *bililights* (given *phototherapy*), but sometimes an *exchange transfusion* is needed.
Refer to Jaundice.

Hypercalcemia (hie-puhr-kal-SEE-mee-uh)
An excessive amount of *calcium* in the blood.
Compare Hypocalcemia.

Hypercapnia (hie-puhr-KAP-nee-uh)
An excessive amount of *carbon dioxide* in the blood stream.
Also known as Hypercarbia.

Hypercarbia (hie-puhr-KAR-bee-uh)
Refer to Hypercapnia.

Hyperextensible (hie-puhr-ik-STEN-si-buhl)
Refer to **Hyperextension.**

Hyperextension (hie-puhr-ik-STEN-shuhn)
A position in which a body part is straightened out (extended) past the normal limit.
Refer to **Extension.**

Hyperglycemia (hie-puhr-glie-SEE-mee-uh)
Abnormally high sugar levels in the blood. Hyperglycemia can occur as a complication of other conditions, such as *diabetes mellitus,* and can result in increased susceptibility to infection.
Compare **Hypoglycemia.**

Hyperkalemia (hie-puhr-kuh-LEE-mee-uh)
Excessive amounts of *potassium* in the blood. Hyperkalemia can be caused by *kidney* dysfunction or adrenal insufficiency, or occur in response to certain types of serious injury or infection. It can produce weakness and *paralysis,* and *heart arrhythmias.*
Compare **Hypokalemia.**

Hyperkinetic (hie-puhr-ki-NET-ik)
Refer to **Hyperactivity.**
Compare **Hypokinetic.**

Hyperlexia (hie-puhr-LEX-ee-uh)
A form of *learning disability* in which the child can read far above what would be considered his normal reading level, but does not comprehend much of what he reads (similar to an English-speaking person sounding out written words in Spanish). For some children with an *autism spectrum disorder* or some children with *mental retardation,* hyperlexia is a *symptom* of their *disorder.* Hyperlexia is an example of a *splinter skill.*

Hypermobility (hie-puhr-moe-BIL-i-tee)
Excessive movement within a *joint.*

Hypernasality (hie-puhr-nay-ZAL-i-tee)
A voice *disorder* that occurs when too much air passes through the nose during speech due to failure of the *soft palate* to close the nasal passages.
Compare **Hyponasality.**

Hypernatremia (hie-puhr-nuh-TREE-mee-uh)
Excessive amounts of *sodium* in the blood.
Compare **Hyponatremia.**

Hyperopia (hie-puhr-OE-pee-uh)
A *refractive error* that causes blurred vision of close objects. Hyperopia occurs when the eye is too short, which makes the *lens* focus close objects *behind* the

retina rather than on it. Prescription lenses can increase the vision in a child with hyperopia.
> *Also known as* **Farsightedness.**
> *Compare* **Myopia.**
> *Refer to* **Aphakia** *and* **Refraction.**

Hyperphagia (hie-puhr-FAY-jee-uh)
Excessive uncontrolled eating.

Hyperplasia (hie-puhr-PLAY-zee-uh)
An increased number of normal *cells* resulting in an enlarged organ or *tissue.* *Gingival hyperplasia* is an example.
> *Compare* **Hypoplasia.**

Hyperproteinemia (hie-puhr-proe-teen-EE-mee-uh)
An *abnormally* high level of protein in the blood.
> *Compare* **Hypoproteinemia.**

Hyperreflexia (hie-puhr-ree-FLEK-see-uh)
An increased response of the *deep tendon reflexes.*

Hyperresponsive (hie-puhr-ree-SPON-siv)
Describes the state of feeling overwhelmed by very small amounts of *sensory stimulation,* which the brain registers too intensely and perceives as reason to withdraw from or react to negatively. For example, a child who is hyper-responsive might react to someone tapping him gently on the shoulder by screaming or running away.
> *Also known as* **Overreactive** *and* **Overresponsive.**
> *Compare* **Hyporesponsive.**
> *Refer to* **Sensory Overload.**

Hypertelorism (hie-puhr-TEL-or-izm)
A *congenital* condition in which there is an *abnormally* wide space between 2 paired organs or body parts, such as the eyes.
> *Compare* **Hypotelorism.**

Hypertelorism-Hypospadias Syndrome
(hie-puhr-TEL-or-izm hie-poe-SPAY-dee-uhs)
> *Refer to* **G Syndrome.**

Hypertension (hie-puhr-TEN-shuhn)
High *blood pressure.* Either a high systolic or high diastolic pressure reading may indicate hypertension.
> *Compare* **Hypotension.**
> *Refer to* **Blood Pressure.**

Hyperthermia (hie-puhr-THUR-mee-uh)
Abnormally high body temperature. It may be caused by heatstroke (a condi-

tion characterized by high fever, cessation of sweating, headache, rapid *pulse* and *respiration rates*, and sometimes high *blood pressure* and *coma*), burn, sweat *gland disorder*, or as a reaction to certain *general anesthetics* in individuals who have *inherited* this *genetic* trait.
  Compare **Hypothermia.**

Hyperthyroidism (hie-puhr-THIE-roid-iz-uhm)
Increased activity of the *thyroid gland*, resulting in increased appetite, weight loss, enlarged thyroid, rapid *heart rate*, intolerance to heat, increased sweating, and sometimes *exophthalmos* (an *abnormal* protrusion of the eyeball).
  Compare **Hypothyroidism.**

Hypertonia (hie-puhr-TOE-nee-uh)
Increased *tone* (stiffness) in the muscles.
  Also known as **Hypertonicity** *and* **High Tone.**
  Compare **Hypotonia.**
  Refer to **Muscle Tone.**

Hypertonic (hie-puhr-TON-ik)
  Refer to **Hypertonia.**

Hypertonicity (hie-puhr-toe-NI-si-tee)
  Refer to **Hypertonia.**

Hypertrichosis (hie-puhr-tri-KOE-sis)
Excessive hair growth, possibly caused by *disease* of the *endocrine glands.*

Hyperuricemia (hie-puhr-yoo-ris-EE-mee-uh)
An elevated level of *uric acid* in the blood.

Hyperventilation (hie-puhr-ven-ti-LAY-shuhn)
An *abnormally* rapid breathing rate or increased volume of air exchanged.
  Compare **Hypoventilation.**

Hypervolemia (hie-puhr-voe-LEE-mee-uh)
An increase in the amount of *intravascular* fluid. It can occur with *congestive heart failure.*
  Compare **Hypovolemia.**

hypo-
A prefix meaning under, below, or less than normal.
  Compare **hyper-.**

Hypoactivity
Abnormally diminished activity. It is usually used to describe diminished peristaltic activity (the progressive wave of *contraction* of certain muscle fibers of tubular organs that propels its contents through the tube, such as with the intestine).
  Compare **Hyperactivity.**

Hypoallergenic (hie-poe-al-uhr-JEN-ik)
Referring to a decreased likelihood for producing an *allergic* reaction.
> *Refer to* **Allergy.**

Hypocalcemia (hie-poe-kal-SEE-mee-uh)
Abnormally low levels of *calcium* in the blood.
> *Compare* **Hypercalcemia.**

Hypoglycemia (hie-poe-glie-SEE-mee-uh)
Abnormally low blood sugar levels. Hypoglycemia may be caused by *pancreatic* dysfunction, *intestinal malabsorption*, injection of an excessive quantity of *insulin*, or *liver* or *endocrine disease*.
> *Compare* **Hyperglycemia.**

Hypogonadism (hie-poe-GOE-nad-izm)
Abnormally low activity of the *gonads* (*testes* or *ovaries*) caused by a *disorder* of the gonads or *pituitary gland*. This condition usually results in retarded growth and sexual development.

Hypokalemia (hie-poe-kuh-LEE-mee-uh)
Too little *potassium* in the blood.
> *Compare* **Hyperkalemia.**

Hypokinetic (hie-poe-ki-NET-ik)
Slow moving or lethargic.
> *Compare* **Hyperkinetic.**

Hyponasality
A voice *disorder* that occurs when too little or no air passes through the nose during speech. It can be caused by blockage of the nasal passages, allergies, and *colds*.
> *Compare* **Hypernasality.**

Hyponatremia (hie-poe-nuh-TREE-mee-uh)
Too little *sodium* in the blood.
> *Compare* **Hypernatremia.**

Hypoplasia (hie-poe-PLAY-zee-uh)
An underdeveloped or incomplete organ or *tissue*, usually due to a decrease in the number of *cells*.
> *Compare* **Hyperplasia.**

Hypoplastic
Underdeveloped.

Hypoplastic Left Heart Syndrome (HLHS)
A nearly always fatal group of *heart* malformations in which the entire left side of the heart is underdeveloped. This causes severe *cyanosis* (a lack of *oxygen* in

the bloodstream that results in a blue color to the skin and *mucous membranes*), and *heart failure*. A heart transplant may save the affected infant's life.

Hypoproteinemia (hie-poe-proe-tee-in-EE-mee-uh)
An *abnormally* low level of *protein* in the blood.
>Compare **Hyperproteinemia.**

Hyporesponsive
Describing the state of underreacting to *sensory stimulation*. The brain fails to register incoming information and, thus, the child does not demonstrate an *adaptive* response. A child who is hyporesponsive may crave or require intensive *sensory input*. She may appear clumsy or aggressive, constantly bumping/running into walls, furniture, or people, and/or touching people or objects in an effort to seek out sensory feedback. A hyporesponsive child may also have a high tolerance to pain.
>*Also known as* **Underreactive** *and* **Underresponsive.**
>Compare **Hyperresponsive.**

Hypospadias (hie-poe-SPAY-dee-uhs)
A *congenital defect* in which the *urethral* canal opens on the undersurface of the penis, before it reaches the tip of the penis. Similarly, the urethra may open into the vagina in a female.

Hypotelorism (hie-poe-TEL-oe-rizm)
A *congenital* condition in which there is an *abnormally* decreased space between two paired organs or body parts, such as the eyes.
>Compare **Hypertelorism.**

Hypotension
Abnormally low *blood pressure.*
>Compare **Hypertension.**
>*Refer to* **Blood Pressure.**

Hypothalamus
A part of the *diencephalon* of the *brain* that activates and controls the part of the *nervous system* that regulates internal body functioning (such as appetite, temperature, sleep, and emotions) and *endocrine* activity, including indirectly regulating the *pituitary gland* (which, in turn, controls many body functions including growth, sexual development, and fertility).

Hypothermia
Abnormally low body temperature. Hypothermia can lead to death.
>Compare **Hyperthermia.**

Hypothyroidism
A condition in which the *thyroid gland* is underactive, resulting in insufficient or no thyroid *hormone*. It is characterized by a lowered *basal metabolic* rate, low *blood pressure*, and lethargy.
>Compare **Hyperthyroidism.**
>Compare **Congenital Hypothyroidism.**

Hypotonia (hie-poe-TOE-nee-uh)
Decreased *tone*, or floppiness, in the muscles, characterized by excessive *range of motion* of the *joints* and little muscle resistance when parts of the body are being moved. Hypotonia requires the child to exert more effort to initiate movement and maintain *posture*. Hypotonia is often observed in babies who are ill due to a *heart defect*, babies with *Down syndrome* or other *chromosomal abnormalities*, babies with certain types of *cerebral palsy*, and *premature infants*. A baby with hypotonia may be referred to as a *floppy infant*.
> *Also known as* **Hypotonicity** *and* **Low Tone.**
> *Compare* **Hypertonia.**
> *Refer to* **Muscle Tone.**

Hypotonic (hie-poe-TON-ik)
> *Refer to* **Hypotonia.**

Hypotonicity (hie-poe-toe-NI-si-tee)
> *Refer to* **Hypotonia.**

Hypoventilation
Underventilation of the *alveoli* of the lungs, resulting in a lower than normal rate of breathing and volume of air exchanged.
> *Compare* **Hyperventilation.**

Hypovolemia (hie-poe-voe-LEE-mee-uh)
An *abnormally* low volume of blood in the body.
> *Compare* **Hypervolemia.**

Hypoxemia (hie-poks-EE-mee-uh)
A condition in which there is too little *oxygen* in the *arterial* blood. Untreated, this leads to *hypoxia*.

Hypoxia (hie-POKS-ee-uh)
A lack of sufficient *oxygen* in the body *cells* or blood. Hypoxia can lead to *brain damage*.

Hypsibrachycephaly (hips-i-brayk-i-SEF-uh-lee)
A *congenital* malformation of the skull in which the head appears long, with a broad forehead.
> *Also known as* **Turribrachycephaly.**

Hypsicephaly (hips-i-SEF-uh-lee)
> *Refer to* **Oxycephaly.**

hystero-
A prefix meaning *uterus*.

Hz
The abbreviation for hertz.

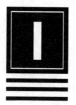

IAC
The abbreviation for indwelling arterial catheter.

IAL
The abbreviation for indwelling arterial line.

I and O
The abbreviation for intake and output or input and outflow (the amount of fluids entering and leaving the body). This includes feedings, *IV* fluid, drawn blood samples, and urine and stool elimination.

-iasis
A suffix meaning condition.

iatr-
A prefix meaning relating to medicine, *physicians*, or medical treatment.

Iatrogenic (ie-at-ruh-JEN-ik)
Referring to an injury, *disease*, or condition induced by medical treatment. An example of an iatrogenic disease is *bronchopulmonary dysplasia*, which is caused by use of a *ventilator*.

Ibuprofin (IE-byoo-proe-fin)
A *nonsteroidal anti-inflammatory drug* used to treat muscle aches and pain. Motrin™ is the brand name of this drug.

ICC
The abbreviation for Interagency Coordinating Council.

ICD
The abbreviation for the International Classification of Diseases.

ICDL
The abbreviation for Interdisciplinary Council on Developmental and Learning Disorders.

ICF
The abbreviation for intermediate care facility.

ICH
The abbreviation for intracranial hemorrhage or intracerebral hemorrhage.

Ichthyosis (ik-thee-OE-sis)
Extremely dry and scaly skin, usually first seen at birth or shortly after. Ichthyosis is any of several *inherited* conditions and may be associated with one of several rare *syndromes*.

ICN
The abbreviation for Intensive Care Nursery.'

Icterus (IK-tuh-ruhs)
Refer to **Jaundice.**

id
1. The abbreviation for the same.
2. The abbreviation for during the day.

IDEA
The abbreviation for Individuals with Disabilities Education Act of 1990.

IDEA 2004
An abbreviation for Individuals with Disabilities Education Act of 2004.
Refer to **Individuals with Disabilities Education Improvement Act of 2004.**

IDEIA
An abbreviation for Individuals with Disabilities Education Improvement Act of 2004.
Refer to **Individuals with Disabilities Education Improvement Act of 2004.**

Identical Twins
Refer to **Monozygotic Twins.**

Identification
The determination that a child should be evaluated as a possible candidate for *early intervention* or *special education* services.

idio-
A prefix meaning peculiar or distinctive.

Idioglossia (id-ee-oe-GLOS-ee-uh)
An inability to articulate sounds correctly, resulting in speech that sounds like an invented or foreign language and is unintelligible. Idioglossia may include

sound omissions, substitutions, distortions, and transpositions. It is often associated with *mental retardation*.
>   *Also known as* **Idiolalia.**

Idiolalia (id-ee-oe-LAY-lee-uh)
>   *Refer to* **Idioglossia.**

Idiopathic (id-ee-oe-PATH-ik)
Referring to a *disease* with an unknown cause.

Idiopathic Epilepsy
Epilepsy that does not have an identified cause.
>   *Also known as* **Primary Epilepsy.**
>   *Refer to* **Epilepsy.**

Idiopathic Seizure
>   *Refer to* **Idiopathic Epilepsy** *and* **Epilepsy.**

IDM
The abbreviation for infant of a diabetic mother.

IEP
The abbreviation for Individualized Education Program.

IFSP
The abbreviation for Individualized Family Service Plan.

Ig
The abbreviation for immunoglobulin.

IL®
The abbreviation for intralipid.

Ileal Conduit (IL-ee-uhl KON-doo-it)
A surgical procedure in which a segment of *ileum* (the third section of the *small intestine*) is used to replace another hollow organ (usually the *bladder*).
>   *Also known as* **Ileal Loop.**

Ileal Loop
>   *Refer to* **Ileal Conduit.**

ileo-
A prefix meaning *ileum.*

Ileostomy (il-ee-OS-toe-mee)
An *ostomy* (surgically created opening) in the *ileum* (the third section of the *small intestine*). A surgical procedure is performed to create an opening in the *abdominal* wall so *fecal matter* can be eliminated from the body.

Ileum (IL-ee-uhm)
The third section of the *small intestine*. It opens into the *large intestine*. (The *duodenum* is the first section and the *jejunum* is the middle section of the small intestine.)
Refer to **Small Intestine.**

Ilium (IL-ee-uhm)
The *superior* (uppermost) part of the *coxae*, or hip bone.

Illocutionary Stage (i-loe-KYOO-shuhn-er-ee)
A preverbal stage of language development in which the infant's attempts at *communication* are intentional but consist mostly of nonverbal forms of *expressive language* (*babbling, gesturing,* and other vocal sounds). This stage typically develops between 8 and 15 months.
Refer to **Locutionary Stage** *and* **Perlocutionary Stage.**

IM
The abbreviation for intramuscular (such as an *intramuscular injection*).

IMH
The abbreviation for Infant Mental Health.

Imipramine Hydrochloride (im-IP-ruh-meen hie-droe-KLOR-ied)
An *antidepressant drug* sometimes used in the treatment of certain *autistic-like behaviors*. It is also used to treat childhood *nocturnal enuresis* (bedwetting). Tofranil™ is the brand name for this drug.

Imitative Play
Copying the actions of another child or an adult. Pretending or attempting to comb one's hair and helping to wipe a table are examples of imitative play. (The imitative play of young children frequently involves copying the actions of daily routines.) Imitative play is an important skill for learning.

Immittance Audiometry (i-MIT-ns aw-dee-OM-uh-tree)
An auditory test that is used to measure *tympanic membrane* mobility or function (which may reflect possible *otitis media*).
Also known as **Tympanometry, Immittance Tympanometry,** *or* **Impedance Audiometry.**

Immittance Tympanometry (im-PEE-dans tim-puh-NOM-uh-tree)
Refer to **Immittance Audiometry.**

Immune Body
Refer to **Antibody.**

Immune System
A collection of *cells* and *proteins* within body *organs* and *tissues* and the *physiological* processes used by the body to identify potentially harmful *microorganisms,* such as *bacteria, fungi,* and *viruses,* and prevent them from harming the body.

Immunity (i-MYOO-ni-tee)
Protection from, or resistance to, certain *diseases* or conditions that is either natural (*inherited*) or *acquired* by having the disease or by injection, inoculation, or vaccination with an *antigen*.
> *Refer to* **Vaccine.**

Immunization
The process by which protection from an infectious *disease* is induced. A *vaccine* may be used.
> *Refer to* **Inoculate** *and* **Vaccine.**

Immunoglobulin (Ig) (im-yoo-noe-GLOB-yoo-lin)
Any of 5 classes of *proteins* that function as *antibodies*.

Impedance Audiometry (im-PEE-dans aw-dee-OM-uh-tree)
> *Refer to* **Immittance Audiometry.**

Imperforate Anus (im-PER-foe-rayt AY-nuhs)
A *congenital defect* in which the anal opening is absent or obstructed, making elimination of stools impossible.
> *Also known as* **Anal Atresia.**

Impetigo (im-puh-TIE-goe or im-puh-TEE-goe)
A *bacterial, inflammatory* skin infection characterized by reddened skin that blisters. When the *lesions* burst, the fluid may dry on the skin creating a characteristic honey-colored crust. Impetigo often initially appears around the nose and mouth but can be spread (usually by the hands), to other parts of the body. Impetigo is highly *contagious* and is common in children.

Impulse (IM-puls)
A sudden, spontaneous, irresistible urge, desire, or action.
> *Refer to* **Nerve Impulse.**

Impulsivity (im-pul-SIV-i-tee)
Behavior characterized by acting on impulse, or without thought or conscious judgment.

in-
A prefix meaning into or not.

Inactivated Poliovirus Vaccine of Enhanced Potency (IPV-E)
An *immunization* against *poliomyelitis* made from an inactivated (by formaldehyde) *polio virus*. The child receives doses at 2 and 4 months, between 6 and 18 months, and before starting school at 4½ to 6 years of age. It is administered by injection. The IPV-E, rather than the orally-administered *OPV* (*Oral Poliovirus Vaccine*), is now recommended.
> *Also known as* **Salk Vaccine.**
> *Refer to* **Poliomyelitis.**

Inborn
Referring to a condition obtained while in the *uterus* (*prenatally*). An inborn condition may be, but is not necessarily, *inherited*.

Inborn Error of Metabolism
A *genetic disorder* caused by an *inherited* deficiency in an important *enzyme*. Many inborn errors of metabolism can be *diagnosed prenatally* in mothers who are known to be at risk. If not detected and treated early, some of these disorders will lead to *mental retardation* and death. Examples of inborn errors of metabolism include *PKU* and *Tay-Sachs Disease*.
> *Refer to* **Metabolism.**

Inborn Lysosomal Disease (lie-suh-SOE-muhl)
> *Refer to* **Lysosomal Storage Disease.**

Incidence
Frequency of occurrence, such as the number of new cases of a *disease* occurring in a given period of time.

Inclusion/Inclusive
Including a child with a *disability* as a full-time member in a center-based program or regular education classroom setting in which children who do not have disabilities participate. (The program or classroom setting would exist even if there were no children with *special needs* enrolled.)
> *Refer to* **Integration, Mainstreaming,** *and* **Natural Environment.**

Incompetent Cervix
A condition in which the mother's *uterus* opens at the *cervix* in mid to late pregnancy, risking a *miscarriage* or premature birth.
> *Also known as* **Cervical Incompetence.**

Incontinence
The inability to control urination or *defecation*.

Incubation Period
> *Refer to* **Latency Period.**

Incubator
An enclosed bed that provides an ill or *premature infant* with the benefits of an environment with controlled temperature, humidity, and *oxygen*.

Incus (ING-kuhs)
The middle of the three small bones of the *middle ear*. (The other two bones are the *malleus* and the *stapes*.)
> *Also known as* **Anvil.**
> *Refer to* **Ear.**

Individualized Education Program (IEP)

A written plan required by the *Individuals with Disabilities Education Improvement Act of 2004* for all children in *special education,* ages 3 years and up. The IEP is reviewed (at least) annually and includes a statement of a child's current level of *development* (abilities and impairments) and an individualized plan of instruction, including the *annual goals,* the specific services to be provided, the people who will carry out the services, the standards and time lines for evaluating progress made, and the amount and degree to which the child will participate with non-disabled peers at school. The IEP is developed by the child's parents and the professionals who evaluated the child.

Individualized Family Service Plan (IFSP)

A written *early intervention* plan describing the infant's (age birth to 3 years) current level of *development;* the family's strengths and needs related to enhancement of the infant's or toddler's development; *annual goals* for the infant and the other family members (as applicable), including the criteria, procedures, and time lines used to evaluate progress (the IFSP should be evaluated and adjusted at least once a year and reviewed at least every 6 months); and the specific early intervention services needed to meet the annual goals (including the frequency and intensity and method of delivering services, the projected date of initiating services, and the anticipated duration of services). The IFSP is developed and implemented by the child's parents and a multidisciplinary early intervention team (for example, the *service coordinator, infant educator, physical therapist, occupational therapist,* or *speech-language pathologist*). The name of the person responsible for implementation of the IFSP should be listed on the IFSP. If it is likely that the child will require *special education* services at age 3, a *transition plan* should also be stated in the IFSP. The Individualized Family Service Plan is required by the *Individuals with Disabilities Act (IDEA)* for all infants receiving early intervention services.

Refer to **Early Intervention.**

Individuals with Disabilities Education Act of 1990 (IDEA) (Public Law 101-476)

A federal law amended in 1997 (*Public Law 105-17*) and reauthorized in 2004 (*Public Law 108-446*) that amends the *Education for All Handicapped Children Act of 1975.* Part C (previously known as Part H) of the law focuses on services to infants and toddlers who are *at-risk* or have *developmental delays.* Part B focuses on services to preschoolers and school-aged children with *developmental disabilities.*

Individuals with Disabilities Education Improvement Act of 2004 (IDEA 2004, IDEIA) (Public Law 108-446)

A federal law that reauthorizes and amends the *Individuals with Disabilities Education Act of 1990 (IDEA).* It is currently referred to as IDEA 2004 or IDEIA.

Refer to **Individuals with Disabilities Education Act of 1990 (IDEA).**

Indomethacin (in-doe-METH-uh-sin)

A drug that is sometimes used to close the *ductus arteriosus.* Indomethacin is also used to reduce pain and *inflammation.*

Indwelling Arterial Catheter (IAC)
Refer to Arterial Catheter and Catheter.

Indwelling Arterial Line (IAL)
Refer to Arterial Catheter and Catheter.

Indwelling Catheter
Refer to Catheter.

Indwelling Thumb
Abnormal fisting of the hand with the thumb next to the palm and the fingers over the thumb holding it tucked in. Holding the thumb against the palm is normal in the first 2 months of life.
Also known as Cortical Thumbing.

Indwelling Venous Catheter (IVC)
Refer to Venous Catheter and Catheter.

Indwelling Venous Line (IVL)
Refer to Venous Catheter and Catheter.

Infant
A child up to 12 months of age.

Infant Development Program
A program of activities designed to promote the development of the infant's basic skills. An *infant educator* or the child's parent/*primary caregiver* may implement the *developmental* activities (often in the form of play activities), which are chosen for and adapted to the individual child based on his areas of strength and *deficit*. The activities may be natural and simple as an adult describing the actions and sensations of an activity the baby is experiencing. For example, as the baby is being dressed, the adult might say, "Now I am putting your arm through the sleeve of your shirt. Where is your hand? There it is! Your blue shirt is so soft and warm!" Infant development activities also include planned experiences. For example, offering the child a sticky ball of brightly-colored masking tape (too large to fit in the mouth) is a planned play activity that incorporates many areas of development. The child experiences *transferring* an object hand-to-hand (the sticky quality encourages the child to pull the ball of tape from one hand to the other); the sensations of stickiness, texture, and color; descriptive language associated with the activity; and the social aspects of cooperative ball play (rolling, tossing, or chasing the ball). The child's infant development program should focus on the child's *developmental age* (the level at which the child is functioning) rather than his *chronological age*. This makes it possible to set appropriate and realistic goals (and implementations designed to help minimize the child's *developmental delays*). The child's health, his family and home environment, his style of learning, and his likes/dislikes are all important considerations for planning the infant development program. Addressing the parents' questions and

concerns is also a critical infant program component. The individualization of the components of the infant development program is usually reflected in the *Individualized Family Service Plan*.

>Also known as **Infant Stimulation Program.**
>Refer to **Individualized Family Service Plan.**

Infant Development Specialist

>Refer to **Infant Educator.**

Infant Educator

A specialist trained to assess infants and young children in the six main areas of *development*: *cognitive, communication* (language), *gross motor, fine motor* (perceptual), *social/emotional*, and *self-help* (*adaptive*) skills, and to plan and implement a program that addresses the infant or young child's developmental needs. The infant educator should have knowledge of how infants and young children typically develop so that appropriate and realistic goals, objectives, and implementations (often in the form of play activities) can be planned. The role of the infant educator varies from one *early intervention* program to the next, but the infant educator should be part of a *multidisciplinary team* that includes other specialists who address specific developmental concerns (such as the *pediatrician*; the *speech-language pathologist*; *occupational, physical*, or *vision therapist*; and the *service coordinator*).

>Also known as **Early Educator, Early Intervention Educator, Early Interventionist, Infant Development Specialist, Infant Specialist,** and **Infant Teacher.**
>Refer to **Infant Development Program.**

Infantile (IN-fuhn-tiel)

Referring to an infant or infancy.

Infantile Acquired Aphasia

>Refer to **Landau-Kleffner Syndrome.**

Infantile Autism

>Refer to **Autistic Disorder.**

Infantile Cerebral Sphingolipidosis (suh-REE-bruhl sfing-goe-lip-id-OE-sis)

>Refer to **Tay-Sachs Disease.**

Infantile Muscular Atrophy (MUS-kyuh-luhr AT-roe-fee)

>Refer to **Werdnig-Hoffmann Disease.**

Infantile Myoclonic Seizures (mie-oe-KLON-ik)

>Refer to **Infantile Spasms.**

Infantile Scoliosis (skoe-lee-OE-sis)

Lateral curvature of the spine that develops in children under 3 years of age.

>Refer to **Scoliosis.**

Infantile Spasms

A rare type of *myoclonic seizure* with onset usually within the first year of life that usually involves *flexion* of the head and trunk (dropping of the head) and flexion of the arms and legs. (Most children have a mixture of *flexor* and *extensor spasms*.) These *seizures* may occur hundreds of times a day, frequently in clusters. The *prognosis* for the child who has infantile spasms varies greatly, depending on whether the seizures are *idiopathic* (there is no known cause) or *symptomatic* (there is an identifiable cause).

Also known as **Infantile Myoclonic Seizures.**
Refer to **Adrenocorticotropic Hormone.**

Infantile Spinal Muscular Atrophy

Refer to **Werdnig-Hoffmann Disease.**

Infant Mental Health (IMH)

The psychological functioning of an infant or young child influenced by the child's relationships and interaction experiences with his primary caregivers; the child's individual differences, including strengths, vulnerabilities, and temperament (and his caregivers' responses to his individual differences); and the family's cultural context. *Zero to Three: National Center for Infants, Toddlers, and Families* describes infant mental health as "synonymous with healthy social and emotional development."

Infant of a Chemically-Dependent Mother

Refer to **Prenatally Exposed to Drugs.**

Infant of a Substance-Abusing Mother (ISAM)

Refer to **Prenatally Exposed to Drugs.**

Infant Specialist

Refer to **Infant Educator.**

Infant Stimulation Program

Refer to **Infant Development Program.**

Infant Teacher

Refer to **Infant Educator.**

Infarct/Infarction (in-FAHRKT/in-FAHRK-shuhn)

Death of small amounts of body *tissue*. Infarction is usually caused by an interruption in the blood supply to the organ or tissue.

Infection

Invasion of the body or a body part by *microorganisms* (*germs*) that multiply and cause *disease*.

Infectious Mononucleosis (mon-oe-noo-klee-OE-sis)

An infection caused by the *Epstein-Barr virus* or *cytomegalovirus* and with *symptoms* including fever, sore throat, swollen *lymph nodes*, enlarged *spleen* and *liver*, bruising, and lethargy.

> *Also known as* **Mono** *and* **Mononucleosis.**

Inferior Pincer Grasp

Grasp of a small object using the thumb and the index finger with the thumb positioned at the side of the bent index finger. The inferior pincer grasp develops between 7½ and 10 months of age.

> *Compare* **Neat Pincer Grasp.**
> *Refer to* **Grasp.**

Inferior Vena Cava (VEE-nuh KAY-vuh)

> *Refer to* **Vena Cava.**

Infiltrate (in-FIL-trayt)

The passing of fluid or *cells* into surrounding *tissues*, such as when an *IV (intravenous) catheter* slips out of a *vein* or when fluid collects in the lungs.

Inflammation (in-fluh-MAY-shuhn)

The body's response to injury, infection, or irritation. Inflammation is a protective reaction and the primary signs are redness, heat, swelling, and pain, often accompanied by loss of function.

Influenza (in-floo-EN-zuh)

A highly *contagious viral* infection, transmitted by airborne particles through direct person-to-person contact and contact with *secretions. Symptoms* include *inflammation* of the *respiratory tract*, sore throat, cough, chills, fever, muscular pains, irritation in the intestinal tract, and weakness.

> *Also known as the* **Flu.**

infra-

A prefix meaning beneath.

Infusion Pump

A device attached to an *intravenous catheter* through which fluids or medications are injected in measured amounts.

Ingestion

The process of taking food, drink, or medication by mouth.

> *Refer to* **Nutrition.**

Inguinal Hernia (ING-gwi-nuhl)

A *hernia* that occurs when part of the intestine protrudes through the *abdominal* wall or into the inguinal canal (the passageway in the groin area that leads to the scrotum in the male, and transmits a *ligament* in the female). Inguinal hernias are usually repaired surgically.

> *Refer to* **Hernia.**

Inherited/Inheritance
Referring to the transmission of traits, via the *genes*, from parents to their baby.
> *Also known as* **Hereditary** *or* **Genetic.**
> *Compare* **Acquired** *and* **Congenital.**

Inhibitive Casting (in-HIB-i-tiv)
Use of a cast that holds the foot in normal alignment (a *neutral position* with toes forward, ankle flexed) and helps to reduce increased *muscle tone* or unwanted *reflexes.*

Innate (in-AYT)
Existing from birth. An innate condition may also be a *congenital* condition, an *inborn* condition, or a *hereditary* condition.

Inner Ear
> *Refer to* **Cochlea, Ear, Labyrinth, Proprioception, Semicircular Canal,** *and* **Vestibular Aparatus.**

Inoculate (i-NOK-yuh-layt)
To introduce into the body *immune serums, vaccines,* or other foreign materials that are capable of causing the production of an *antibody* to prevent or cure *disease. Immunity* is achieved when the body produces antibodies that defend the body from the *bacteria, virus,* or other *microorganism* which causes the disease. A *vaccine* may be used.
> *Refer to* **Immunization** *and* **Vaccine.**

Input
Information that a person receives through any of the *sensory* systems (sight, *hearing,* touch, *taste,* smell, *vestibular,* and *proprioceptive*).
> *Refer to* **Sensory Integration** *and* **Sensory Processing.**

Insistence on Sameness
A tendency in many children with an *autism spectrum disorder* to become upset when familiar routines or environments are changed.

In Situ (in-SIE-too or in-SIT-oo)
1. In the natural, original, or usual place.
2. Describing a *cancer* that has not spread to other *tissues.*

Insulin (IN-soo-lin or IN-syuh-lin)
A *hormone* produced by the *pancreas* to regulate the *metabolism* of *blood sugar* and to maintain proper blood sugar levels. Insulin can also be prepared synthetically or obtained from animals for the treatment of *diabetes.*

Integration
Including children with *special needs* in classroom or school activities with *typically developing* peers. There are degrees of integration. Some children with special needs may be integrated only into nonacademic activities such

as recess, physical education, and lunch, while others may be integrated into all school activities.

Refer to **Inclusion** *and* **Mainstreaming.**

Integrity
1. The quality of being unbroken or unimpaired.
2. Honesty.

Intellectual Disability (ID)
Cognitive impairment or *mental retardation.*

Intelligence
The ability to acquire, retain, understand, and apply knowledge. Intelligence is measured using a standardized *intelligence test,* and the results are expressed numerically. (This is the *intelligence quotient,* or IQ). 100 is considered to be the average IQ. Based on IQ test scores, the following levels have commonly been used to describe a child's intelligence:

- Normal Intelligence—An IQ *score* between 85 and 116. (Above 130 is considered gifted.)
- Borderline Intelligence—An IQ score between 70 and 84. Scoring in this range does not mean the child has *mental retardation*; skills may be acquired at a slower rate, but the child is able to learn independent living skills.
- Mild Mental Retardation—An IQ score between 50 and 69. The child learns more slowly but, as an adult, is typically able to work and/or live independently or with some assistance. Many adults with mild mental retardation marry.
- Moderate Mental Retardation—An IQ score between 35 and 49. The child is able to learn basic skills for coping with daily living. As an adult, he usually needs living assistance and may be able to work in a supervised setting.
- Severe Mental Retardation—An IQ score between 20 and 34. The child also often has other *disabilities* such as *seizures, cerebral palsy,* or speech problems. As an adult, he usually needs to live in a supervised setting and may be able to participate in a supervised workshop or activity center.
- Profound Mental Retardation—An IQ score below 20. The child also often has other disabilities such as *seizures, cerebral palsy,* or speech problems. As an adult, he will need to live in a supervised setting and may learn skills to care for some of his basic needs.

The above terminology describing the levels of mental retardation has been phased out in favor of new terminology to describe intellectual functioning. The new levels, as defined by the *American Association on Mental Retardation,* identify the level of support a person needs. The level of support can be identified once an individual receives a *diagnosis* of mental retardation and his need for support is classified. (The diagnosis of mental retardation is made if the individual is 18 years or younger with an IQ score below 70-75 and significant *disability* in two or more *adaptive skill* areas. Classification of an individual's need for support is based on intellectual functioning and adaptive skills, psychological and emotional considerations, health and physical considerations, and environmental considerations.) The four levels of support include:

- Intermittent—The individual only requires support on a short-term basis for special circumstances, such as help in finding a new job.
- Limited—The individual has a consistent need for certain supports, such as handling finances or job training.
- Extensive—The individual requires consistent support in certain aspects of daily living, such as long-term job support.
- Pervasive—The individual requires constant support for all aspects of life.

Intelligence Quotient (IQ)
A numerical test score that describes the relationship between a child's *mental age* and *chronological age*. The average IQ is considered to be 100. On several scales, the IQ is determined by dividing the child's mental age (based on the results of *standardized test* scores) by the chronological age and multiplying the result by 100.

Intelligence Test
A *standardized test* that measures the child's *mental age*.
> *Refer to* **Intelligence Quotient.**

Intensive Care Nursery (ICN)
> *Refer to* **Neonatal Intensive Care Unit.**

Intensive Special Care Nursery (ISCN)
> *Refer to* **Neonatal Intensive Care Unit.**

Intensive Special Care Unit (ISCU)
> *Refer to* **Neonatal Intensive Care Unit.**

inter-
A prefix meaning between.

Interactive Disorder
A *disorder* in which the primary challenge to the child originates from the infant- or child-caregiver interaction patterns and related family and environmental patterns. *Symptoms* can include disruptive *behavior, anxiety*, depression, and eating disturbances. Interactive disorder is one of the five main categories of primary *diagnoses* (Axis 1) listed in the *Interdisciplinary Council on Developmental and Learning Disorders' (ICDL's) Diagnostic Manual for Infancy and Early Childhood.*
> *Refer to* **Diagnostic Manual for Infancy and Early Childhood.**

Interagency Coordinating Council (ICC)
A state council comprised of parents and representatives from local, state, and federal agencies that provide *early intervention* services to infants and toddlers with *special needs*. The Council members are appointed by the governor.

Intercostal (in-tuhr-KOS-tuhl)
Pertaining to the space between two ribs.

Interdisciplinary Council on Developmental and Learning Disorders (ICDL)
A group of professionals representing all the disciplines that work with infants and children with *developmental* and learning *disorders* and their families. The ICDL's mission statement includes its goal "to integrate knowledge from the different disciplines and improve the prevention, *assessment, diagnosis,* and treatment of these *disorders*." Dr. Stanley I. Greenspan and Dr. Serena Weider are co-chairs of the ICDL.

Interdisciplinary Team
A group of professionals who each represent areas of expertise useful in planning and implementing the educational, therapeutic, and/or medical treatment programs of children with *special needs*. The team periodically evaluates the child, and, with the child's parents, determines the child's areas of strength and *deficit*. Based on the evaluation, a plan for addressing the child's needs is developed, as well as a determination of the professionals who will implement the plan. Members of the interdisciplinary team may include a *service coordinator, infant educator, physical* or *occupational therapist, speech-language pathologist, social worker, physician, psychologist,* and the parents.
    Compare **Multidisciplinary Team** and **Transdisciplinary Team**.

Intermediate Care Facility (ICF)
A residential institution for people who have *disabilities* and are unable to live independently.

Intermittent Positive Pressure Breathing (IPPB) Machine
A type of *ventilator* used to help a baby breathe by intermittently forcing pressurized air into the lungs. The baby then relieves the pressure by exhaling.
    Refer to **Ventilator.**

Intern
A doctor in the first postgraduate year from medical school who is in supervised training.

Internal Auditory Canal
    Refer to **Auditory Canal.**

Internalization
A *cognitive* process that enables the child to remember an action or experience (internalize it) and repeat it at a later time, in a new situation. He doesn't have to experiment all over again, but can draw on past experience. For example, if the child is playing with nesting cups, he will be able to immediately place the small cup in the large cup rather than need to experiment to see how they fit together.
    Also known as **Internal Representation.**

Internal Representation
Refer to **Internalization.**

International Classification of Diseases (ICD)
The manual used in place of the *DSM* in countries other than the United States for *diagnosing* medical *disorders*.

Internist
A medical doctor who specializes in the *diagnosis* and treatment of adult *diseases* of the internal organs.

Interstitial Emphysema (in-tuhr-STISH-uhl em-fuh-SEE-muh)
Refer to **Pulmonary Interstitial Emphysema.**

Intervention
Treatment to repair or help relieve an *abnormality* or *deficit* in mental, emotional, or physical function.
Refer to **Early Intervention.**

Intestinal Disorder
Refer to **Gastrointestinal Disorder.**

Intestinal Ostomy
Refer to **Ostomy.**

Intestine
Also known as **Bowel.**
Refer to **Large Intestine** *and* **Small Intestine.**

Intoeing
Refer to **Toeing In.**

intra-
A prefix meaning inside or within.

Intracerebral (in-truh-SER-uh-bruhl)
Referring to within the *cerebrum*.

Intracerebral Hemorrhage (ICH) (in-truh-SER-uh-bruhl HEM-or-ij)
Bleeding in or around the *brain* caused by a *stroke*, loss of *integrity* of the *blood vessels*, injury to the head, or a lack of *oxygen*. A small amount of bleeding may resolve without serious complications, but a large bleed can result in *brain damage* or death.
Compare **Intraventricular Hemorrhage, Periventricular Hemorrhage,** *and* **Subarachnoid Hemorrhage.**

Intracranial (in-truh-KRAY-nee-uhl)
Referring to within the skull.

Intracranial Hemorrhage (ICH) (in-truh-KRAY-nee-uhl HEM-or-ij)
Bleeding within the *cranium.*
> *Refer to* **Intracerebral Hemorrhage.**

Intralipid (IL)® (in-truh-LIP-id)
An *intravenous,* calorie-rich fat solution that may be used during *total parenteral nutrition* to help the infant gain weight.

Intramuscular Injection
An injection into a muscle to administer medication.

Intraocular (in-truh-OK-yuh-luhr)
Referring to within the eye.

Intraocular Pressure (IOP)
The pressure of the fluid within the eye.

Intrauterine Growth Retardation (IUGR) (in-truh-YOO-tuhr-in)
Insufficient *fetal* growth that results in a baby who is *small for gestational age* (SGA). IUGR can be *symmetric* or *asymmetric,* depending on whether the infant's height, weight, and *head circumference* are all involved. (The head circumference will be the last to be affected; head circumference involvement occurs when IUGR is most severe.) IUGR may be caused by *genetic* factors, a fetal defect, fetal *malnutrition, maternal disease,* or maternal cigarette smoking or alcohol consumption. The impact of the IUGR depends on the severity of the factors causing the IUGR as well as the time during *prenatal* life that the factors were present. For example, an infant affected later in gestational life will be born at a lower weight, but not necessarily smaller in length or head circumference.
> *Refer to* **Birth Length, Birth Weight, Head Circumference,** *and to* the **CDC Growth Charts** *in the Appendix.*

Intravascular (in-truh-VAS-kyuh-luhr)
Pertaining to the inside of a *blood vessel.*

Intravenous (IV) (in-truh-VEE-nuhs)
1. Referring to within a *vein.*
2. Referring to a tube or needle placed into a vein for injecting drugs or fluids into the blood stream.

Intravenous Feeding
> *Refer to* **Hyperalimentation.**

Intravenous Immunoglobulin (IVIG)
(in-truh-VEE-nuhs im-yoo-noe-GLOB-yoo-lin)
An *immunoglobulin* administered *intravenously.*

Intravenous Pyelogram (IVP) (in-truh-VEE-nuhs PIE-uh-loe-gram)
An *x-ray* picture of the organs within the urinary system, including the *kid-*

neys, ureters, and *bladder.* The x-rays are taken after a contrast material has been injected into the bloodstream to determine whether there are any problems within or damage to these organs.

Intraventricular Hemorrhage (IVH)
(in-truh-ven-TRIK-yuh-luhr HEM-or-ij)
Bleeding into the fluid-filled chambers (*ventricles*) of the *brain.* IVH may be caused by rupture of *blood vessels* due to *oxygen* deprivation, abrupt fluctuations in *blood pressure,* improper blood flow, or *trauma* to the head. The IVH is graded by severity, from Grade I (also known as a *subependymal hemorrhage*), which refers to slight leaking of blood within brain *tissue* (but not so severe that the blood enters the ventricles of the brain), to Grade IV, which indicates such severe bleeding into the ventricles that it pushes blood back into surrounding brain tissue. Intraventricular hemorrhage does not always have a serious or fatal outcome. The location, amount, and cause of bleeding determine whether *disability* or death will result. Some problems that can occur due to IVH include *hydrocephalus, mental retardation,* visual or *auditory impairment,* and *cerebral palsy.* Neurological damage usually results with a Grade IV hemorrhage.
> *Also known as* **Brain Bleed.**
> *Compare* **Periventricular Hemorrhage, Intracerebral Hemorrhage,** *and* **Subarachnoid Hemorrhage.**

Intraverbal Exchange
A back-and-forth communicative exchange between people. For example, when a child says, "I like Mickey Mouse," and his parent responds, "I like Mickey, too! He's funny!" they are having an intraverbal exchange.

Intubation (in-tyoo-BAY-shuhn)
The insertion of a tube into the *trachea* to deliver air, *oxygen,* or *anesthetic* gas to the lungs. The tube may be inserted through the nose or mouth, or through a *tracheostomy.*
> *Compare* **Extubation.**

In Utero (in-YOO-tuhr-oe)
Referring to within the womb, or *uterus.*

Inversion
1. A *chromosomal abnormality* in which a section of a chromosome breaks off then reattaches in reverse direction.
2. An *abnormal* condition in which an organ is turned inside out.
3. The turning of a body part toward *midline,* such as turning the foot inward.
> *Compare* **Eversion.**

Involuntary Movements
Movements made without conscious control or direction, such as *automatic reflexes* or *athetosis.*

Iodine

An essential trace element primarily found in the *thyroid gland*.

IOP

The abbreviation for intraocular pressure.

Ipecac Syrup (IP-uh-kak)

A drug taken orally to induce vomiting. The practice of using ipecac syrup as a treatment for accidental poisoning is now contraindicated since a poison that has been swallowed can cause further damage to the body during regurgitation.

IPPB

The abbreviation for intermittent positive pressure breathing.

IPV-E

The abbreviation for Inactivated Poliovirus Vaccine of Enhanced Potency.

IQ

The abbreviation for intelligence quotient.

IQ Score

> *Refer to* **Intelligence Quotient.**

Iris

The clear *tissue* of the eye under which are pigment *cells* that give the eye its color. The iris sits between the *cornea* and the *lens*. The iris is made up of circular muscular fibers surrounding the *pupil* which function to dilate the pupil. (This is how the amount of light entering the eye is regulated.)
> *Refer to* **Eye.**

Iron (Fe)

A common *mineral* component of *hemoglobin* and certain *enzymes*. A medication used to treat iron-deficiency *anemia*.

is-

A prefix meaning equal.

ISAM

The abbreviation for infant of a substance-abusing mother.

Ischemia (is-KEE-mee-uh)

A decreased supply of *oxygenated* blood to an organ or part. It results from *disease* or damage which causes obstruction (usually a narrowing) of a *blood vessel* supplying the organ or part. Pain and organ disease may result.

Ischemic (is-KEE-mik)

Relating to *ischemia*.

Ischium (IS-kee-uhm)
The inferior back part of the hip bone. It joins the *ilium* and the *pubis* to form the *acetabulum*.

ISCN
The abbreviation for Intensive Special Care Nursery.

ISCU
The abbreviation for Intensive Special Care Unit.

iso-
A prefix meaning equal or like.

Isochromatic (ie-soe-kroe-MAT-ik)
Of the same color throughout.

Isolette™
A brand of *incubator*.

Isomil™
A milk-free formula made with soy *protein* used with infants sensitive to milk.

Isoxsuprine Hydrochloride (ie-SOK-suh-preen hie-droe-KLOR-ied)
A vasodilator drug (a medicine that causes dilation, or an increase in the diameter of *blood vessels*) that may be used to suppress *uterine contractions* of premature *labor*.

-itis
A suffix meaning *inflammation*.

IUGR
The abbreviation for intrauterine growth retardation.

IV
The abbreviation for intravenous.

IVC
The abbreviation for indwelling venous catheter.

IVH
The abbreviation for intraventricular hemorrhage.

IVIG
The abbreviation for Intravenous Immunoglobulin.

IVL
The abbreviation for indwelling venous line.

IVP
The abbreviation for intravenous pyelogram.

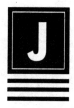

Jabbering

Referring to the talk of the toddler as she plays or experiments with words and the sound of her own voice. Around 18 months of age, the child begins to "practice" talking and to expand on the ways she can control her environment with speech.

*Compare **Babbling, Cooing,** and **Jargon.***

Jargon

The vocal play of the child between 18 and 22 months of age in which she "talks" to herself (or to someone else) using a string of *consonant* sounds (and occasional actual words). Jargon sounds similar to adult speech because of the inflection and rate used.

*Compare **Babbling, Cooing,** and **Jargon.***

Jaundice (JAWN-dis)

A yellowing of the skin, the *mucous membranes,* and the whites of the eyes (and deeper eye *tissues*) caused by too much *bilirubin* (a pigment byproduct of the breakdown of *red blood cells*) in the blood. Jaundice is common in newborns, but untreated jaundice (an extremely high level of bilirubin) can result in a form of *brain damage* known as *kernicterus.*

*Also known as **Icterus.***
*Refer to **Hyperbilirubinemia.***

Jaw Deviation

Pulling of the jaw to one side or the other.

jejuno-

A prefix meaning *jejunum.*

Jejunostomy (jee-joo-NOS-toe-mee)

An *ostomy* (surgically created opening) in the *jejunum* (the middle section of the *small intestine*).

Jejunum (juh-JOO-nuhm or jee-JOO-nuhm)

The middle section of the *small intestine.* (The *duodenum* is the first section

and the *ileum* is the third section of the small intestine.)
   Refer to **Small Intestine.**

Jervell and Lange-Nielsen Syndrome
A very rare *autosomal recessive disorder* characterized by *bilateral conductive hearing impairment, seizures* that cause loss of consciousness, *heart anomalies,* and *syncopal* attacks (fainting, or periods of brief unconsciousness) that may result in sudden infant death. If the infant survives these attacks, they become less frequent as the child grows older.

Joint
An *articulation,* or point of connection between two bones.

Joint Attention
   Refer to **Shared Attention and Meaning.**

Joint Compression
   Refer to **Compression.**

Joint Contracture
An *abnormal* condition in which the *joint* is bent with decreased *range of motion* due to permanent shortening of muscle fibers.
   Refer to **Contracture.**

Joint Fusion
   Refer to **Arthrodesis.**

Joint Stability
Referring to the support of a *joint* provided by the surrounding muscles and *ligaments* which enable the joint to successfully perform *motor* responses.

Jugular Shunt
   Refer to **Ventriculojugular Shunt and Shunt.**

Jugular Vein
One of three *veins* on each side of the neck that returns *deoxygenated* blood to the *heart* from the head and neck.

Jumping
Movement in which both feet propel the child's body into the air and then land at the same time.

Juvenile Spinal Muscular Atrophy
   Refer to **Kugelberg-Welander Disease.**

juxta-
A prefix meaning next to or near.

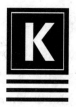

k
1. The abbreviation for constant.
2. The abbreviation for kilo, or 1000.

K
The chemical symbol for potassium.

KABC
The abbreviation for Kaufman Assessment Battery for Children.

Kabuki Make-up Syndrome (kuh-BOO-kee)
A *sporadically* occurring rare *congenital disorder* characterized by *craniofacial anomalies*, including long *palpebral fissures* (the opening between the upper and lower eyelids) that turn out at the outer third of the lower eyelids (resembling the make-up of the actors of Kabuki, a traditional Japanese theater form). Other craniofacial anomalies include large ears, tooth *abnormalities*, arched eyebrows, a short nasal *septum*, a depressed nasal tip, and, frequently, a *cleft palate*. *Mild* to *moderate mental retardation*; skeletal abnormalities of the hands, *vertebrae*, and hips; *hypotonia*; *joint hyperextensibility*; *short stature*; and often *cardiac* defects may also be present.

KAFO
The abbreviation for knee-ankle-foot orthosis.

Kanamycin Sulfate (kan-uh-MIE-sin SUL-fayt)
A type of *antibiotic drug* used for treating some severe infections.

Kangaroo Care
Caring for the newborn *premature infant* with prolonged skin-to-skin contact by his parent.

Kanner's Syndrome
> *Refer to* **Autistic Disorder.**

Karyotyping (KER-ee-oe-tie-ping)
A type of *genetic* test in which *cells* are photographed through a microscope *lens* in order to examine the *chromosomes'* size, shape, number, and arrangement. A normal karyotype shows 23 pairs of chromosomes. *Chromosomal abnormalities* can be detected both before and after birth using this procedure.

Kaufman Assessment Battery for Children (KABC)
A *norm-referenced intelligence test* used to evaluate the intelligence and academic achievement of the 2½- to 12½-year-old. The KABC is useful in detecting *learning disabilities*. Typically, the Kaufman is administered by a professional with a minimum of a bachelor's degree.

Keflex™ (KEF-leks)
Refer to **Cephalexin.**

Keppra™ (KEP-ruh)
Refer to **Levetiracetam.**

kerato-
A prefix meaning *cornea* or horny *tissue.*

Kernicterus (ker-NIK-tuhr-uhs)
A *disorder* that is caused by an *abnormally* high level of *bilirubin* in the *central nervous system*. It can result in *brain damage, choreoathetoid cerebral palsy, auditory impairment,* and *mental retardation* if it is not caught in time. Without treatment, kernicterus is fatal.

Ketoacidosis (kee-toe-a-si-DOE-sis)
A form of *metabolic acidosis* caused by an excessive accumulation of *ketone bodies* in the blood, as in *diabetes* or starvation. (Ketone bodies are substances that increase in the blood as a result of faulty *carbohydrate metabolism*. An example of a ketone body is acetone, a chemical found in solvents such as nail polish remover.)
Refer to **Acidosis.**

Ketogenic Diet (kee-toe-JEN-ik)
A diet high in *fats* and low in *carbohydrates*, and carefully prescribed *protein* for body maintenance and growth. It is sometimes used in the treatment of uncontrollable *seizure disorders* when there has not been a good response to *drug therapy*. The goal is to achieve *ketosis*, which raises the *seizure threshold*. The ketogenic diet can be difficult to maintain because foods need to be carefully weighed, there is not a lot of variety in the diet, and the diet must be strictly followed. The ketogenic diet is also sometimes prescribed for certain *metabolic* disorders.

Ketone Body (KEE-toen)
A substance that increases in the blood as a result of faulty *carbohydrate metabolism*. An example of a ketone body is acetone, a chemical found in solvents such as nail polish remover.

Ketosis (kee-TOE-sis)
A condition in which there is an increased production of *ketone bodies* in the body, such as in *diabetes mellitus* or starvation.

kg
The abbreviation for *kilogram*.

Kidney
One of two organs located on each side of the *spine*, in back below the ribs. The kidneys filter waste products from the blood (in the form of urine) so it can be eliminated from the body.

Kidney Failure
> *Refer to* **Renal Failure.**

Killer Cell
A small *lymphocyte* without B or *T cell* markers that destroys certain *abnormal cells*.
> *Refer to* **Lymphocyte.**

Killer T Cell
A *T cell* that secretes chemical compounds essential to the *immune system*, assists B cells in destroying foreign *protein*, and appears to play a significant role in fighting *cancer*.
> *Refer to* **T Cell.**

Kilogram (kg)
The unit of weight of the metric system that equals 1000 grams or 2.2 pounds.

Kindling
The "learned" response of the *cells* in the *brain* to have more *seizures*.

Kinesthesia (kin-is-THEE-zee-uh)
The muscle sense by which the child is aware of his body position and his movements in relation to the environment.

Kinesthetic (kin-is-THET-ik)
Related to *kinesthesia*.

Kinesthetic Learner
A child who learns best through movement and touch. For example, playing a game of "follow the leader" that involves climbing in a box and *crawling* under a table might be an activity that would help the kinesthetic learner understand what the prepositions "in" and "under" mean.
> *Also known as an* **Active Learner.**

Kinney Sticks™
Crutches that include *bands* around the forearms.

Klebsiella (kleb-see-EL-uh)
A kind of *bacteria* frequently associated with *respiratory* infections, such as infection that can cause *pneumonia*.
Refer to **Pneumonia.**

Klinefelter Syndrome (KLIEN-fel-tuhr)
A *genetic disorder* in which a boy is born with at least one extra *X chromosome*. The disorder is characterized by low to *normal intelligence*, small penis and *testes*, sterility, female-like breasts, usually minimal tendency toward obesity, long *limbs* with relatively tall stature, and chronic *pulmonary disease*. The more X chromosomes there are, the greater the number of *congenital defects* and the more severe the *mental retardation*.
Also known as **XXY Syndrome** *and* **47, XXY Syndrome.**

Klonopin™ (KLON-oe-pin)
Refer to **Clonazepam.**

Knee-Ankle-Foot Orthosis (KAFO)
A long leg *brace* used to passively stretch muscles and to stabilize *joints*.
Refer to **Orthosis.**

Knee Jerk Reflex
Refer to **Patellar Reflex.**

Knee Joint Hyperextensibility
Refer to **Genu Recurvatum.**

Kneel-Stand Position
To stand on the knees.

Knock Knees
Refer to **Genu Valgum.**

Kugelberg-Welander Disease
The mildest form of *spinal muscular atrophy* (a *disorder* characterized by weakness and wasting of muscle caused by *spinal cord nerve* defect). This *autosomal recessive disorder* progresses slowly, and usually the patient is still able to walk 20 years after onset. Onset is typically late childhood or adolescence. *Intervention* such as *physical therapy* and *orthopedic* care can help the child develop or maintain *motor skills*.
Also known as **Juvenile Spinal Muscular Atrophy.**
Refer to **Spinal Muscular Atrophy.**

Kwashiorkor (kwah-shee-OR-kor)
Severe *protein malnutrition* that primarily affects children between 1 and 3 years of age who are suddenly weaned onto a *nutritionally* insufficient diet. It results in stunted growth, *edema* (fluid retention that causes swelling), weakness, lethargy, skin disorder, enlargement of the *liver*, *dehydration*, and loss of resistance against serious infection. The condition may lead to death.

Kyphoscoliosis (kie-foe-skoe-lee-OE-sis)

An exaggerated curve of the upper part of the *spine* creating a "humped" appearance in addition to a lateral curve of the spine.

*Refer to **Scoliosis** and **Kyphosis**.*

Kyphosis (kie-FOE-sis)

An exaggerated curve of the upper part of the *spine*, creating a rounded back. Kyphosis can be caused by a disorder of the spine, a *tumor*, a fracture, or poor *posture*.

*Compare **Scoliosis** and **Lordosis**.*

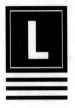

L
The abbreviation for left.

L1 Syndrome
An X-linked *recessive disorder* characterized by *hydrocephalus* with *stenosis* (constriction) of the *cerebral acqueduct, mental retardation, hypotonia* progressing to *spasticity, adducted* thumbs, *agenesis of corpus callosum,* and *aphasia.* Boys are affected by this disorder (girls can be *carriers* of L1 syndrome), and the characteristics of the disorder can range from severe to mild.

Labeling
1. Naming objects or actions the child encounters, such as by saying to the child, "Here comes the red ball! You caught it!"
2. Identifying someone by her *disability,* such as by describing an infant as a "mentally retarded baby." Although identifying a child's *at-risk* factors or disability is a necessary step in determining her eligibility for *early intervention* or *special education* services, using *people first language* (i.e., "a baby with mental retardation") is the current and preferred custom.

labi-/labio-
A prefix meaning lip.

-labial
A suffix meaning lip.

Labile (LAY-biel)
Unstable or changing.

Labiodental Speech Sound
Sound that is produced by the contact of the lower lip and the upper teeth, such as the /v/ sound.

Labor
The process of childbirth from dilation of the *cervix* to delivery of the infant and *placenta.*

Labor Contraction
Refer to **Uterine Contraction.**

Labyrinth (LAB-uh-rinth)
The *inner ear*, which contains the three ring-shaped structures called the *vestibular apparatus* (which function to provide the sense of *balance* and position), and the *cochlea* (which makes *hearing* possible).
Refer to **Ear.**

Labyrinthitis (lab-uh-rin-THIE-tis)
Inflammation of the *inner ear* which causes *vertigo* (a feeling that one's surroundings or one's own body is spinning) and loss of *balance*. Labyrinthitis is usually caused by a *bacterial* or *viral* infection.

Laceration (las-uh-RAY-shuhn)
A wound resulting from the tearing of the skin.

Lacrima (LAK-ri-muh)
Tears, or fluid, from the eye.

Lacrimal Bone (LAK-rim-uhl)
A small bone of the skull located in the front and *medial* part of the *orbit* (the bony socket that contains the eye) near the tear *duct* opening.

Lacrimal Duct (LAK-ri-muhl DUKT)
One of two channels through which tears pass from the eyes.

Lacrimal Duct Stenosis (LAK-ri-muhl DUKT sti-NOE-sis)
A narrowing, or blockage, of the *lacrimal duct*. It can result in irritation and infection in the eye.

Lacrimal Gland (LAK-ri-muhl)
The *gland* that *secretes* tears.

Lactation
The production of milk by the breasts.

Lactic Acid (LAK-tik)
A chemical made of 3 *carbons* that is produced by the body. (It is also found in certain *bacteria*.)

Lactic Acidosis (LAK-tic as-i-DOE-sis)
A condition that develops when *lactic acid* accumulates in the blood. It occurs most often due to insufficient *oxygen* in body *tissue* but can be the result of other organ *disease* or impairment.

Lactose
Sugar found in milk.

Lactose Intolerance

Inability to digest milk and some dairy products, which may be a *congenital* condition or develop in later years due to a deficiency in the *enzyme* lactase, which is necessary for *absorption* of *lactose*. Treatment is by dietary restrictions.

-lalia

A suffix meaning a *disorder* of speech.

Lallation

Repetitive, unintelligible utterances. Sometimes the term lallation is used to describe an infant's normal *babbling*, but more frequently it is used to describe the unintelligible speech sounds of a person with *severe mental retardation* or *schizophrenia*.

Landau-Kleffner Syndrome (LKS) (LAHN-dou KLEF-nuhr)

A form of *acquired aphasia* with accompanying controllable *seizures* (in 80 percent of cases). Children with this *syndrome* lose the ability to understand and use spoken language (*verbal auditory agnosia*). LKS can develop gradually or suddenly, between 3-7 years of age, either after the first seizure or with the onset of language difficulties. Children with LKS seem as if they have lost the ability to hear, but actually, *hearing* is intact. The cause is unknown; however, all children with LKS have *abnormal* electrical *brain* activity. Most children with LKS have *normal intelligence*. Some children improve or even recover, and most children are seizure-free by 15 years of age.

> *Also known as* **Acquired Childhood Epileptic Aphasia, Acquired Epileptic Aphasia,** *and* **Infantile Acquired Aphasia.**
> *Refer to* **Aphasia.**

Landau Reflex (LAN-dou)

A normal response in children 6 months to 2½ years old of straightening out the *spine* and legs (the legs slightly flexed) and the head raised (maintaining a convex arc position) when held *prone*, mid-air, with support around the trunk. This *reflex* is normally not present in children younger than 6 months and older than 2½ years. The reflex is exaggerated in a baby with *hypertonia* and poor in a baby with *hypotonia*.

> *Refer to* **Primitive Reflex.**

Landouzy-Déjérine Muscular Dystrophy

> *Refer to* **Fascioscapulohumeral Muscular Dystrophy.**

Language

> *Refer to* **Expressive Language** *and* **Receptive Language.**

Language Disorder

An inability to or difficulty with expressing, understanding, or processing language (oral or written information). Language disorders often occur in children who have other *disorders*, including *cerebral palsy*, a *chromosomal* or *genetic* disorder, or a structural *anomaly* of the speech or *hearing* systems.

A child can have a language disorder without any other apparent condition. *Aphasia* is an example of a language disorder.

> Compare **Speech Disorder.**

Lanugo (la-NOO-goe)
Fine, downy hair that covers the body of the *fetus*. It is almost all shed by the ninth month of *gestation*.

Large for Gestational Age (LGA)
A newborn infant who is above the 90th percentile in weight for her *gestational age*.

> Compare **Appropriate for Gestational Age** and **Small for Gestational Age.**
> Refer to the **CDC Growth Charts** in the Appendix.

Large Intestine
The portion of the *digestive tract* made up of the *cecum* (the chamber at the beginning of the large intestine); the *appendix*; the ascending, transverse, descending, and *sigmoid colons*; and the *rectum*.

> Refer to **Bowel** and **Small Intestine.**

laryngo-
A prefix meaning *larynx*.

Laryngologist (ler-in-GOL-oe-jist)
A medical doctor who specializes in the care of the *larynx* (voice box).

Laryngomalacia (ler-ing-goe-muh-LAY-shee-uh)
Softening of the *tissues* of the *larynx* that may result in *stridor* (an *abnormal* high-pitched breath sound). It is typically a *congenital* condition and, if so, is usually outgrown in 2 years.

Laryngopharynx (ler-in-goe-FER-ingks)
The lowest portion of the *pharynx*, or throat. It lies below the *hyoid* bone (the bone lying at the base of the tongue).

> Refer to **Pharynx.**

Laryngoscope (ler-IN-goe-skope)
A long, lighted tube that allows the doctor to see the vocal cords during the process of *intubation*, and to perform *diagnostic* and surgical procedures such as removal of a *tumor* on the *larynx*.

Laryngotracheobronchitis (le-ring-goe-tray-kee-oe-brong-KIE-tis)
> Refer to **Croup.**

Larynx (LER-ingks)
The voice box. The larynx is located in the throat and functions to produce voice.

Lasix™ (LAY-siks)
Refer to **Furosemide.**

Latency Period (LAY-tuhn-see)
1. The period of time between contact with a *pathogen* (any *microorganism* capable of causing *disease*) and onset of *symptoms*.
2. The time between a *stimulus* and a response, such as the time between when an infant's foot is touched and when she looks at or touches the same spot.
   Also known as **Incubation Period.**

Late Onset Autistic Disorder
Refer to **Childhood Disintegrative Disorder.**

later-/latero-
A prefix meaning side.

Lateral (LAT-uh-ruhl)
Relating to the side.
   Compare **Bilateral.**

Laterality
1. Internal awareness of the right and left sides of the body and their differences.
2. The tendency to use preferentially the organs on one side of the body (having a sidedness), especially when engaging in voluntary movement. This is determined by dominance of one *cerebral hemisphere* over the other. Preferring to use the right hand to catch a ball and the right foot to kick a ball is an example of laterality.
   Refer to **Hand Preference.**

Lateralization (lat-uh-ral-ie-ZAY-shuhn)
Affecting one side of the body, such as one *hemisphere* of the *brain*.

Lateral Pinch
Grasp of a tiny object using the thumb and the side of the index finger.
   Compare **Neat Pincer Grasp.**

Lateral Rotation
A turning away from the *midline* of the body, such as when twisting the arm outward.
   Compare **Medial Rotation.**

Laurence-Moon Syndrome (LAW-rens MOON)
An *autosomal recessive disorder* characterized by *retinitis pigmentosa*, underdeveloped *genitals*, *abnormally* decreased functional activity of the *gonads*, *mild* to *moderate mental retardation*, and *spastic paraplegia*.

Lax/Laxity
Loose or slack.

Laxative
A substance that is used to treat *constipation* by increasing the bulk of the *feces*, by softening the stool, or by lubricating the intestinal wall.

LBW
The abbreviation for low birth weight.

LD
The abbreviation for learning disability.

LE
The abbreviation for lower extremity.

LEA
The abbreviation for Local Education Agency.

Lead Agency
The state agency responsible for the provision of *early intervention* services. The lead agency (or an agency with which it contracts) provides intake, *assessment*, referral to services needed by the child and/or family, and service coordination.

Lead Poisoning
Illness caused by ingesting or inhaling lead that can result in *anemia* and damage to many organs, including the *brain, kidneys, liver*, and *gastrointestinal* system. *Seizures, brain damage, paralysis*, and death can also result.

Lead Wires
Wires that lead from *electrodes* placed on the body to a monitoring device (such as an *electrocardiograph*, or *EKG*, machine) that records the body's electrical activity.

LEAP
*The abbreviation for **Learning Experiences…An Alternative Program for Preschoolers and Parents**.*

Learning Disability (LD)
As defined in the *Individuals with Disabilities Education Improvement Act of 2004* (formerly *Education for All Handicapped Children Act, PL 94-142*), "…a *disorder* in one or more of the basic psychological processes involved in understanding or in using language, spoken or written, which may manifest itself in an imperfect ability to listen, speak, read, write, spell, or do mathematical calculations." Children with learning disabilities may have problems with learning for a variety of reasons, including *hyperactivity* and *dyslexia*. These children have average or above average *intelligence* and learning potential.

Learning Experiences...An Alternative Program for Preschoolers and Parents (LEAP)

An *inclusive* preschool program, located in Pittsburgh, Pennsylvania, for 3- to 5-year-olds who have an *autism spectrum disorder* and their non-disabled peers. LEAP uses a *developmentally* based early childhood curriculum and provides supplemental activities that address the social, language, and *adaptive behavior* needs of the students with *ASD*. The *typically developing* students interact with the children with ASD in naturalistic play and teaching activities, as well as in small group play activities in which the typically developing children have been trained to facilitate the learning of the children with ASD (peer mediated learning).

Learning Style

The way in which a child best acquires knowledge or processes information. For example, some children learn best by listening (*auditory learners), and others by doing (kinesthetic learners*).

Learning Support Assistant

*Refer to **Paraprofessional**.*

Least Restrictive Environment (LRE)

The educational setting that permits a child with *disabilities* to derive the most educational benefit while participating in a regular educational environment to the maximum extent appropriate. LRE is a requirement under *IDEA 2004*.

*Refer to **Education for All Handicapped Children Act of 1975** and **Individuals with Disabilities Education Improvement Act of 2004**.*

Lecithin (LES-ith-in)

A group of *fats*, rich in *phosphorus*, found in plants and animals. Lecithin is also one of the components of *surfactant*.

Legally Blind

*Refer to **Blindness**.*

Leigh Disease (LEE)

A serious *mitochondrial disease* characterized by *brain damage, hypotonia, seizures, cognitive* dysfunction, inability to eat due to lack of appetite, vomiting, delayed *development*, and eye and breathing *disorders*. The disease is usually fatal before age 3.

*Also known as **Subacute Necrotizing Encephalomyelopathy** and **Subacute Necrotizing Encephalopathy**.*

Lens

1. The part of the eye that functions to focus an image on the *retina*. The lens is located between the *iris* of the eye and the *vitreous humor* (the gel-like substance of the eye).
2. A curved, transparent piece of glass or plastic that is formed to produce *refraction* in a specific way, as in eyeglasses or microscopes.

   *Also known as **Crystalline Lens**.*

   *Refer to **Eye**.*

Lesch-Nyhan Syndrome (LNS) (lesh-NI-uhn)

An *X-linked recessive metabolic disorder* characterized by *hyperuricemia* (an *abnormal* level of *uric acid* in the blood); *pyramidal cerebral palsy; choreoathetosis; mental retardation;* and *self-injurious behavior* to the point of self-mutilation. The hyperuricemia is caused by absence of an *enzyme* (*HGPRT*, or *hypoxanthine guanine phosphoribosyltransferase*) necessary for controlling production of uric acid. The *motor* problems result in *hypertonia*; jerky, *involuntary movements*; and, usually, the inability to walk or sit independently. The self-injurious behavior typically consists of biting the lips or fingers to the point of destruction, requiring the child to be restrained. (Some behavioral interventionists feel this is a more comfortable option since the child experiences pain from the biting *behaviors*.) Lesch-Nyhan syndrome is a rare *disorder* that only affects males. Boys with LNS may live into their teens.

Lesion (LEE-zhen)

Any wound or injury, or *pathologic* change in body *tissue*.

leuk-, leuko-

Prefixes meaning white.

Leukemia (loo-KEE-mee-uh)

Any of several types of *cancer* in which there is proliferation (rapid reproduction) of *white blood cells* in the *bone marrow*. This leads to an excessive number of leukemic *cells* accumulating in the blood and in body organs, such as the *brain, liver, spleen,* and *lymph nodes,* and to dysfunction of these organs. In addition, the production of leukemic cells causes the production of *red blood cells, platelets,* and normal white blood cells to be impaired. Leukemias are classified as either acute or chronic types. Chronic leukemia rarely develops in children. A type of acute leukemia called acute lymphoblastic leukemia is the most common type in children. It appears to result from *mutation* of a single white blood cell. Treatment is by anticancer drugs, blood and platelet transfusion, and, sometimes, *radiation therapy*. Bone marrow transplantation may also be considered. Treatment may provide a cure.

Leukocyte (LOO-koe-siet)

*Refer to **White Blood Cell**.*

Leukomalacia (loo-koe-muh-LAY-shuh)

*Refer to **Periventricular Leukomalacia**.*

Levetiracetam (lev-uh-ter-AS-uh-tam)

An *antiepileptic drug* used to treat *complex partial seizures*. Keppra™ is the brand name of this drug.

Levothyroxine Sodium (lee-voe-thie-ROK-seen SOE-dee-uhm)

A thyroid replacement *hormone* used to treat *hypothyroidism*. Synthroid™ is the brand name for this drug.

Lexical Syntactic Syndrome (LSS) (LEK-si-kuhl sin-TAK-tik)

A type of *developmental language disorder* characterized by *dysfluent speech*, *paraphasias* (forms of *aphasia* in which the child does not correctly use spoken words or word groupings), immature *syntax*, normal phonologic skills, and intelligible speech. Comprehension is usually adequate, although there are frequently difficulties with higher-level *receptive language* skills.

Lexicon

The words in a language.

LGA

The abbreviation for large for gestational age.

Lice

1. Parasitic insects that can be found in the hair or on the body of humans. *Secretions* from the bites can result in a *rash* which, if scratched, can become infected with *bacteria*. (Infestation with lice commonly causes itching.) Lice are transmitted via direct contact with infected persons and indirect contact with the infected person's belongings, such as a hair brush or hat.
2. Plural of louse.
   Refer to **Pediculosis** *and* **Nits.**

Licensed Practical Nurse (LPN)

A *nurse* who is trained in basic nursing techniques and who provides care to patients under the supervision of *registered nurses* and doctors.
   Compare **Licensed Vocational Nurse** *and* **Registered Nurse.**

Licensed Vocational Nurse (LVN)

A *licensed practical nurse* who is permitted by license to practice in certain states.
   Compare **Registered Nurse.**

Life Support Machine

   Refer to **Ventilator.**

Ligament (LIG-uh-muhnt)

One of many *bands* of *fibrous tissue* that binds *joints* together and connects bones and *cartilage*. Ligaments are flexible and help facilitate body movements.

Ligation (lie-GAY-shuhn)

A surgical procedure to close, or tie off, a *duct* or *blood vessel*. Ligation is sometimes required to close a *patent ductus arteriosus*.

Light Perception (LP)

The ability to distinguish light from dark.

Limb (LIM)

An *extremity* of the body, such as an arm or leg.

Limb Girdle Muscular Dystrophy
An *autosomal recessive* form of *muscular dystrophy* characterized by weakness in the muscles of the hips and shoulders.

Limbic System (LIM-bik)
A group of structures within the *brain* associated with various emotions such as fear, sadness, pleasure, and anger.

Linear Growth
Height gain.

Lingua (LING-gwuh)
The tongue.
> *Also known as* **Glossa.**

Lingual
Pertaining to the tongue.

Lingual Frenulum (FREN-yoo-lum)
> *Refer to* **Lingual Frenum.**

Lingual Frenum (FREE-nuhm)
Mucous membrane that attaches the tongue to the floor of the mouth.
> *Also known as* **Lingual Frenulum.**
> *Refer to* **Ankyloglossia** *and* **Frenum.**

Linguistics
The study of the origin and structure of language.

Linkage Analysis
A method for *diagnosing* a *genetic disorder* for which a specific *gene* change has not yet been identified. *DNA* samples from both affected and unaffected family members are needed and the goal is to compare *genetic* variations between affected and unaffected family members and, sometimes, to be able to trace a gene's transmission. Linkage analysis sometimes helps scientists discover specific *disease* genes so that *Direct DNA analysis* can be utilized.

Lioresal™ (lie-OR-uh-sahl)
> *Refer to* **Baclofen.**

lip-
A prefix meaning fat (as in *lipid*).

Lip Closure
Bringing the lips together. Lip closure is necessary for many functions, including production of certain speech sounds (/m/, /b/, and /p/) and drinking from a cup.

Lipid (LIP-id)
Fatty substances in *tissue*.

lipo-
A prefix meaning fat.

Lipodystrophy (lip-oe-DIS-troe-fee)
A condition caused by *abnormal metabolism* of *fats* in the body, in which the fat deposits under the skin disappear in patches and sometimes build up in other areas.

Lipreading
>   Refer to **Speechreading**.

Lisp
A type of speech delay in which the child substitutes the "th" sound for the "s" and "z" sounds. For example, the child may say "toyth" instead of "toys."

Lissencephaly (lis-en-SEF-uh-lee)
A rare malformation in which the *fetal* brain fails to develop, resulting in a smooth *brain* surface. (A "smooth brain surface" means that the normal *convolutions* in the *cerebral cortex* of the brain do not develop and the brain remains small in size.) Lissencephaly is characterized by *microcephaly*; *failure to thrive*; initial *hypotonia* that is later replaced by *hypertonia*; *seizures*; finger and toe *anomalies*; *cardiovascular* anomalies; and *severe mental retardation*. Some children with lissencephaly also have other *disorders* such as *Miller-Dieker syndrome* or *Zellweger syndrome*. Children with lissencephaly usually do not live beyond early childhood.
>   *Also known as* **Agyria**.

lith/litho-
A prefix meaning stone.

Liver
The largest internal organ, located on the right beneath the *diaphragm*. The liver has many functions, including producing *proteins* and metabolizing proteins, sugars, and *fats*; producing *bile* and purifying the blood; and storing sugars and fats.

LKS
The abbreviation for Landau-Kleffner Syndrome.

LLE
The abbreviation for left lower extremity.

LNS
The abbreviation for Lesch-Nyhan Syndrome.

Local Anesthesia/Anesthetic (an-es-THEE-zee-uh/an-es-THET-ik)
Refer to Anesthesia.

Local Education Agency (LEA)
The agency responsible for providing *special educational* services on the local (school district, city, and county) level.

Localization
Limitation to one place or part.

Localize
The ability to "find" a sensation one is experiencing, such as touching or looking at the foot when it is touched, or turning the head and eyes to the source of a voice or sound.

Local Seizure
An older term for a *partial seizure.*
Refer to Partial Seizure and Epilepsy.

Loci (LOE-sie or LOE-kee)
Plural of *locus.*

Lockjaw
Refer to Tetanus and Trismus.

Locomotion
The educational term for movement from one place to another.

Locomotor
Referring to *locomotion.*

Locus (LOE-kuhs)
A specific place, such as the locus (position) of a particular *gene* on a *chromosome.*

Locutionary Stage (loe-KYOO-shuhn-er-ee)
A verbal stage of language *development* in which the young child uses words and sentences intentionally. It typically emerges around 15 months.
Refer to Perlocutionary Stage and Illocutionary Stage.

Lofstrand Crutches™
Crutches that have a *band* around the forearm and a handle.

Longitudinal (lon-juh-TOO-duh-nuhl)
Referring to a study in which the same group of children are tested repeatedly on the same items as they get older.

Long Leg Sitting
Sitting with the legs extended to the front and slightly apart.

Lorazepam (lor-A-zuh-pam)

A *psychotropic drug* used to treat *seizures*. It is also used to sedate and to treat *anxiety disorders*. Ativan™ is the brand name of this drug.

Lordosis (lor-DOE-sis)

An exaggerated *curvature of the spine*. Lordosis is most often noted in the lower *spine*, creating a swayback appearance. Weak *abdominal* muscles and poor *posture* contribute to excessive lordosis, as can *neuromuscular disease*.

> *Also known as* **Swayback.**
> *Compare* **Kyphosis** *and* **Scoliosis.**

Lorenz Night Splint™

A *splint* that is usually worn during sleep to separate the child's legs to stretch the *adductors* and prevent *hip dislocation*.

Louis-Bar Syndrome

> *Refer to* **Ataxia-Telangiectasia.**

Louse (LOUS)

Singular of *lice*.

Lovaas Method (LOE-vahs)

An intensive behavioral *intervention* approach (a form of *discrete trial instruction*) used to teach the young child with an *autism spectrum disorder*, developed by Dr. O. Ivar Lovaas.

Low Birth Weight Infant (LBW)

A baby who weighs less than 2500 grams (approximately 5 pounds, 8 ounces) at birth. Low birth weight can result from prematurity (and may be average for the baby's *gestational age*) or from *intrauterine growth retardation* (and be *small for gestational age*).

> *Compare* **Birth Weight, Very Low Birth Weight Infant,** *and* **Extremely Low Birth Weight Infant.**
> *Refer to* **Premature Infant.**

Low Blood Sugar

> *Refer to* **Hypoglycemia.**

Lower Extremity (LE)

One of either leg.

Lower GI

Pertaining to the lower *gastrointestinal tract* (the *jejunum* and *ileum* of the *large* and *small intestines*.) Lower GI is commonly used to refer to the *barium enema* test.

Lower Respiratory Tract Infection (LRI)

An infection affecting the *trachea, bronchi*, or the lungs.

> *Compare* **Upper Respiratory Infection.**

Lowe Syndrome

An *X-linked recessive disorder* characterized by *failure to thrive, hypotonia*, eye *abnormalities* including *cataracts* and *blindness, kidney* abnormalities, *cryptorchidism (undescended testes)*, diminished or absent *deep tendon reflexes, hyperactivity*, and *mental retardation*.

Also known as **Oculocerebrorenal Syndrome**.

Low Tone/Low Muscle Tone

Refer to **Hypotonia**.

Low Vision

A *label* used by many school systems to describe children with corrected *visual acuity* of less than 20/70 in the better eye. Low vision may be enhanced by *optical* aids, such as magnifying devices and special *lenses*.

Low Vision Aid

A device that helps people to see. These *optical* aids are used when prescription *lenses* do not help, or in addition to prescription lenses to magnify things such as words on a page.

LP

1. The abbreviation for lumbar puncture.
2. The abbreviation for light perception.

LPN

The abbreviation for licensed practical nurse.

LRE

The abbreviation for least restrictive environment.

LRI

The abbreviation for lower respiratory tract infection.

LSO

The abbreviation for lumbar-sacral orthosis.

L/S Ratio

The relative proportions between *lecithin* and *sphingomyelin* (components of *surfactant*) in the *amniotic fluid*. A higher amount of L in relation to S indicates the maturity of the unborn baby's lungs. This is because lecithin levels increase after 35 weeks *gestation*.

LUE

The abbreviation for left upper extremity.

Lumbar (LUM-bahr)

Referring to the lower back or to the part of the body between the *thorax* (the chest) and the *pelvis*. The last 5 *vertebrae* are the lumbar vertebrae.

Lumbar Puncture (LP)
A procedure involving the insertion of a hollow needle in between the *vertebrae* of the lower back to withdraw *cerebrospinal fluid* or to inject drugs, contrast (to perform an *x-ray* study), or an *anesthetic*.
> Also known as a **Spinal Tap**.

Lumbar-Sacral Orthosis (LSO)
A *brace* that counteracts spinal deformities such as *scoliosis*, *kyphosis*, and *lordosis*.
> Refer to **Orthosis**.

Luminal™ (LOO-mi-nahl)
> Refer to **Phenobarbital**.

Lungs
The organs located in both sides of the chest which function to supply the body with *oxygen* from air that is inhaled, and to rid the body of *carbon dioxide* with the air that is exhaled.

LVN
The abbreviation for licensed vocational nurse.

Lymph (LIMF)
A body fluid that plays an important role in the *immune system* and in absorbing *fats* from the *intestine*. Lymph provides a defense against local *infection*.

Lymphatic System (lim-FAT-ik)
A vast, complex network of tubes, *nodes*, organs, and *valves* that produces, filters, and conveys *lymph*; produces various *blood cells*; transports *fats*, *proteins*, and other substances to the blood system; and restores the majority of the fluid that is filtered during normal *metabolism*.

Lymph Node
One of many small *glands* clustered throughout the body that fight infection by housing the *white blood cells* that produce *antibodies* and filter out and destroy *bacteria*.

Lymphocyte (LIM-foe-siet)
One of two principal kinds of *white blood cells*: *B cells* and *T cells*. B cells primarily function to produce *antibodies*. T cells are principally responsible for initiating and regulating the *immune system*.

Lymphoid (LIM-foid)
Pertaining to *lymph* or the *lymphatic system*.

-lysis
A suffix meaning breakdown, separation, or destruction.

Lysis (LIE-sis)
Destruction of a *cell* by damage to its outer *membrane*.

Lysosomal Storage Disease (lie-suh-SOE-muhl)
Any of a group of *diseases* caused by a defective lysosomal *enzyme* and, as a result, the *lysosome* stores rather than metabolizes *biochemicals* in the body. *Niemann-Pick disease* is an example of a Lysosomal Storage Disease.
    *Also known as **Inborn Lysosomal Disease.***

Lysosome (LIE-soe-soem)
A small structure within a *cell* that contains *enzymes* that break down large molecules and are capable of metabolizing certain chemicals in the body.

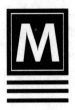

M
The abbreviation for male.

MA
The abbreviation for mental age.

Macrencephaly (mak-ren-SEF-uh-lee)
An *abnormally* large size of the *brain*. (The organ itself is larger than usual, rather than being enlarged due to *tumor* growth.)
    Compare **Megalencephaly.**

macro-
A prefix meaning long or large.

Macrocephaly (mak-roe-SEF-uh-lee)
An *abnormally* large head size in relation to the body. Macrocephaly may be *congenital* or *acquired*. *Mental retardation* is sometimes associated with this *congenital anomaly*.

Macroglossia (mak-roe-GLOS-ee-uh)
An *abnormally* large tongue.

Macrognathia (mak-roe-NAY-thee-uh)
An *abnormally* large jaw.

Macroorchidism (MAK-roe OR-kid-izm)
Abnormally large *testes*. This condition is common in males with *Fragile X syndrome*.

Macrophage (MAK-roe-fayj)
A type of large *white blood cell* found in *tissue* that destroys foreign substances which have entered the body.

Macrosomia (mak-roe-SOE-mee-uh)
An *abnormally* large body size.

Macrostomia (mak-roe-STOE-mee-uh)
A very large mouth.

Macule (MAK-yool)
A small, flat skin discoloration, such as a freckle.
Compare **Papule.**

Magnesium Sulfate (mag-NEE-see-uhm SUL-fayt)
A drug used in the treatment of *toxemia* and in stopping pre-term *labor*. It is also used to stimulate the production of *bowel movements*.

Magnetic Resonance Imaging (MRI)
A *diagnostic* procedure that involves creating cross-sectional images of body organs and structures. MRI is done by exposing the patient to a magnetic field while lying inside a large magnet structure. Images or "maps" are created when the body's hydrogen ions move (the movement is caused by exposure to radio waves), producing a radio signal that is detected and changed by computer to an image. Body *tissue* that contains a large amount of hydrogen will produce a bright image. Body tissue that contains little or no hydrogen is dark. No radiation is used in MRI.

Mainstreaming
Placing a child with *disabilities* in a general education classroom or in the educational setting that is as close to typical as possible. Mainstreaming may allow the child with disabilities to be a member of a regular classroom, even though supplemental resource services may be needed and provided.
Refer to **Inclusion** *and* **Integration.**

mal-
A prefix meaning *abnormal*, bad, or poor.

Malabsorption (mal-uhb-SORP-shuhn)
A condition in which the *absorption* of nutrients from the *gastrointestinal tract* is impaired. It occurs in a variety of diseases, such as *celiac disease* and may result from conditions such as *malnutrition* or an *inborn error of metabolism*.
Compare **Absorption** *and* **Reabsorption.**

malac-, malaco-
Prefixes meaning soft.

Malacia (muh-LAY-shee-uh)
An *abnormal* softening in an organ due to *degeneration* of its *tissues*.

Malar (MAY-lar)
Refer to **Zygomatic Bone.**

Malecot Tube™
A *gastrostomy tube*.

Malignancy/Malignant (muh-LIG-nuhn-see/muh-LIG-nuhnt)
A condition (often a *tumor*) that becomes progressively worse and will likely result in death. Malignancy frequently refers to *cancer* that is invasive or spreading to other organs.
>   *Compare* **Benign.**

Malleable (MAL-ee-uh-buhl)
Referring to something that is soft or easily molded.

Malleolus (muhl-EE-oe-luhs)
A rounded bone, such as those on each side of the ankle.

Malleus (MAL-ee-uhs)
One of the three small bones of the *middle ear*. (The other two bones are the *incus* and the *stapes*.)
>   *Also known as* **Hammer.**
>   *Refer to* **Ear.**

Malnutrition
Nutritional disorders that develop for a variety of reasons, including an unbalanced diet (usually lacking in *carbohydrate* or *protein*), a diet consisting of too little food or too much food, or the improper body utilization of foods.
>   *Compare* **Nutrition.**

Malocclusion (mal-uh-KLOO-zhuhn)
An *abnormal* relationship of the teeth of the upper jaw with the teeth of the lower jaw based on their contact or the bite. (For example, teeth may meet improperly, overlap too much, or not overlap at all). Malocclusion is usually the result of *heredity*. It may also result from thumb-sucking.

mammo-
A prefix meaning breast.

Mand
A request or instruction. For example, "please sit down" is a mand. Mand is derived from the word "com*mand*" or "de*mand*," and is a concept developed by American psychologist B.F. Skinner as he studied the functions of how people use language to communicate.

Mandated Reporter
Any professional who is required by law to report cases of child abuse or *neglect*. The professional needs only to have reasonable suspicion of abuse or neglect. Individuals who are considered to be mandated reporters include child care custodians (such as teachers, administrative officers, *social workers*, foster parents, and certificated pupil personnel employees) and health practitioners (such as *physicians*, *nurses*, *psychologists*, dentists, and counselors).
>   *Refer to* **Child Abuse and Neglect** *and* **Emotional Abuse.**

Mandible (MAN-di-buhl)
The lower jaw bone.

Mandibulofacial Dysostosis (man-dib-yuh-loe FAY-shuhl dis-os-TOE-sis)
Refer to Franceschetti Syndrome and Treacher Collins Syndrome.

Mantoux Test (man-TOO)
A test to determine the presence of tuberculous infection.
Refer to Tuberculosis.

Manual Alphabet
An alphabet of hand-signs that are used to spell out words. Each letter of the alphabet has its own sign.
Refer to Fingerspelling and Sign Language.

Manual Sign
Refer to Sign Language.

Manual Thrust
Refer to Heimlich Maneuver.

MAP
Abbreviation for Miller Assessment for Preschoolers.

Maple Syrup Urine Disease
Refer to Branched Chain Ketoaciduria.

Marasmus (muhr-AZ-muhs)
Severe *protein* calorie *malnutrition* that is primarily seen in young children with *failure to thrive* and in starving people.

Marfan Syndrome
A *connective tissue disorder* that affects many body systems, including the *musculoskeletal system* (underdeveloped muscles, *lax ligaments, joint hypermobility*, bone elongation), the *cardiovascular system*, and the eyes. It results in a tall and lanky body build, *scoliosis*, cardiovascular problems, and eye problems such as *nearsightedness* and *dislocation* of the *lens*. Marfan syndrome affects both males and females. With proper medical management, the *prognosis* and lifespan are greatly improved. Most often, Marfan syndrome occurs as an *autosomal dominant disorder*, but approximately one-quarter of the cases occur as a result of a spontaneous *genetic mutation*.
Refer to Arachnodactyly.

Marking Time Pattern
Refer to Non-reciprocal Gait.

Maroteaux-Lamy Syndrome (mah-roe-TOE lah-MEE)
An *autosomal recessive disorder* of *carbohydrate metabolism* (it is a *mucopolysaccharidosis*) with 3 clinical forms (severe, intermediate, and mild). It is

characterized by *coarse facial features*, irregular *dentition*, *visual impairment*, *small stature*, *kyphosis*, *genu valgum* (knock knees), finger *abnormalities*, tendency toward bone fractures and, typically, *normal intelligence*.

Also known as **Mucopolysaccharidosis VI** or **MPS VI**.

Marrow

Refer to **Bone Marrow.**

Marshall-Smith Syndrome

A rare, *sporadically* occurring *disorder* characterized by accelerated skeletal *maturation* (for example, a 2-week-old affected infant might have the wrist "bone age" of a 3- to 4-year-old). Other characteristics include accelerated early linear (length) growth with *failure to thrive* in weight followed by growth failure; chronic *respiratory disease* and *respiratory tract anomalies*; *dysmorphic* facial features, including prominent forehead and eyes, bluish *sclerae* (the normally white *membrane* starting at the edges of the *cornea* and covering most of the back of the eyeball), an upturned nose, small jaws, and low nasal bridge; *umbilical hernia*; bone *abnormalities* of the fingers or toes; *hypotonia*; *hypertrichosis* (excessive hair growth); and *mental retardation*. Children with Marshall-Smith Syndrome typically do not survive early childhood due to respiratory complications.

Martin-Bell Syndrome

Refer to **Fragile X Syndrome.**

masto-

A prefix meaning breast.

Mastoiditis (mas-toid-IE-tis)

A serious *inflammation* of the air *cells* of the mastoid bone behind the ear. Mastoiditis may result when *middle ear infection* spreads to the mastoid bone. It can cause *conductive hearing impairment*.

Maternal

1. *Inherited* or received from the mother.
2. Motherly in *behavior*.

Maturation (mach-uh-RAY-shuhn)

Referring to the process of becoming an adult or fully developed.

Maxilla (mak-SIL-uh)

One of a pair of bones that forms the upper jaw.

Maxillary

Pertaining to the upper jaw.

MBD

The abbreviation for minimal brain dysfunction.

McCarthy Scales of Children's Abilities
A *norm-referenced evaluation* tool used to assess the verbal, perceptual, quantitative, memory, *motor*, and *cognitive* abilities of children between 2½ and 8 years of age. Typically, the McCarthy is administered by a professional with a doctoral in psychology (Ph.D.) or education (Ed.D.) and/or has significant, relevant experience and training.

M-CHAT
The abbreviation for the Modified Checklist for Autism in Toddlers.

MD
The abbreviation for the Latin words meaning doctor of medicine.

MDR
The abbreviation for minimum daily requirement.

Mean
The average of a group of values (numbers). The mean is obtained by adding all of the values given and dividing by the number of items which were added.

Mean Length of Utterance (MLU)
The average number of *morphemes* per utterance (sentence or phrase).

Measles
A highly *contagious, viral* illness. *Symptoms* include high fever, runny nose, cough, *conjunctivitis*, discomfort, and an itchy red *rash*. Measles is spread by nasal *secretions*. Patients with measles may be sick enough to be hospitalized and may even die.
> *Also known as* **Rubeola.**
> *Compare* **Rubella (German Measles).**
> *Refer to* **Measles, Mumps, and Rubella Vaccine.**

Measles, Mumps, and Rubella Vaccine (MMR)
An *immunization* against *measles*, mumps, and *rubella* made from live, weakened strains of the 3 *viruses*. An injection of this *vaccine* is given to children between 12-15 months of age and again before starting school at 4½ to 6 years of age.

Meatus (mee-A-tuhs)
An opening or passageway in the body.

Mebaral™ (MEB-uh-rahl)
> *Refer to* **Mephobarbital.**

Meconium (mee-KOE-nee-uhm or me-KOE-nee-uhm)
A greenish-black material that collects in the *fetal* intestinal tract before birth and is usually passed during the first day or 2 after birth. Meconium passed before birth into the *amniotic fluid* (meconium staining) can indicate fetal dis-

tress. *Physicians* caring for the meconium-stained newborn must do all they can to prevent the baby from inhaling the meconium while taking his first breaths (meconium *aspiration*), because this can result in blocked airways.

Meconium Aspiration
> *Refer to* **Meconium.**

Meconium Plug
A solid plug of *meconium* blocking the *colon* of a newborn infant. A meconium plug may be identified when the newborn is unable to defecate within 48 hours after birth, or if the infant has vomiting or *abdominal* distention. It can be caused by a deficiency of certain necessary *secretions*. The meconium plug must be removed.
> *Refer to* **Meconium.**

Meconium Staining
> *Refer to* **Meconium.**

MED
The abbreviation for minimum effective dose.

med-/medi-
A prefix meaning middle.

Medial (MEE-dee-uhl)
Referring to a position toward the middle of the body.

Medial Rotation
A turning toward the middle of the body, such as the arm turning inward.
> *Compare* **Lateral Rotation.**

Median Plane
The vertical plane that divides the body into right and left halves.

Medicaid
A federally funded program that supports individual state programs in providing medical assistance to people who qualify for *Supplemental Security Income (SSI).*

Medically Fragile
Referring to an infant or child whose health status either is unstable, or renders him *at-risk* for *developmental delay* (often due to poor health or limitations on the infant's ability to participate in normal activities). Examples of infants who may be medically fragile include those who were *premature*, have *chronic lung disease*, or were *prenatally exposed to drugs.*

Medicare
A federal health insurance program that funds medical care for adults who are over 65 years old and for children and adults who are permanently disabled.

Medicine
Refer to **Drug**.

Medulla (muh-DUL-uh)
The innermost part of a body structure or organ.

Medulla Oblongata (muh-DUL-uh ob-long-GAH-tuh)
The lower part of the *brainstem* through which *nerve* fibers from higher *brain* centers pass on their way to the *spinal cord*. The *heart, blood vessel,* and breathing centers of the brain are contained in the medulla oblongata, and the nerve fibers of the *pyramidal tract* cross over in the medulla oblongata.
Refer to **Brain**.

mega-
A prefix meaning great or large.

Megalencephaly (meg-uhl-en-SEF-uh-lee)
A condition characterized by *disease* to the functional parts of the brain resulting in an *abnormally* large size of the brain. Usually, children with megalencephaly also have some level of *mental retardation*.
Compare **Macrencephaly**.

megalo-
A prefix meaning great or large.

Megalocephaly (meg-uh-loe-SEF-uh-lee)
An enlargement of the head that is most commonly caused by increased *intracranial* pressure with *hydrocephalus*. It may also be caused by excessive *brain* growth. Megalocephaly may be present at birth or be *acquired*. People with megalocephaly usually have *mental retardation*.

-megaly
A suffix meaning enlargement.

Megavitamin Therapy
Treatment with doses of *vitamins* greater than the amounts needed to prevent deficiency (per the RDA, or recommended daily allowance, suggested level). Extremely high doses of vitamins have been tried as an alternative therapy to treat *developmental disabilities* such as *autism spectrum disorders* and *Down syndrome*. The ability of megavitamin therapy to produce a desired effect on a child's *developmental disability* is unproven.
Compare **Orthomolecular Therapy**.

Meiosis (mie-OE-sis)
Division of sex *cells* (before fertilization occurs) into *daughter cells,* each containing half of the number of *chromosomes* (23) of regular cells. When egg and *sperm* cells unite, a total of 46 chromosomes are again present, producing a unique child with half of his *inherited genetic* material from his mother and half from his father.
Compare **Mitosis**.

Meiotic Division (mei-OT-ik)
*Refer to **Meiosis.***

melan-
A prefix meaning black.

Melatonin (mel-uh-TOE-nin)
A *hormone* produced by the human body that influences the sleep-wake cycle. Melatonin is also produced synthetically and is sometimes prescribed to treat sleeplessness.

Mellaril™ (MEL-uh-ril)
*Refer to **Thioridazine Hydrochloride**.*

Melnick-Fraser Syndrome
*Refer to **Branchio-Oto-Renal Syndrome**.*

Membrane
A thin layer of *tissue* that covers a body surface, divides a space or organ, or lines a cavity.

mening-
A prefix meaning *membrane*. It usually refers to the membranes covering the *brain* and *spinal cord*.

Meninges (men-IN-jez)
The *membranes* surrounding the *brain* and *spinal cord*. There are three layers of meninges, the *dura mater*, the *arachnoid*, and the *pia mater*.

Meningitis (men-in-JIE-tis)
Inflammation of the *meninges*, which is usually caused by either a *viral* or *bacterial* infection. Viral meningitis is usually mild and the infected child suffers no *brain damage*. Bacterial meningitis requires prompt medical attention, in the form of large doses of *antibiotic drugs*. Children with bacterial meningitis typically recover without brain damage if they receive immediate medical assistance.

Meningocele (men-IN-goe-seel)
A *congenital anomaly* in which the *meninges* (the *membranes* surrounding the *spinal cord*) protrude through an opening in the *spinal column* under the skin. This form of *spina bifida* must be surgically repaired, but the child usually suffers no functional problems such as the *paralysis* common to *myelocele*.
    Compare *Myelocele* and *Myelomeningocele*.
    *Refer to **Spina Bifida**.*

Meningoencephalitis (men-in-goe-en-sef-uh-LIE-tis)
An *inflammation* of both the *brain* and the *meninges*, usually caused by a *bacterial* infection. Meningoencephalitis can lead to serious illness, and, depending on the type of bacteria that caused the infection, can be fatal.

Meningoencephalocele (men-in-goe-en-SEF-uhl-oe-seel)
A *congenital anomaly* in which *brain tissue*, *cerebrospinal fluid*, and the *meninges* protrude through an opening in the skull. This condition usually results in *brain damage*.
>Also known as **Encephalomeningocele**.

Meningomyelocele (men-in-goe-mie-EL-oe-seel)
>Refer to **Myelomeningocele**.

mens-
A prefix meaning month.

Mental Age (MA)
The age level at which a child functions *cognitively*.
>Compare **Developmental Age**.

Mental Deficiency
>Refer to **Mental Retardation**.

Mental Handicap
In Canada, the preferred term for *mental retardation*.

Mental Health
>Refer to **Infant Mental Health**.

Mental Retardation (MR)
According to the *American Association on Mental Retardation* (1992), "mental retardation refers to substantial limitations in present functioning. It is characterized by significantly subaverage intellectual functioning, existing concurrently with related limitations in two or more of the following applicable *adaptive skill* areas: *communication*, self-care, home living, *social skills*, community use, self-direction, health and safety, functional academics, leisure, and work. Mental retardation manifests before age 18." In other words, someone with mental retardation performs significantly below his age level in both intellectual functioning (*intelligence*) and *adaptive behavior*. Mental retardation is the most common *developmental disability*, affecting about 2 to 3 percent of the population.
>Refer to **Intelligence** and **Oligophrenia**.

Mephobarbital (mef-oe-BAR-bi-tol)
A drug used to treat *seizure disorders* and *anxiety*. Mebaral™ is the brand name of this drug.

Mercury
A heavy, silver metal that is liquid at room temperature. Mercury is produced commercially and is used in many industries. Because it is highly poisonous, in 1999 it was determined that mercury-based preservatives should no longer be used in routine childhood *vaccines*.
>Refer to **Thimerosal**.

Mesencephalon (mes-en-SEF-uh-lon)
Refer to **Midbrain.**

meso-
A prefix meaning middle.

meta-
1. A prefix meaning beyond, after, or next.
2. A prefix meaning change or exchange.

Metabolic
Pertaining to *metabolism*.

Metabolic Acidosis
An excess of acid in the blood and body *tissues* that may develop due to illness, such as *respiratory distress syndrome* of the *premature infant, renal failure, diabetes mellitus,* or severe diarrhea. This can lead to a disruption of the chemical processes within the body.
Compare **Respiratory Acidosis.**

Metabolism
All the chemical processes carried out by the *cells* in the body that are necessary for sustaining life.
Refer to **Inborn Error of Metabolism.**

Metacarpals (met-uh-KAR-puhlz)
The five bones of the hand to which the finger bones are attached.

Metachromatic Leukodystrophy
(met-uh-kroe-MAT-ik loo-kuh-DIS-truh-fee)
An *autosomal recessive disorder* of *lipid metabolism* (a *sphingolipidosis*) in which the body does not produce enough of the *enzyme* cerebroside sulfatase. Deficiency of this enzyme results in an accumulation of metachromatic lipids, which leads to progressive *disease* of the *white matter* of the *brain*. It results in *ataxia, motor* problems, *dementia,* and *optic atrophy* with *symptoms* beginning by 2 years of age, and death by 3 to 8 years of age.
Also known as **Sulfatide Lipidosis.**

Metaproterenol Sulfate (met-uh-proe-TER-uh-nol SUL-fayt)
A *bronchodilator drug* used to treat *bronchospasm* associated with chronic *bronchitis* and *asthma*. Alupent™ is the brand name of this drug.

Metatarsal (met-uh-TAR-suhl)
1. Any one of the five bones of the *metatarsus*.
2. Pertaining to the *metatarsus*.

Metatarsus (met-uh-TAR-suhs)
The part of the foot consisting of the 5 bones to which the toe bones are attached. This area forms the *forefoot*.

Metatarsus Adductus (met-uh-TAR-suhs a-DUKT-uhs)
Refer to **Metatarsus Varus.**

Metatarsus Valgus (met-uh-TAR-suhs VAL-guhs)
A *congenital orthopedic* condition in which the baby's *forefoot* turns outward
(but the ankle and heel are in normal positions).

Metatarsus Varus (met-uh-TAR-suhs VAY-ruhs)
A *congenital orthopedic* condition in which the baby's *forefoot* turns inward
(but the ankle and heel are in their normal positions), possibly due to *fetal*
positioning in the *uterus.*
> *Also known as* **Metatarsus Adductus.**
> *Compare* **Toeing In.**

Methicillin (meth-uh-SIL-in)
An *antibiotic drug* given mostly in the treatment of severe *penicillin*-resistant
staphylococcal infections.

Methsuximide (meth-SUK-si-mied)
An *antiepileptic drug.* Celontin™ is the brand name of this drug.

Methylmalonic Acidemia (meth-uhl-muh-LON-ik as-i-DEE-mee-uh)
A group of *disorders* characterized by the inability to metabolize methylmalonic acid (a chemical important to the *metabolism* of *fatty acids*), or by a defect
in the metabolism of *vitamin* B12. Methylmalonic Acidemia is a rare *autosomal recessive inborn error of metabolism* occurring in approximately 1 out of
50,000 live births. Methylmalonic Acidemia can be *diagnosed prenatally*, and
treatment is possible for B12 responsive Methylmalonic Acidemia. Treatment
in infants includes strict dietary management. The death rate in infancy is
high, and children who do survive may have *mental retardation*, growth retardation, *convulsions*, and illness caused by *fungal* infections.
> *Refer to* **Inborn Error of Metabolism.**

Methylmalonic Aciduria (meth-uhl-muh-LON-ik as-id-YOO-ree-uh)
A form of *methylmalonic acidemia.*
> *Refer to* **Methylmalonic Acidemia.**

Methylphenidate Hydrochloride (MPH)
(meth-uhl-FEN-i-dayt hi-droe-KLOR-ied)
A *psychostimulant drug* that enhances the *brain's* ability to focus and is sometimes used to treat certain *behaviors* associated with *attention-deficit/hyper-
activity disorder*, such as inattention, *hyperactivity, impulsivity*, and distractibility. Methylphenidate is also known by the brand names *Ritalin*™ and *Con-
certa*™. It is typically prescribed for children over 6 years of age.

Metoclopramide Hydrochloride
(met-oe-kloe-PRAM-ied hie-droe-KLOR-ied)
A drug used to treat nausea and vomiting and to stimulate motility of the upper *gastrointestinal tract*. It is commonly used for treating *gastroesophageal
reflux*. Reglan™ is the brand name of this drug.

Metopic (mee-TOP-ik)
Relating to the forehead.

metro-
A prefix meaning *uterus*.

micro-
A prefix meaning small.

Microbe (MIE-kroeb)
A microscopic *germ*.

Microbrachycephaly (mie-kroe-brayk-ee-SEF-uh-lee)
A small, short, and broad shape to the head.

Microcephaly (mie-kroe-SEF-uh-lee)
An *abnormally* small head size, resulting in poor *brain* growth. Microcephaly is nearly always due to a small brain size associated with *prenatal* factors such as intrauterine infection (from *congenital rubella, toxoplasmosis, AIDS, herpes simplex 2*), *PKU, fetal alcohol syndrome*, radiation exposure, and *chromosomal abnormalities*, or due to conditions occurring at or soon after birth, such as *brain injury* or *disease* (often associated with *anoxia*, or insufficient *oxygen*). There is also a rare form of microcephaly that may be caused by an *autosomal recessive disorder*. Babies with microcephaly usually have *mental retardation* and may have *cerebral palsy* and *seizures*.

Microdeletion
Deletion of *genetic* material, which is not visibly detectable using a microscope, along an often normal-appearing *chromosome*. *Diagnosis* of a microdeletion requires that *DNA* be analyzed at the molecular level using *FISH (fluorescent in situ hybridization.)* Microdeletions account for an increase in some diagnosed *syndromes*, due to the availability of FISH and its ability to detect even submicroscopic deletions. *Velocardiofacial syndrome* is the most commonly known microdeletion *disorder*.
> *Refer to* **Fluorescent In Situ Hybridization.**
> *Compare* **Chromosomal Deletion.**

Micrognathia (mie-kroe-NAY-thee-uh)
Small, underdeveloped jaws, especially the lower jaw.

Microorganism (mie-kroe-OR-gan-izm)
Any minute (microscopic) plant or animal *organism* such as *bacteria, fungi*, and *viruses*. Some microorganisms cause *disease*.
> *Refer to* **Organism.**

Microphthalmia (mie-krof-THAL-mee-uh)
> *Refer to* **Microphthalmos.**

Microphthalmos/Microphthalmus (mie-krof-THAL-muhs)
An *abnormally* small eyeball present at birth.
> *Also known as* **Microphthalmia.**

Micropremie/Micropreemie (MIE-kroe-pree-mee)
A baby born earlier than 26 weeks *gestation.* Micropremies typically weigh less than 750 grams (approximately 1 pound, 10½ ounces) at birth. Twenty-five to 50 percent of babies born so early now survive due to advances in *neonatal* care. Long-term health and *development* concerns including *chronic lung disease* and neurologic and visual problems are present for over half of micropremies.
> *Compare* **Premature Infant.**

Microsomia (mie-kruh-SOE-mee-uh)
The condition of having an unusually small and underdeveloped yet normally formed body, including normal and proportionate relationships of the various parts.

Microtia (mie-KROE-shee-uh)
Congenital abnormal smallness of the *external ear.*

Midbrain
The highest part of the *brainstem*, which connects the *pons* and the *cerebellum* with the *hemispheres* of the *cerebrum.*
> *Also known as* **Mesencephalon.**
> *Refer to* **Brain.**

Middle Ear
> *Refer to* **Auditory Ossicles, Ear, Eustachian Tube, Hearing, Incus, Malleus, Stapes,** *and* **Tympanum.**

Midface
The middle of the face.

Midline
The vertical center line of the body.

Midsupination (mid-soo-pin-AY-shuhn)
A position in which the forearm is turned so that the little finger is down and the thumb is up. Normal reaching and *grasping* are done in midsupination.

Mild Mental Retardation (MMR)
> *Refer to* **Educable** *and* **Intelligence.**

Miller Assessment for Preschoolers (MAP)
An *evaluation* tool used to assess the preacademic, *motor* coordination, language, and *cognitive development* of children between 2 years, 9 months and 5 years, 8 months. Typically, the Miller is administered by a professional with a minimum of a master's degree.

Miller-Dieker Syndrome (MIL-ur DEE-kur)

A rare, *contiguous gene deletion syndrome* involving *chromosome* 17 (usually there is loss of part of the short arm). It is characterized by incomplete development of the *brain* (often resulting in *lissencephaly*, or a smooth brain surface); *cardiac* defect; *severe mental retardation*; *hypotonia* initially; *failure to thrive*; *seizures*; *opisthotonos* (severe, continuous *hypertonic* muscle *spasm* causing the back to arch backward); *heterotopias* (development of normal *tissue* in parts of the body where that tissue isn't normally found); and *craniofacial abnormalities* including *microcephaly*, vertical ridging and furrowing in the center of the forehead, vertical furrowing of a thin upper lip (especially when crying), a long *philtrum*, a small nose, upslant to the *palpebral fissures*, *micrognathia*, low set and/or unusually shaped outer ears, and a small lower jaw. Most children with Miller-Dieker syndrome do not survive early childhood.

Mineral

A naturally occurring element of the earth. Minerals are necessary nutrients for the regulation of many body functions, including *electrolyte* balance and *hormone* production required for normal growth.

Mineral Oil

A *laxative* used to treat *constipation*. Mineral oil is also used as a skin softener.

Minimal Brain Dysfunction (MBD)

A term previously used to describe children with *behaviors* such as those associated with *attention-deficit/hyperactivity disorder*, with *learning disabilities*, and with *language disorders*.

Minimum Daily Requirement (MDR)

The daily requirement of nutrients that human beings need for health.

Misarticulation

Producing the sounds of speech incorrectly. Misarticulations include substituting, omitting, and adding sounds, as well as sound distortion. Young children frequently misarticulate sounds, but persistent misarticulations may be caused by *auditory impairment* or a structural malformation such as *cleft palate*.

Miscarriage

A spontaneous end of pregnancy before the middle of the second *trimester* (prior to the *fetus* being able to survive on its own outside of the *uterus*). Miscarriage often occurs for unknown reasons. Known causes of miscarriage include defects of the fetus or uterus, exposure to *toxins* such as *x-rays* or drugs, and *maternal* infection.

Also known as **Spontaneous Abortion.**

Misdiagnosis

An incorrect *diagnosis*.

Compare **Diagnosis.**

Mist Tent
Refer to **Tent.**

Mitochondria (mie-toe-KON-dree-uh)
Plural of *mitochondrion.*

Mitochondrial Disease (mie-toe-KON-dree-uhl)
One of many *diseases* of the mitrochondrion (the principal energy source of the *cell*), caused by *DNA mutation.* A mitochondrial disease can be *inherited* or acquired. Examples include *Reye syndrome* and certain forms of *cardiomyopathy.*

Mitochondrion (mie-toe-KON-dree-uhn)
The principal energy source of the *cell.*

Mitosis (mie-TOE-sis)
The simplest type of *cell* division. It results in two identical cells (*daughter cells* with the same *chromosomes,* or *genetic* material) being formed. Mitosis occurs so that the body can make new cells to replace dead cells.
Compare **Meiosis.**

Mitral Valve (MIE-truhl)
One of four *valves* in the *heart* that open and close with each heartbeat to control the flow of blood. Blood exits each chamber of the heart through one of the valves. The mitral valve is located between the left *atrium* and the left ventricle. It usually has two cusps (small flaps) and may have some additional smaller cusps, which close to force blood from the left ventricle to the *aorta.* The mitral valve is the only valve that typically has just two cusps. (The other valves each have three cusps.)
Also known as the **Bicuspid Valve.**
Compare **Aortic Valve, Pulmonary Valve,** *and* **Tricuspid Valve.**

Mixed Hearing Impairment
Auditory impairment that involves a combination of both *conductive hearing impairment* and *sensorineural hearing impairment.* Mixed hearing impairment can occur *congenitally* or be *acquired.*
Compare **Conductive Hearing Impairment** *and* **Sensorineural Hearing Impairment.**
Refer to **Auditory Impairment.**

Mixed-Type Cerebral Palsy
A form of *cerebral palsy* in which both *spasticity* and *choreoathetoid movements* are present. Mixed-type cerebral palsy results when there is damage to both the *pyramidal* and *extrapyramidal* areas of the *brain.*

MLU
The abbreviation for mean length of utterance.

MMR
1. The abbreviation for Measles, Mumps, and Rubella Vaccine.
2. The abbreviation for mild mental retardation.

Mobility Aid
A piece of *adaptive* equipment that offers support, makes movement easier, or provides *balance* and stability. Mobility aids include *wedges, scooter boards, wheelchairs*, and *walkers*.

Mobility Specialist
An individual trained to teach the children or adults with *developmental disabilities* or *visual impairments* how to move about independently. Initially, the child is taught how to move about within familiar environments and then, as his skills develop, he may be taught how to travel beyond familiar areas.

Mobius (or Moebius) Syndrome (MEE-bee-uhs)
A condition characterized by *palsy* (partial *paralysis*) of several of the cranial *nerves*. Patients have facial paralysis (resulting in difficulty with using the upper lip such as for smiling or for speech), droopy eyelids that may not close completely, and inability to move the eyes away from *midline*. This *syndrome* is associated with *webbing* of the neck, fingers, and toes; extra fingers or toes; and sometimes *mental retardation, deafness, cleft palate*, and a small mouth and jaw. Children with Mobius syndrome may also have *nutritional* difficulty (which can affect body growth), due to the paralysis and deformities of the facial and oral structures.
> *Also known as* **Congenital Facial Diplegia** *and* **Congenital Oculofacial Paralysis.**

Modality
Any *sensory* pathway, such as vision, *taste*, or touch, through which information may be received.

Model
To provide an example for imitation, such as pronouncing a word to be repeated.

Moderate Mental Retardation
> *Refer to* **Intelligence.**

Modified Checklist for Autism in Toddlers (M-CHAT)
A 23 question checklist designed to identify toddlers who are *at-risk* for a *diagnosis* of an *autism spectrum disorder*. It is an expanded version of the questionnaire developed in the U.K. and consists of 23 yes/no items that the parent or caregiver answers.
> *Compare* **Checklist for Autism in Toddlers.**

Modulation
> *Refer to* **Sensory Modulation.**

Moebius Syndrome (MEE-bee-uhs)
    Refer to **Mobius Syndrome.**

Molecular Probe
A short piece of *DNA* with a known sequence of *nucleotides* that laboratory scientists can reproduce. It can be used to study DNA and to determine a *diagnosis* for *genetic disorders*. The scientist places the DNA that is being analyzed with the molecular probe that has been "tagged" with a radioactive or fluorescent chemical to distinguish it from the DNA sample. The DNA probe then searches for its complementary sequence among the DNA being analyzed and will combine with it if it finds it present. An *abnormality* in a particular *gene* can be detected and diagnosis of some *inherited* disorders can be made, such as *fragile X syndrome* and *cystic fibrosis*.
    Refer to **Deoxyribonucleic Acid (DNA).**

Molluscum Contagiosum (muh-LUS-kuhm kuhn-tay-jee-OE-suhm)
A *viral* infection consisting of a skin *rash* (small, light-colored, waxy-appearing bumps) that is transmitted by direct contact with the *lesions*. Molluscum contagiosum is generally harmless and usually heals without treatment.

Mongolian Spot (mong-GOE-lee-uhn)
A harmless, blue-black spot most commonly appearing on the lower back or buttocks of some newborns. (A Mongolian spot may also be on the whole back, legs, etc.) It is caused by an accumulation of pigment-producing *cells* and usually disappears by 3 or 4 years of age. (The Mongolian spot should be carefully documented so it is not confused with abuse.)

Mongolism (MONG-guh-liz-uhm)
A formerly used and no longer accepted name for *Down syndrome*.

Monilia (moe-NIL-ee-uh)
    Refer to **Candida Albicans.**

mono-
A prefix meaning one or single.

Mono
    Refer to **Infectious Mononucleosis.**

Mononucleosis (mon-oe-noo-klee-OE-sis)
    Refer to **Infectious Mononucleosis.**

Monoplegia (mon-uh-PLEE-jee-uh)
A form of *cerebral palsy* in which only one *extremity* (an arm or leg) is affected. The child's movements may only be mildly impaired and his *motor* abilities frequently improve.
    Refer to **Pyramidal Cerebral Palsy.**

Monoploid (MON-uh-ploid)
    Refer to **Haploid.**

Monosomy (MON-uh-soe-mee)
Any *chromosome disorder* that occurs when one chromosome from a particular pair of chromosomes is missing in the *cells* of the body. (There is one copy of the chromosome rather than the usual two copies.) Most pregnancies that produce a monosomic *embryo* end during the early *embryonic* stage.
Compare **Trisomy.**

Monosomy X
Refer to **Turner Syndrome.**

Monozygotic Twins (mon-oe-zie-GOT-ik)
Two infants born of the same pregnancy from one fertilized egg that splits into equal halves. Monozygotic twins may have their own *placentas*, are the same sex, have the same *genetic* traits, and look very much alike.
Also known as **Identical Twins.**
Compare **Dizygotic Twins.**

Mood Lability (MOOD lay-BIL-i-tee)
Emotional states that shift or change without an apparent environmental cause and that influence a child's perception of his environment.

Morbidity (mor-BID-i-tee)
Disease or illness.

Moro Reflex/Response (MOR-oe)
A startle reaction normal in infants up to 4 months of age. The moro response is observed when the infant reacts to a sudden change of body or head position by opening his hands and rapidly extending and *abducting* his arms briefly, then more slowly bringing them and the legs back close to his body into a flexed and adducted (embrace) position. This response appears to be a protective reaction for the young infant.
Compare **Startle Reflex.**
Refer to **Primitive Reflex.**

morph-, morpho-
Prefixes meaning shape or form.

Morpheme (MOR-feem)
The smallest unit of meaning in language, such as a root word, prefix, or suffix. For example, both the word "cat" (which is a root word), and the ending "s" on the word "cats" (which changes the meaning of the root word) are morphemes.

Morphological (mor-foe-LOJ-i-kuhl)
Pertaining to *morphology*.

Morphology (mor-FOL-uh-jee)
The science of the shape and structure of living *organisms*, both plants and animals.

Morquio Syndrome (mor-KEE-oe)
A *disorder* of *carbohydrate metabolism* (a *mucopolysaccharidosis*) characterized by growth deficiency, *coarse facial features*, skeletal *anomalies* including *kyphoscoliosis* (an exaggerated curve of the upper part of the *spine* creating a "humped" appearance in addition to a *lateral* curve of the spine) and *knock knees*, an enlarged *liver, hearing impairment*, and occasionally *mental retardation*.
> *Also known as* **Mucopolysaccharidosis IV** *or* **MPS IV.**

Mosaicism (moe-ZAY-i-sizm)
A condition in which there are two *genetically* different types of *cells* in a child's genetic makeup. Mosaicism is probably caused by faulty early cell division and is one process by which *chromosomal abnormalities*, such as *Down syndrome* and *Turner syndrome,* can occur. When a child is mosaic for these conditions, his genetic makeup includes some normal and some *abnormal* cells. This is because a portion of cells divided normally and continue to have the correct amount and structure of *chromosomes*, while another portion of cells divided incorrectly. The percentages of normal and abnormal cells depend upon how early in development the faulty division occurred. These percentages also determine the features associated with the *disorder*. Frequently, features in children with mosaicism will be less noticeable than in children who developed the disorder due to chromosomal abnormality in all cells. Sometimes a child's genetic makeup can include two separate chromosomal disorders, such as Down syndrome and Turner syndrome occurring in the same child.

Motor
Referring to movement produced by a muscle or *nerve*.

Motor Control
The ability to voluntarily engage muscles in purposeful movement.

Motor Cortex
The area within the *cerebral cortex* of the *brain* that controls motor activity.
> *Refer to* **Cerebral Cortex.**

Motor Nerve
Any *nerve* composed of motor fibers. Motor *nerves* are primarily responsible for stimulating muscles and *glands*.
> *Refer to* **Peripheral Nervous System.**

Motor Pattern
A sequence of movements.

Motor Planning
The ability to organize *sensory* information in order to plan and carry out the appropriate sequence of movements required to complete a task (for example, climbing stairs).
> *Also known as* **Motor Praxis.**
> *Refer to* **Dyspraxia.**

Motor Praxis
Refer to **Motor Planning.**

Motor Skill
Referring to the learned ability to perform movements, such as holding the body in an upright position to sit, using the hands to manipulate small toys, scooping food onto a spoon and bringing the spoon to the mouth, and moving the lips and tongue to articulate different sounds.
Refer to **Gross Motor** *and* **Fine Motor.**

Motrin™
Refer to **Ibuprofin.**

Mottling (MOT-l-ing)
A condition of spotting or variability of coloration without a distinct pattern, such as on the skin.

Mouthing
Placing objects into the mouth for oral exploration. This *behavior* usually emerges between 3 and 6 months of age. Mouthing safe objects helps infants learn about, and develop tolerance for, different textures, temperatures, sizes, and shapes. Oral play can help to decrease an excessive *gag reflex*, and is also an important experience needed for the development of speech.
Also known as **Oral Exploration** *and* **Oral Play.**
Refer to **Oral Stimulation.**

Mouth-to-Mouth
Referring to the mouth-to-mouth *respiration* technique used with *cardiac massage* to perform *cardiopulmonary resuscitation*.
Refer to **Artificial Respiration** *and* **Cardiopulmonary Resuscitation.**

MP Finger Joint
The Metacarpal Phalangeal *joint* between the finger and the hand.

MPH
1. The abbreviation for Methylphenidate Hydrochloride.
2. The abbreviation for Master's Degree in Public Health.

MPS
The abbreviation for mucopolysaccharidosis.

MPS I
The abbreviation for mucopolysaccharidosis I.
Refer to **Hurler Syndrome.**

MPS II
The abbreviation for mucopolysaccharidosis II.
Refer to **Hunter Syndrome.**

MPS III
The abbreviation for mucopolysaccharidosis III.
*Refer to **Sanfilippo Syndrome.***

MPS IV
The abbreviation for mucopolysaccharidosis IV.
*Refer to **Morquio Syndrome.***

MPS V
The abbreviation for mucopolysaccharidosis V.
*Refer to **Scheie Syndrome.***

MPS VI
The abbreviation for mucopolysaccharidosis VI.
*Refer to **Maroteaux-Lamy Syndrome.***

MPS VII
The abbreviation for mucopolysaccharidosis VII.
*Refer to **Sly Syndrome.***

MR
The abbreviation for mental retardation.

MRI
The abbreviation for magnetic resonance imaging.

MSEL
The abbreviation for Mullen Scales of Early Learning.

muco-
A prefix meaning *mucus.*

Mucopolysaccharidosis (MPS) (myoo-koe-pol-ee-sak-uh-rie-DOE-sis)
One of several *inherited disorders* of *carbohydrate metabolism* in which carbohydrate substances collect in a variety of body *tissues* due to an *enzyme* deficiency. The characteristics depend upon the exact enzyme deficiency but can include variable degrees of *mental retardation*, growth deficiency, bone *abnormalities*, an enlarged *liver* and *spleen*, and *coarse facial features*. Typically, there is also a shortened life expectancy. Examples of MPS disorders include *Hunter syndrome* and *Hurler syndrome.*

Mucopolysaccharidosis I (MPS I)
*Refer to **Hurler Syndrome.***

Mucopolysaccharidosis II (MPS II)
*Refer to **Hunter Syndrome.***

Mucopolysaccharidosis III (MPS III)
*Refer to **Sanfilippo Syndrome.***

Mucopolysaccharidosis IV (MPS IV)
Refer to **Morquio Syndrome.**

Mucopolysaccharidosis V (MPS V)
Refer to **Scheie Syndrome.**

Mucopolysaccharidosis VI (MPS VI)
Refer to **Maroteaux-Lamy Syndrome.**

Mucopolysaccharidosis VII (MPS VII)
Refer to **Sly Syndrome.**

Mucous Membrane (MYOO-kuhs MEM-brayn)
Any one of four major kinds of thin sheets of *tissue cells* that cover or line various parts of the body, such as the mouth, and the *digestive, respiratory,* and *genitourinary tracts.*
Refer to **Mucus.**

Mucus (MYOO-kuhs)
The slippery, sticky *secretions* of *mucous membranes* and *glands.*
Compare **Phlegm.**

Mullen Scales of Early Learning (MSEL)
A comprehensive tool used to measure development in young children. The test generates scores in *gross motor,* visual reception, *fine motor, receptive language,* and *expressive language.*

Multicystic (mul-tie-SIS-tik)
Of, or pertaining to, many *cysts.*

Multidisciplinary Team
A team of two or more professionals from different disciplines who draw upon their areas of expertise to provide *assessment* and treatment to children with *developmental disabilities.*
Compare **Interdisciplinary Team** *and* **Transdisciplinary Team.**

Multifactorial Disorder
A *disorder* caused by the interaction between *genetic* and environmental factors. Sometimes the environmental factors can be identified, such as *maternal* drug use during pregnancy, but often they are unknown, as with *spina bifida* or *cleft palate.*
Compare **Chromosomal Abnormalities** *and* **Unifactorial Disorder.**

Multi-handicapped
Referring to a child who has impairments in more than one area of *development,* such as a child who has *orthopedic* and visual *disabilities.*

Multipara (mul-TIP-uh-ruh)
Referring to a woman who has had two or more pregnancies which resulted in *viable fetuses.*

Multiple Birth
Referring to carrying and delivering more than one infant per single pregnancy.

Mumps
A *viral* infection resulting in swelling of the salivary, and sometimes other, *glands*. Many children show no *symptoms* or just mild symptoms of discomfort. Swelling under the jaw line, fever, and headache are the usual symptoms in more severe cases. Mumps infection of mature males can affect the *testes*, causing *inflammation*, pain, and swelling.
> *Refer to* **Measles, Mumps, and Rubella Vaccine.**

Murmur
> *Refer to* **Heart Murmur.**

Muscle
A type of *tissue*, or body structure, composed of bundles of *cells* capable of *contraction* and relaxation. Muscles function to effect movement of a part of the body or an organ. There are three types of muscle: skeletal muscle (also called striated muscle because of the stripes marking the muscle fibers), smooth muscle (non-striated muscle), and *cardiac* muscle. The movement response of skeletal muscle is voluntary; the movement of smooth muscle and cardiac muscle is not under conscious control. Skeletal muscles move body parts up and down, and toward and away from the body, and extend and flex at the *joints*. Another type of skeletal muscle is *sphincter*, or constrictor muscle, which closes off certain body openings, such as the anal sphincter. Smooth muscle is found in the internal organs, such as in the *digestive tract*, the *respiratory* passages, and the urinary *bladder*. Cardiac muscle (also called *myocardium*) enables the *heart* to contract.

Muscle Biopsy
A *diagnostic* procedure in which a small amount of muscle *tissue* is surgically removed and examined under the microscope. Muscle biopsy is done using a *local anesthetic*.

Muscle Enzyme Test
A *diagnostic* procedure to determine the existence of muscle *disease* or muscle *abnormality*. The test involves obtaining and studying a blood sample for its level of specific muscle *enzymes*.

Muscle Lengthening
A surgical procedure that lengthens a muscle and releases muscle *contractures*.

Muscle Relaxant
A drug given to relax *hypertonic* muscles. Sometimes muscle relaxants are referred to as *antispastic medications*.

Muscle Tone
A muscle's level of *tension* while at rest, or its resistance to passive movement. Muscle tone reflects the condition of the muscle and the *nerves* which sup-

ply it. *Abnormal* muscle tone may be described as *hypertonic* (stiff), *hypotonic* (floppy), or combination (*fluctuating tone*).
> *Refer to* **Tonus.**

Muscular Dystrophy (mus-kyuh-luhr DIS-troe-fee)
A group of *inherited, degenerative* muscle *disorders* characterized by progressive weakness and wasting. There are several forms of muscular dystrophy, each of which varies in age of onset, the pattern of *inheritance*, the speed of *disease* progression, and the level of resulting *disability*. The most common form of muscular dystrophy is *Duchenne muscular dystrophy*.

Musculoskeletal System (mus-kyoo-loe-SKEL-uh-tuhl)
All of the muscles, bones, *joints*, and related structures, such as the *tendons* and *connective tissue*. The musculoskeletal system functions in the movement of body parts and organs.

Mutation
An alteration in *genetic* information. A *gene* can be affected by a mutation, as can a piece of or a whole *chromosome*. A mutation can occur due to outside influence (such as *x-rays*, which could modify the genetic material), or spontaneously, without outside influence. A mutation can be passed from parent to child. *Achondroplasia* is an example of a *disorder* that usually occurs due to a mutation.

Mutism (MYOO-tiz-uhm)
A condition of being unable to speak due to *organic disability* (such as *paralysis*), structural disability (such as *deafness*), or emotional disability (such as certain types of *schizophrenia*).
> *Compare* **Selective Mutism.**

-myces
A suffix meaning *fungus*.

myco-
A prefix meaning *fungal*.

Mycostatin™ (MIE-koe-stat-in)
> *Refer to* **Nystatin.**

Myelin (MIE-uh-lin)
The fatty *protein* material that forms the *myelin sheath*.
> *Refer to* **Myelin Sheath.**

Myelinization (mie-el-in-ie-ZAY-shun)
The process of acquiring layers of *myelin* to form a sheath that wraps around various *nerve* fibers.
> *Also known as* **Myelinogenesis.**

Myelinogenesis (mie-el-in-oe-JEN-uh-sis)
Refer to **Myelinization.**

Myelin Sheath (MIE-uh-lin)
The layers of *myelin* that wrap around the fibers of *nerve cells* (neurons) that conduct electrical impulses away from the nerve cell. The myelin sheath also provides electrical insulation and increases the velocity of impulse transmission of neurons (nerve cells).

myelo-
A prefix meaning *bone marrow* or *spinal cord.*

Myelocele (MIE-uh-loe-seel)
A *congenital anomaly* in which the *spinal cord* protrudes through an opening in the *spinal column.*
      Compare **Myelomeningocele** *and* **Meningocele.**
      Refer to **Spina Bifida.**

Myelomeningocele (mie-uh-loe-muh-NING-goe-seel)
A *congenital anomaly* in which the *meninges* (the *membranes* surrounding the *brain* and *spinal cord*), the spinal cord, and *cerebrospinal fluid* protrude through an opening in the *spinal column*, exposing the *nerves*. With this form of *spina bifida*, the child has some (partial to total) degree of loss of sensation and *paralysis* below the area of the spinal cord protrusion, and often other *symptoms*/conditions such as *hydrocephalus, scoliosis, visual impairment, learning disabilities,* and/or *seizures.*
      Also known as **Meningomyelocele.**
      Compare **Meningocele** *and* **Myelocele.**
      Refer to **Spina Bifida.**

myo-
A prefix meaning muscle.

Myocardiopathy (mie-oe-kar-dee-OP-uh-thee)
Refer to **Cardiomyopathy.**

Myocardium (mie-oe-KAR-dee-uhm)
The layer of muscle *cells* that forms most of the *heart* wall (heart muscle).

Myoclonic Seizure (mie-oe-KLON-ik)
A form of *generalized seizure* characterized by brief, involuntary jerking of muscles. Myoclonic seizures can affect a limited area, such as an arm or leg, or they can involve jerking of the entire body. A brief loss of consciousness may, but does not always, occur.
      Refer to **Generalized Seizure** *and* **Epilepsy.**

Myoclonus (mie-OK-luh-nuhs)
A muscle jerk (*spasm*) or spasm of a group of muscles.

Myofascial Release (mie-oe-FASH-ee-uhl)
Refer to Soft Tissue Release.

Myopathy (mie-OP-uh-thee)
A *disease* or *disorder* of muscle (but not *nerve* dysfunction), resulting in wasting and weakness, and sometimes progressing to complete *paralysis*. *Muscular Dystrophy* is an example of a myopathy.

Myopia (mie-OE-pee-uh)
Blurred vision of distant objects. Myopia occurs when the eyeball is too long (which makes the *lens* focus distant objects in front of the *retina* rather than on it), or due to a problem with the lens or *cornea*. Prescription lenses can improve the vision in a child with myopia.
Also known as **Nearsightedness.**
Compare **Hyperopia.**
Refer to **Refraction.**

Myositis (mie-uh-SIE-tis)
Inflammation of muscle *tissue* caused by infection, *trauma*, or *parasite* infestation. The inflammation usually affects skeletal (voluntary) muscle tissue.

Myositis Ossificans (mie-uh-SIE-tis uh-SIF-uh-kans)
A rare, *inherited* progressive *disease* that begins early in life in which muscle *tissue* is converted into bony tissue. Medication may prevent bone replacement of muscle tissue, but the process cannot be reversed.
Compare **Myositis.**

Myotomy (mie-OT-oe-mee)
A surgical procedure in which muscle is cut to release muscle *contractures*, such as to relieve *constriction* in the *sphincter.*

Myotonia (mie-oe-TOE-nee-uh)
A condition in which muscles do not relax promptly after contracting.

Myotonic Muscular Dystrophy (mie-oe-TON-ik DIS-troe-fee)
An *autosomal dominant* form of *muscular dystrophy* characterized by strong muscle *contraction* with poor muscle relaxation, and floppy *muscle tone*. Myotonic muscular dystrophy begins in infancy and affects the muscles of the hands, feet, neck, and face. The affected person has a great deal of difficulty using the facial muscles for speech and for expressing emotion due to facial muscle weakness. Associated features that develop over the years include *mental retardation*, *cataracts*, and *endocrine* problems.
Refer to **Muscular Dystrophy.**

Myotubular Myopathy (mie-oe-TOOB-yoo-luhr mie-OP-uh-thee)
A rare *genetic syndrome* characterized by moderate to severe *hypotonia;* severe *respiratory* problems; *cardiac abnormalities*; decreased muscle mass (with the majority of muscle fibers resembling *fetal* muscle fibers); *paralysis* of the mus-

cles of the eyes; swallowing *disorder*; and facial *myopathy* (muscle *disease*), resulting in an expressionless face. If the respiratory or cardiac abnormalities are severe, the child may not survive infancy. In milder cases, the syndrome may not be identified until adulthood.

Also known as **Centronuclear Myopathy.**

Myringotomy (mir-in-GOT-oe-mee)
A surgically created opening in the *tympanic membrane* to allow drainage from the *middle ear* and to relieve pressure. Sometimes a tube (an *ear tube*) will be placed in the opening to keep fluid draining. The tube usually falls out on its own when the hole closes up. Myringotomy can prevent *hearing impairment* that can occur due to persistent fluid accumulation in the middle ear.

Myringotomy Tube
Refer to **Ear Tube** *and* **Myringotomy.**

Mysoline™ (MIE-soe-leen)
Refer to **Primidone.**

myx-
A prefix meaning *mucus*.

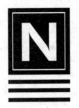

N
The abbreviation for normal.

Na
The chemical symbol for *sodium*.

NA
The abbreviation for not applicable.

Nager Acrofacial Dysostosis
(NAY-guhr ak-roe-FAY-shuhl dis-os-TOE-sis)
A rare *genetic disorder* characterized by *craniofacial* differences, including underdevelopment of the lower jaw and cheekbones, ear defects with *conductive hearing impairment*, extension of hair growing along the upper side of the cheeks, *cleft palate*, downward slanting *palpebral fissures* (the opening between the upper and lower eyelid), and partial to total absence of lower lid eyelashes; thumb, and sometimes, forearm bone *anomalies*; and initial feeding difficulties. Nager Acrofacial Dystosis usually occurs *sporadically*, but *autosomal dominant* and *autosomal recessive inheritance* patterns have also been suggested. Children with Nager Acrofacial Dysostosis generally have *normal intelligence*.
    *Also known as **Acrofacial Dysostosis, Nager Type** and **Nager Syndrome.***

Nager Syndrome
    *Refer to **Nager Acrofacial Dysostosis.***

NaHCO₃
The chemical symbol for *sodium bicarbonate*.

Narcotic Drug
A very potent type of prescribed controlled drug that relieves pain. Morphine™ and Demerol™ are examples of prescribed narcotic drugs.

Nares (NER-eez)
Plural of *naris*.

Naris (NER-is)
The nostril.

Nasal Bones
The bones of the nose.

Nasal Consonants
The /m/, /n/, and /ing/ speech sounds.
    Refer to **Consonant.**

Nasal CPAP
The delivery of *oxygen* and air pressure via *Continuous Positive Airway Pressure* through a small tube inserted in the nose to help keep the patient's airways and *alveoli* (the tiny air sacs in the lungs) from collapsing. CPAP oxygen delivery can also be administered through a tube inserted in the mouth.
    Refer to **Continuous Positive Airway Pressure.**

Nasal Regurgitation
The passing of swallowed food back out through the nose.
    Refer to **Regurgitate.**

naso-
A prefix meaning nose.

Nasogastric Tube (NG Tube) (nay-zoe-GAS-trik)
A small, flexible tube inserted through the nose and *esophagus*, and into the stomach. It is used to remove digestive juices and gas and to *gavage* feed (feed liquids through a tube). Feeding through an NG tube can be done by allowing formula to flow down the tube over a period of approximately 15 to 20 minutes or it can be administered with a syringe. For infants who cannot tolerate a large volume of food all at once, a continuous drip method is used to deliver formula over a few hours (or continuously), with the use of a machine called an *infusion pump*.

Nasojejunal Tube (NJ Tube) (nay-zoe-juh-JOO-nuhl)
A small, flexible *feeding tube* inserted through the nose, *esophagus*, and stomach, and into the *jejunum* (the middle section of the *small intestine*). Placing the tube in the intestine allows for feeding that bypasses the stomach.

Nasolacrimal Duct (nay-zoe-LAK-ri-muhl)
A structure that empties tears (*lacrima*) *secreted* from the *lacrimal gland*.

Nasopharynx (nay-zoe-FER-ingks)
The part of the throat behind the nose. It lies above the *soft palate* and extends to the *oropharynx* (the central portion of the *pharynx*, or throat) below.
    Refer to **Pharynx.**

Natal (NAY-tuhl)
Pertaining to birth.
    Refer to **Neonatal Period, Perinatal,** *and* **Prenatal.**

Natural Environment
A home or community setting, such as a child care/*development* program, in which children without *disabilities* participate. The setting would exist even if there were no children with *special needs* present. The *Individuals with Disabilities Education Improvement Act of 2004* mandates that infants and toddlers with special needs be served in natural environments.

Natural Killer Cell
A *lymphocyte* that is capable of destroying *virus*-infected *cells* and some *tumors*.
> *Refer to* **Lymphocyte**.

Navane™
> *Refer to* **Thiothixene**.

Navel
> *Refer to* **Umbilicus**.

Navicular Bone (nuh-VIK-yuh-luhr)
A small bone of the wrists and ankles.
> *Also known as* **Scaphoid Bone**.

NBAS
The abbreviation for Brazelton Neonatal Behavioral Assessment Scale.

NBIC
The abbreviation for Newborn Intensive Care.

NBICU
The abbreviation for Newborn Intensive Care Unit.

NDRC
The abbreviation for neurodevelopmental disorder of relating and communicating.

NDT
The abbreviation for neurodevelopmental treatment/therapy.

Nearsightedness
> *Refer to* **Myopia**.

Near Vision
The ability to perceive objects distinctly at normal reading distance (usually about 14 inches from the eye).

Neat Pincer Grasp
Grasp of a tiny object using the tip of the thumb and the tip of the index finger. A neat pincer grasp typically develops between 10 and 12 months of age.
> *Also known as* **Precise Finger Opposition**.
> *Compare* **Inferior Pincer Grasp** *and* **Lateral Pinch**.
> *Refer to* **Grasp**.

Nebulizer (NEB-yoo-lie-zer)
A device used to administer medications in mist form for inhalation. A nebulizer may use humidified *oxygen* and/or air, creating a mist that is delivered through a mask over the nose and mouth, in a *mist tent* (a tent erected over the patient's bed), or through a device placed in the mouth.

NEC
The abbreviation for necrotizing enterocolitis.

Neck Righting Reflex
A normal response in infants between 2 and 10 months of age. When the infant is *supine* (on her back) and her head is turned to one side, this *reflex* causes her shoulders and trunk to turn to the same side as the head.
    Refer to **Primitive Reflex.**

necro-
A prefix meaning dead.

Necrosis (ne-KROE-sis)
The death of *tissue cells* in a small, *localized* area. Causes may include an inadequate blood supply to the tissue (which can result in gangrene, or tissue death that may spread), infection, or damage to tissue cells caused by exposure to certain harmful chemicals, excessive *x-rays*, or extreme heat or cold.

Necrotizing Enterocolitis (NEC)
(NEK-roe-tie-zing en-tuh-roe-koe-LIE-tis)
An *inflammation* of the *bowels* of *premature* or *low birth-weight* infants that can result in a gangrene-like condition (*necrosis*) in the walls of the intestinal tract. The inflammatory *disease* causes decreased blood flow to the intestines, which results in *tissue* death. The exact cause is not known, but is probably related to other medical problems of the premature or low birth-weight infant. Treatment may include cessation of oral feedings, *antibiotic drugs*, and, if the condition is advanced, surgical removal of the segment of dead bowel tissue.

Negative Reinforcement
    Refer to **Reinforcement.**

Neglect
Failure by the parent/guardian to provide the necessary physical and emotional care to his child (under age 18); i.e., food, clothing, shelter, medical attention, safety, and recognition of and response to the child's emotional needs, including that of a secure and nurturing *attachment*.

Neomycin Sulfate (nee-oe-MIE-sin SUL-fayt)
An *antibiotic drug* used to treat infections.

Neonatal (nee-oe-NAY-tuhl)
    Refer to **Neonatal Period.**

Neonatal Abstinence Syndrome
A constellation of *symptoms* seen in an infant during the first 6 weeks of life caused by a sudden withdrawal of drugs she experienced as a *fetus*. Symptoms may include irritability, *tremors or seizures*, tonal problems (stiffness and jerkiness), difficulty with eating and sleeping, and incessant crying/inconsolability. Drug withdrawal can be fatal to newborns. (Some of the symptoms of drug withdrawal, such as *seizure disorders* and *muscle tone abnormalities*, may remain after infancy.)
> *Refer to* **Prenatally Exposed to Drugs.**

Neonatal Behavioral Assessment Scale (NBAS)
> *Refer to* **Brazelton Neonatal Behavioral Assessment Scale.**

Neonatal Intensive Care Unit (NICU)
The hospital unit staffed with specially trained medical practitioners who care for critically ill newborns, both premature babies and sick full-term babies. The NICU is supplied with special equipment, including *isolettes* that help the baby regulate her temperature; monitors to track and record the baby's *vital signs*; *respiration* aids such as an *oxygen hood* and *ventilator*; *bililights* to treat *jaundice*; and *catheters* (tubes) to provide food and medication, and to withdraw blood.
> *Also known as* **Intensive Care Nursery, Intensive Special Care Nursery, Intensive Special Care Unit,** *and* **Newborn Intensive Care Unit.**

Neonatal Period
The first 4 weeks of life.

Neonate
A baby during the first 4 weeks of life.
> *Also known as a* **Newborn.**

Neonatologist (nee-oe-nay-TOL-uh-jist)
A *pediatrician* who has received extra training in the care of premature and/or sick *neonates*.

Neoplasm (NEE-oe-plazm)
An *abnormal* growth of new *tissue* that negatively affects normal healthy tissue. A *tumor* is an example of a neoplasm (whether *cancerous* or *benign*).

nephr-, nephro-
Prefixes meaning *kidney*.

Nephrectomy (nuh-FREK-toe-mee)
Surgical removal of a *kidney*.

Nephritis (nuhf-RIE-tis)
Kidney disease characterized by *inflammation* and impaired function. There are many types of nephritis with varying causes.

Nephrocalcinosis (nef-roe-cal-sin-OE-sis)
A condition in which *calcium phosphate* deposits form in *kidney tissue.*

Nephrologist (nef-ROL-uh-jist)
A *physician* who specializes in treating *diseases* of the *kidney.*

Nerve
A bundle of fibers consisting of many *neurons* (*nerve cells*) that carry signals between the *brain* and the *spinal cord* (the *central nervous system*) and other parts of the body (by way of the *peripheral nervous system*).
> *Refer to* **Autonomic Nervous System, Central Nervous System, Nerve Tract,** *and* **Peripheral Nervous System.**

Nerve Block Anesthesia (an-es-THEE-zee-uh)
An injection of a *local anesthetic* into a specific *nerve* to inhibit pain in the areas supplied by the nerve. Nerve blocks are also done on some children who have *cerebral palsy* to reduce *spasticity.*
> *Refer to* **Anesthesia/Anesthetic.**

Nerve Cell
> *Refer to* **Nerve** *and* **Neuron.**

Nerve Conduction Study
A procedure that records the speed and patterns of electrical conductivity of a *nerve.* It is used as a *diagnostic* measure to determine whether a child's condition is caused by muscle *disease* or nerve damage, and if nerve damage, the type.

Nerve Impulse
The process involved in the transmission of *nerve cell* signals.
> *Refer to* **Impulse** *and* **Nerve.**

Nerve Tract
A collection of *nerve* fibers within the *central nervous system* (the *brain* and the *spinal cord*).
> *Compare* **Nerve.**
> *Refer to* **Central Nervous System.**

Nervous System
> *Refer to* **Autonomic Nervous System, Central Nervous System,** *and* **Peripheral Nervous System.**

Neural Tube (NOOR-uhl)
A tube of *nerve*-like *tissue* that develops along the back of the *embryo.* As the *fetus* develops, the neural tube differentiates into the *brain, spinal cord,* and other parts of the *nervous system.*

Neural Tube Defect (NTD)
Any *congenital anomaly* of the *brain* and *spinal cord* caused by failure of the *neural tube* to close during *embryonic* growth. Examples of neural tube defects include *spina bifida* and *anencephaly.*

Neurectomy (noo-REK-toe-mee)
A surgical procedure involving cutting out a part of a *nerve*, usually done to reduce *spasticity* of the muscle group that the nerve is supplying.

neuro-
A prefix meaning *nerve*.

Neuroblastoma (noor-oe-blas-TOE-muh)
A highly *malignant tumor* that originates in the *sympathetic nervous system* (the division of the *autonomic nervous system* that regulates involuntary body functions including acceleration of the *heart rate, constriction* of *blood vessels,* and raising of *blood pressure*). Treatment with surgery, irradiation, and *chemotherapy* may be successful if done prior to the spread of tumor *cells* to other parts of the body. Spontaneous *remission* may also occur.
> *Refer to* **Cancer** *and* **Malignancy.**

Neurocutaneous Disorder (noo-roe-kyoo-TAY-nee-uhs)
One of several *inherited disorders* of the *central nervous system* that is also characterized by skin *abnormalities*. Examples of neurocutaneous disorders include *neurofibromatosis* and *tuberous sclerosis*.
> *Also known as* **Phakomatosis** *or* **Phacomatosis.**

Neurodevelopmental (noor-oe-duh-vel-uhp-MEN-tuhl)
Pertaining to a *physiological* condition that is present early in *development*, probably *prenatally*; is *symptomatic* in early childhood; and affects the development and function of the *brain*.

Neurodevelopmental Disorder of Relating and Communicating (NDRC)
Any of a group of *disorders* in which the primary challenge to the child involves a developmental disorder (such as an *autism spectrum disorder*), with *symptoms* such as *perseveration* (seemingly purposeless repeated *behavior*) and dysfunction of the child's capacity to relate, communicate, and think. NDRC is one of the five main categories of primary *diagnoses* (Axis 1) listed in the *Interdisciplinary Council on Developmental and Learning Disorders Diagnostic Manual for Infancy and Early Childhood*.
> *Refer to* **Diagnostic Manual for Infancy and Early Childhood.**

Neurodevelopmental Treatment/Therapy (NDT)
An approach to therapy, used by some *physical* and *occupational therapists* and *speech-language pathologists*, that focuses on the development of normal movement patterns and function while inhibiting *abnormal reflexes, postures,* and movements.
> *Also known as* **Bobath Therapy.**

Neurofibroma
> *Refer to* **Neurofibromatosis.**

Neurofibromatosis (NF) (noo-roe-fie-broe-muh-TOE-sis)

An *autosomal dominant disorder* characterized by many fibrous growths (neu-rofibromas, or *benign tumors*) of the *central nervous system, nerves,* and skin; *café au lait spots* on the skin; bone *lesions* and *curvature of the spine*; occasional *seizures; learning disability* in nearly all of the children *diagnosed*; and, some-times, varying degrees of *mental retardation* and growth *abnormality*. When a neurofibroma grows along the *optic nerve* or *auditory nerve,* visual or *auditory impairment* may result. Neurofibromas are usually benign but may need to be removed if they press on adjacent body structures and cause pain. The *gene* for neurofibromatosis is on *chromosome* 17.

    *Also known as **Recklinghausen Disease** or **von Recklinghausen Disease.***

Neurogenic Bladder (noo-roe-JEN-ik)

A *disorder* characterized by loss of voluntary control of the urinary *bladder.* This can result in either *incontinence* or retention. It is caused by *nerve* damage or a *nervous system tumor.*

    *Refer to **Vesicostomy.***

Neurogenic Bowels

A *disorder* characterized by loss of voluntary control of the *bowel.* This can re-sult in either *incontinence* or retention. It is caused by *nerve* damage or a *ner-vous system tumor.*

Neuroleptic Drug (noo-roe-LEP-tik)

A medication that produces a sedating or tranquilizing effect.

Neurological Disorder (noo-roe-LOJ-i-kuhl)

A *disorder* of the *nervous system.* Examples include *epilepsy, ataxia,* and *neurofibromatosis.*

Neurologist (noo-ROL-uh-jist)

A *physician* who specializes in *diagnosing* and treating *disorders* of the *brain* and *nervous system.*

Neuromotor

    *Refer to **Neuromuscular.***

Neuromuscular (noo-roe-MUS-kyoo-luhr)

Referring to the *nerves* and the muscles and their relationship.

    *Also known as **Neuromotor.***

Neuromuscular Disorder

Disease that affects the *nerves* and/or muscles. Examples of neuromuscular disorders include *Werdnig-Hoffmann disease* and *muscular dystrophy.*

Neuron (NOOR-on)

A *nerve cell.* Neurons transmit electrical impulses which signal other neurons and organs of the body to function. Neurons that receive *stimuli* and transmit them to the *brain* are called *afferent*, or *sensory*, neurons. Neurons that carry impulses away from the brain and other nerve centers to muscles are called *efferent*, or *motor* neurons.

Neuronal Ceroid Lipofuscinosis
(noo-ROE-nuhl/NOOR-uh-nuhl SIR-oid lip-uh-fus-i-NOE-sis)
> *Refer to* **Batten Disease.**

Neuropathy (noor-OP-uh-thee)
Disease or *degeneration* of the *peripheral nerves* (the nerves that branch out from the *central nervous system*).

Neurosurgeon (NOOR-oe-sur-juhn)
A medical doctor who specializes in performing surgery on the *brain*, *spinal cord*, or *nerves*.

Neurotransmitter
A chemical substance that is released from one *nerve cell* and either stimulates or inhibits a response from the next nerve cell. Examples of neurotransmitters include *norepinephrine* and *acetylcholine*.

Neutral Position
1. Referring to the normal arm position when the child is standing (arms down, relaxed at the sides of the body with the palms facing the body).
2. Referring to the normal position of the legs when the child is standing (knees and toes are pointing forward and the feet are flat).

Neutral Rotation
Moving a leg or arm to the *neutral position* (so that it is turned neither toward or away from the *midline* of the body).

Nevus Flammeus (NEE-vuhs FLAM-ee-uhs)
> *Refer to* **Port Wine Stain.**

Newborn
> *Refer to* **Neonate.**

Newborn Intensive Care Unit (NBICU)
> *Refer to* **Neonatal Intensive Care Unit.**

NF
The abbreviation for neurofibromatosis.

NG Tube
> *Refer to* **Nasogastric Tube.**

NICU
The abbreviation for Neonatal Intensive Care Unit.

Niemann-Pick Disease (NPD) (NEE-muhn pik)
An *inherited* (usually *autosomal recessive*) *disorder* of *lipid metabolism* (a *sphingolipidosis*) in which "Niemann-Pick" *cells*, or cells filled with *sphingomyelin* (a substance found in *nervous system tissue* and in the *lipids*, or fatty substances, in the blood), collects in the *bone marrow, spleen, liver*, lungs, and *lymph nodes*. It is characterized by *failure to thrive, mental retardation*, and an enlarged liver and spleen. The *disease* is usually fatal within a few years of onset of *symptoms*. Niemann-Pick disease is classified by types A, B, C, and D and is a *Lysosomal Storage Disease.*

Night Splint
A *splint* worn while sleeping. Night splints are most commonly used to prevent *contractures* and to stretch tight muscles.

Nipple Flow Rate
The rate liquid flows or drips out of a baby bottle nipple. Nipples that allow fluids to flow out quickly do not require the infant to suck to obtain the food.

Nippling
Sucking on a baby bottle.

Nissen Fundoplication
> *Refer to* **Fundoplication.**

Nits
The eggs of *lice*.
> *Refer to* **Lice.**

NJ Tube
> *Refer to* **Nasojejunal Tube.**

NL
The abbreviation for normal.

NLP
The abbreviation for no light perception.

Noack Syndrome (NOE-ahk)
An *autosomal dominant disorder* characterized by a *congenital* malformation of the skull caused by premature closure of certain *sutures* (resulting in a head that appears pointed at the top); webbed, or fused, fingers and/or toes; and extra fingers and/or toes. *Intelligence* is usually normal.
> *Also known as* **Acrocephalopolysyndactyly, Type I.**

Nocturnal Enuresis (en-yoo-REE-sis)
Bedwetting.
> *Refer to* **Enuresis.**

Node

A small rounded *tissue* mass.
Refer to **Lymph Node.**

No Light Perception (NLP)

Lacking the ability to distinguish light from dark (total *blindness*).

Nonambulatory

Referring to the child who has not yet learned to walk or is unable to walk.
Compare **Ambulate/Ambulatory.**

Noncategorical Placement

Placement of a child who is *at-risk* or has *developmental delays* in a class setting of children with a variety of *special needs*. This type of environment is useful for observing and testing the individual child until a determination can be made regarding the type of program that would best meet the child's needs, such as a class for children who are primarily delayed in the language and *cognitive* areas versus a class for children who have *visual impairments*. A noncategorical class setting may provide an opportunity for the child with *disabilities* to be placed with nondisabled children.
Compare **Categorical Placement.**

Nonconvulsive Seizure

A *seizure* without *convulsions*. An *absence seizure* is an example of a nonconvulsive seizure.

Nondisjunction

Refer to **Chromosomal Nondisjunction.**

Nondisjunction Trisomy 21

Refer to **Down Syndrome.**

Non-immune

Not protected from a particular *disease*.

Nonketotic Hyperglycemia (non-kee-TOT-ik hie-per-glie-SEE-mee-uh)

A usually fatal *autosomal* recessive *metabolic disorder* in which the *amino acid* glycine accumulates in body fluids. It is usually *diagnosed* in the newborn period and is characterized by seizures, lack of *cerebral* development, muscle jerks, and, often, *respiratory failure* and *coma*.

Non-Reciprocal Gait

A marking time pattern of walking. This is accomplished by stepping forward on one foot, then placing the second foot next to it, followed by moving the second foot forward, then placing the other foot next to it. (Typically, walking is accomplished in a reciprocal manner: stepping forward on one foot, then stepping forward on the second foot, placing it ahead of the first foot.) A non-reciprocal gait is most commonly seen on ascending and descending stairs and is usually used until 2½ to 3 years of age (or later), when the ability to alternate feet while climbing up and down stairs develops.

>Also known as **Marking Time Pattern.**
>Refer to **Gait** and **Reciprocal Movement.**

Nonsteroidal Anti-inflammatory Drug (NSAID)
(NON-stir-oid-uhl an-tie-in-FLAM-uh-tor-ee)
A drug that is used to alleviate pain and reduce *inflammation* in *joints* and *soft tissues*. *Indomethacin* is an example of a NSAID.

Nontropical Sprue (NON-trop-i-kuhl SPROO)
>Refer to **Celiac Disease.**

Nonverbal Communication
Information expressed without the use of words. *Gestures*, facial expressions, pictures, and *sign language* are examples of nonverbal communication.

Nonverbal Learning Disability (NVLD)
A pattern of strengths and weaknesses that includes relatively better verbal abilities than nonverbal abilities (which can be quite impaired), as well as difficulties with social and *motor skills*. NVLD appears to be common in individuals with *Asperger's disorder*, but is not synonymous with Asperger's disorder.

Noonan Syndrome
An *autosomal dominant disorder* with a *multifactorial* pattern of *inheritance* characterized by *congenital heart disease*, often *mild mental retardation* or *learning disabilities, short stature, epicanthal folds, ptosis* (drooping down) of the eyelids, *myopia*, low-set ears, small lower jaw, *webbing* of the neck, *cryptorchidism* (undescended testes), *anomalies* of the fingers and *vertebrae, hirsutism* (excessive body hair), and skeletal problems.

NORD
The abbreviation for the National Organization for Rare Disorders.

Norepinephrine (nor-ep-i-NEF-rin)
A *hormone* released by the *adrenal glands*, along with *epinephrine*, that helps the *heart* maintain a constant *blood pressure* and regulate various *behaviors*.

Normal Intelligence
>Refer to **Intelligence.**

Normocephalic (nor-moe-se-FAL-ik)
Referring to normalcy of the head.

Normotensive (nor-moe-TEN-siv)
Normal *blood pressure*.

Norm-Referenced Test
A *standardized test* that compares a child's test score (performance) to the average score of a group of children who are representative of that child. The *Bayley Scales of Infant and Toddler Development*™ is an example of a norm-referenced test.
Compare **Criterion-Referenced Test** and **Screening Test**.

Norrie Disease (NOR-ee)
A rare *X-linked recessive* condition affecting only boys, characterized by total *blindness* at birth (with many eye defects including *abnormally* small eyes that shrink by the age of 10); *mental retardation* in most affected children; and, frequently, progressive *sensorineural hearing impairment* that develops at around age 20. All children with Norrie Disease experience blindness and eye problems, but the other characteristics of the *disorder* can range from mild (with *normal intelligence* and growth) to profound (with mental retardation and *deafness*).

Nortriptyline Hydrochloride (nor-TRIP-ti-leen hie-droe-KLOR-ied)
An *antidepressant drug* sometimes used in the treatment of certain *behaviors* demonstrated by some children with *autism spectrum disorders*. Pamelor™ is the brand name of this drug.

nos-, noso-
A prefix meaning *disease*.

NPD
The abbreviation for Niemann-Pick disease.

NPO/npo
The abbreviation for the Latin words (nil per os) meaning nothing by mouth. This means the child will be fed *intravenously*.

NSA
The abbreviation for no significant *abnormality*.

NSAID
The abbreviation for nonsteroidal anti-inflammatory drug.

NTD
The abbreviation for neural tube defect.

Nucleotides (NOO-klee-uh-tied)
One of the many molecules of which *DNA* is made.

NUK™ Nipple
A synthetic nipple made to resemble the shape of a mother's nipple. It is designed to make it easier for the baby to compress the nipple to obtain formula.

Nurse

A health care professional whose duties may vary from simple patient-care tasks (such as administering medications) to expert techniques (such as assisting with surgical procedures, responding to acute life-threatening situations, or managing a nursing staff and overseeing the care provided to the patients of a particular hospital unit), depending on the type of health care setting and the particular staff position.

> Refer to **Licensed Practical Nurse, Licensed Vocational Nurse,** and **Registered Nurse.**

Nutramigen™

A *hypoallergenic* formula for infants sensitive to milk and *lactose* (milk sugar). It contains hydrolyzed *protein* and is used for easy digestibility.

Nutrition

The sum of the processes involved in taking in nutrients and assimilating and utilizing them. The body requires nutrients for maintenance, growth, and energy. Nutrition involves *ingestion, digestion, absorption, assimilation,* and *excretion.*

> Compare **Malnutrition.**

Nutritionist

A specialist who studies *nutrition* and assists patients with issues regarding food intake.

NVLD

The abbreviation for *Nonverbal Learning Disability.*

Nystagmus (nis-TAG-muhs)

A *disorder* involving involuntary, rapid, rhythmic movement of the eyes. The eye movement is usually horizontal, but can be vertical or rotary. The cause of nystagmus is variable, but, when *congenital,* the cause is usually unknown.

Nystatin (nie-STAT-in or NIS-tuh-tin)

An *antifungal drug* for treatment of skin, intestinal, and *mucous membrane fungal* infections. Mycostatin™ is the brand name of this drug.

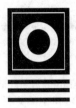

ō
The abbreviation for no.

O
The chemical symbol for *oxygen*.

O$_2$
The chemical symbol for *oxygen* molecule.

O$_2$ Sat
Refer to **Oxygen Saturation.**

OAE
The abbreviation for otoacoustic emissions.

OAV Syndrome
Refer to **Goldenhar Syndrome.**

OB
The abbreviation for obstetrician.

Objective
Refer to **Annual Goal.**

Object Permanence (Constancy)
The understanding that an object still exists even when it is not in sight. Children typically grasp this concept between 8 and 12 months of age.

Obsession
A persistent, recurring thought that a child's mind is involuntarily preoccupied with, and that reasoning does not eliminate. Obsessions often result in *compulsions*. For example, if a child has obsessive thoughts about germs making him sick, he may try to relieve his *anxiety* by repeatedly washing his hands.
Refer to **Obsessive-Compulsive Behavior, Obsessive-Compulsive Disorder,** *and* **Compulsion.**

Obsessive-Compulsive Behavior (OCB)

An act (*compulsion*) that a child performs repeatedly or ritualistically to relieve *anxiety* about an *obsession* or recurring thought or image. For example, if the child is obsessed with *germs,* he may repeatedly wash his hands.
> *Refer to **Obsessive-Compulsive Disorder (OCD).***

Obsessive-Compulsive Disorder (OCD)

A *disorder* that causes *anxiety* due to *abnormal,* recurring thoughts or images that the child can only dispel by performing a specific act.
> *Refer to **Obsessive-Compulsive Behavior (OCB).***

Obstetrician (OB) (ob-stuh-TRISH-uhn)

A medical doctor who specializes in *obstetrics.*

Obstetrics (ob-STET-riks)

The branch of medicine dealing with pregnancy and childbirth.

Obstructive Malformation

Any defect characterized by blockage. *Imperforate anus* is an example of an obstructive malformation.

OCB

The abbreviation for obsessive-compulsive behavior.

Occipital (ok-SIP-i-tuhl)

Referring to the back part of the base of the head.

Occipital Horn Syndrome (OHS) (ok-SIP-i-tuhl)

A rare *inherited* form of *cutis laxa syndrome* characterized by skin that loses its elasticity (possibly due to *abnormal elastin metabolism* causing decreased elastin in the skin), and skeletal and *genitourinary* tract abnormalities.
> *Also known as **X-Linked Recessive Cutis Laxa Syndrome.***
> *Refer to **Cutis Laxa Syndrome.***

Occipital Lobe

> *Refer to **Cerebral Hemisphere.***

Occiput (OK-si-puht)

The back part of the base of the head.

Occlusive Pulmonary Vascular Disease (OPVD)

A serious *heart* condition in which the *pulmonary blood vessels* become so narrow from thickening (due to *pulmonary hypertension*) that not enough blood can flow through to sustain life. In severe cases, the OPVD results in *Eisenmenger syndrome.* OPVD and Eisenmenger syndrome are especially prevalent in children with *Down syndrome.*

Occupational Therapy/Therapist (OT)

Therapeutic treatment aimed at helping children who are ill, injured, or disabled develop and improve *self-help* skills and *adaptive behavior* and play. The occupational therapist also addresses the young child's *motor, sensory,* and postural *development* with the overall goals of preventing or minimizing the impact of impairment and *developmental delay,* and promoting the acquisition of new skills to increase the child's ability to function independently.

OCD

The abbreviation for Obsessive-Compulsive Disorder.

ocul-, oculo-

Prefixes meaning eye.

Ocular (OK-yoo-luhr)

Referring to the eyes or vision.

Oculoauriculovertebral Dysplasia

(ok-yoo-loe-or-ik-yoo-loe-VER-tuh-bruhl dis-PLAY-zee-uh)
> *Refer to* **Goldenhar Syndrome.**

Oculocerebrorenal Syndrome (ok-yoo-loe-ser-uh-broe-REE-nuhl)
> *Refer to* **Lowe Syndrome.**

Oculomotor (ok-yoo-loe-MOE-tuhr)

Related to eye movements.

Oculus Dexter (OD)

The Latin words meaning right eye.

Oculus Sinister (OS)

The Latin words meaning left eye.

Oculus Unitas (OU)

The Latin words meaning both eyes together.

Oculus Uterque (OU) (yoo-TUR-kwee)

The Latin words meaning each eye.

OD

The abbreviation for oculus dexter (right eye).

ODD

The abbreviation for oppositional defiant disorder.

odyn-, odyno-

Prefixes meaning pain.

-odynia
A suffix meaning pain.

Office of Special Education Programs (OSEP)
The US federal government's department that administers the *Individuals with Disabilities Education Act* (*IDEA*). OSEP is dedicated to ensuring that the rights of people with *disabilities* 0 through 21 years old and their parents are protected.

Off-Task Behavior
The *behavior* of a child who is not engaged in any appropriate activity. For example, when a child is engaged in a *stereotypic behavior* (such as *hand flapping*) instead of playing with a toy purposefully, he is considered to be off-task.
    Compare **On-Task Behavior.**

OG Tube
    Refer to **Oral Gastric Tube.**

OHS
The abbreviation for Occipital Horn Syndrome.

-oid
A suffix meaning resembling.

Olanzapine (oe-LAN-zuh-peen)
An *antipsychotic drug*. Zyprexa™ is the brand name of this drug.

-ole
A suffix meaning small.

Olfactory
Referring to the sense of smell.

oligo-
A prefix meaning few or little.

Oligohydramnios (ol-ig-oe-hie-DRAM-nee-oes)
Too little *amniotic fluid*.
    Compare **Hydramnios.**

Oligophrenia (ol-i-goe-FREE-nee-uh)
A previously-used clinical term for *mental retardation*.

Ollier Disease (ol-ee-AY)
    Refer to **Enchondromatosis.**

-ology
A suffix meaning study of.

-oma
A suffix meaning *tumor* or swelling.

omphal-, omphalo-
Prefixes meaning *navel*.

Omphalocele (om-FAL-oe-seel)
A *congenital defect* in which a segment of the intestines protrudes through an opening in the *abdominal* wall into the base of the *umbilical cord*.
> *Also known as* **Exomphalos.** (This is a lesser-used term.)

On-Task Behavior
The *behavior* of a child who is attending to or engaged in an appropriate, purposeful activity.
> *Compare* **Off-Task Behavior.**

onych-, onycho-
Prefixes meaning nail.

oophor-, oophoro-
Prefixes meaning ovary.

-opathy
A suffix meaning *disease* or *disorder*.

Operant Level
> *Refer to* **Baseline.**

ophth-, ophthal-, ophthalmo-
Prefixes meaning eye.

Ophthalmologist (of-thuhl-MOL-oe-jist)
A medical doctor who specializes in *diagnosing* and treating *disorders* of the eye. The ophthalmologist also prescribes corrective *lenses* and medications and performs surgery.
> *Compare* **Optometrist** *and* **Optician.**

Ophthalmoplegia (of-thal-moe-PLEE-jee-uh)
Paralysis of one or more of the eye muscles.

-opia
A suffix meaning vision.

Opisthotonos (oe-pis-THOT-uh-nuhs)
A severe, continuous *hypertonic* muscle *spasm* causing the back to arch backward (the head and heels bend backward) with the front of the body bowing forward. (The spasm forces the child, as he is lying on his back, into a position with his weight on his head and heels.) This type of *tonic* spasm can occur in children with *tetanus*, severe cases of *meningitis* and, sometimes, severe *cerebral palsy*.

Opitz-Frias Syndrome (OE-pits FREE-ahs)
Refer to **G Syndrome.**

Opitz-Kaveggia Syndrome
Refer to **FG Syndrome.**

Opitz Syndrome (OE-pits)
Refer to **G Syndrome.**

Opponens Splint (oe-POE-nens or o-POE-nens)
A *splint* that holds the thumb in correct alignment.

Opposition Movement
The ability to touch the tip of the thumb to the tip of any finger on the same hand.
Also known as **Finger Opposition.**

Oppositional Defiant Disorder (ODD)
A *psychiatric disorder* characterized by recurrent negativistic, defiant, disobedient, and hostile *behavior* toward authority figures, and a tendency to deliberately annoy others. Many of the behaviors seen in ODD are typical in toddlers, such as refusing to comply with the adult's rule or losing one's temper (and *transient* oppositional behavior is common in preschool children and adolescents), but older children (who are *diagnosed* with ODD) continue to exhibit negative, defiant behavior, and often are diagnosed with a *comorbid* (second) disorder, such as *attention-deficit/hyperactivity disorder*, an *anxiety disorder*, or depression. Behaviors associated with ODD are almost invariably present in the home setting, but may not be present at school or in the community.

optic-
A prefix meaning eye or vision.

Optic/Optical (OP-tik/OP-ti-kuhl)
Pertaining to the eye or to vision.

Optic Atrophy (OP-tik AT-roe-fee)
A condition characterized by wasting away of the *optic nerve* fibers due to *heredity, disease*, or injury of the optic nerve. *Visual impairment* results.

Optic Glioma (OP-tik glie-OE-muh)
A *malignant tumor* of the *optic nerve.*

Optic Hypoplasia (OP-tik hie-poe-PLAY-zee-uh)
A *congenital defect* in which the *optic nerve* fibers are underdeveloped, causing *visual impairment* ranging from very slight to severe.
Refer to **Hypoplasia.**

Optician
A technician who fits and makes corrective *lenses.*
Compare **Ophthalmologist** and **Optometrist.**

Optic Nerve
The bundle of *nerve* fibers leading from the *retina* at the back of each eye to the *brain*. Visual impulses are transmitted along the two optic nerves for *binocular vision*.
> *Refer to* **Eye.**

Optometrist
A nonmedical specialist who tests vision and prescribes corrective *lenses*. Optometrists are not *physicians* and thus do not treat eye *disease* or prescribe medication, although they may *diagnose* eye disease and then refer patients to an *ophthalmologist* for further care.
> *Compare* **Ophthalmologist** *and* **Optician.**

OPV
The abbreviation for oral poliovirus vaccine.

OPVD
The abbreviation for Occlusive Pulmonary Vascular Disease.

OR
The abbreviation for operating room.

Oral Defensiveness
> *Refer to* **Oral Tactile Defensiveness.**

Oral Exploration
> *Refer to* **Mouthing.**

Oral Gastric Tube (OG Tube)
A small flexible *feeding tube* inserted through the mouth and *esophagus*, and into the stomach.
> *Refer to* **Nasogastric Tube.**

Oral Motor
Referring to the movements and *sensory* function of the mouth.

Oral Motor Skills
Skills involving muscles in and around the mouth, including *chewing*, swallowing, and forming speech sounds.

Oral Play
> *Refer to* **Mouthing.**

Oral Poliovirus Vaccine (OPV)
An *immunization* against *poliomyelitis* made from a live, weakened *polio virus*. The *Inactivated Poliovirus Vaccine of Enhanced Potency (IPV-E)* rather than the OPV is now recommended.
> *Also known as the* **Sabin Vaccine.**
> *Refer to* **Inactivated Poliovirus Vaccine of Enhanced Potency** *and* **Poliomyelitis.**

Oral Reflex
>*Refer to* **Rooting Reflex, Suck Reflex, Bite Reflex, and Gag Reflex.**

Oral Stimulation
Referring to the natural *mouthing* of toys that emerges in the infant between 3 and 6 months of age, or to the specific activities (such as massaging the *gums* or lips) designed to help the child with *oral tactile defensiveness* tolerate having things placed in his mouth. The child fed through a tube often needs oral stimulation so he does not develop an aversion to food taken orally.
>*Refer to* **Oral Tactile Defensiveness.**

Oral Tactile Defensiveness
An increased sensitivity, and often intolerance, to touch around the mouth. The child may also have intolerance for having things placed in the mouth.
>*Refer to* **Oral Stimulation.**

Oral Temperature
The body's temperature reading when the thermometer is placed under the tongue. A child's oral temperature is normally around 98.6°.
>*Compare* **Axillary Temperature, Rectal Temperature, and Tympanic Membrane Temperature.**

Orap™
>*Refer to* **Pimozide.**

Orbit (OR-bit)
One of a pair of bony sockets in the skull that contains the eyes and related structures.

orchi-
A prefix meaning testicle.

Ordinal Scales of Infant Development
>*Refer to* **Assessment in Infancy Ordinal Scales of Psychological Development.**

Organ
A somewhat independent part of an *organism* that performs one or more special functions. For example, the *heart* and lungs are organs.

Organic
1. Relating to an organ or body structure.
2. Denoting any impairment, such as an illness or *genetic disorder*, that results from a structural alteration or weakness of the *organism*.

Organism (OR-guhn-iz-uhm)
A composition of *cells* capable of carrying on life functions, such as a human being, plant, or animal.
>*Refer to* **Microorganism.**

Organomegaly (or-ga-noe-MEG-uh-lee)
Enlargement of an internal organ, usually one of the *abdominal* organs.

Orientation (or-ee-uhn-TAY-shuhn)
The process by which a child with *visual impairment* develops awareness and knowledge about his environment (i.e., a "mental map"), in order to relate effectively to the environment. For example, the child can orient himself to the playground by using all of his senses (especially his auditory and *tactile* sensations) to help him move from place to place. Specifically, he may learn that the path to the sand box is a gradually-sloping grassy area, and that when he hears the leaves on the tree above him rustle and feels the cool shade of the tree, he is almost to the sandbox.

Orienting
Locating and turning toward a sound or light *stimulus*.

Orifice (OR-i-fis)
The entrance or outlet of any body cavity.

Oropharynx (or-oe-FER-ingks)
The central portion of the *pharynx*, or throat (the part behind the mouth). It lies between the *soft palate* and the *hyoid* bone (the bone lying at the base of the tongue).
    Refer to **Pharynx.**

Orphan Drug
A drug that is effective for treating certain (usually rare) *diseases*, but has little commercial value for pharmaceutical companies. For example, the drug *Pimozide*, which is used to treat *Tourette syndrome*, was considered an orphan drug until it had a commercial sponsor to help cover the costs of needed research and development.

orth-, ortho-
A prefix meaning straight, normal, or correct.

Orthodontist
A dentist who specializes in correcting irregular tooth placement (such as teeth that are crooked, crowded, or unevenly spaced), through the use of braces or other appliances.

Orthomolecular Therapy (or-thoe-muh-LEK-yuh-lur)
An approach to medicine in which patients are treated by attempting to restore the naturally occurring chemical constituents of the body to normal. Doctors of orthomolecular medicine view *biochemical* individuality and the *nutrition* of the individual as critical factors for attaining health. Thus, they believe that by normalizing the balance of *vitamins, minerals, amino acids,* and other similar substances, health can be regained. Orthomolecular regimes have been tried as an alternative therapy to treat *developmental disabilities* such as *au-*

tism spectrum disorders. However, the ability of orthomolecular therapy to produce a desired effect on a child's *developmental disability* is unproven.
Compare **Megavitamin Therapy.**

Orthopedically Impaired (or-thoe-PEE-dik-lee)
Referring to a child who has a *disability* involving *locomotor* structures of his body (such as the bones, *joints,* muscles, and *fascia,* or fibrous *membrane*), which affects his ability to perform in other *developmental* areas. *Cerebral palsy* and *clubfoot* are examples of conditions that may be classified as *orthopedic* disabilities.

Orthopedic Appliance
Adaptive equipment used to correct *abnormal* or maintain normal body *positioning,* to inhibit unwanted *postures* or *reflexes,* and to maintain *range of motion.* Examples of orthopedic appliances include *braces,* splints, casts, *traction,* shoe inserts, and custom seating and standing devices.

Orthopedics
The branch of medicine concerned with the prevention and correction of *disorders* involving form and function of the bones, *joints,* muscles, *tendons, ligaments, cartilage,* and *fascia.*

Orthopedic Specialist
Refer to **Orthopedist.**

Orthopedist
A medical doctor who specializes in *orthopedics.*
Also known as an **Orthopedic Specialist** and **Orthopod.**

Orthopod
Refer to **Orthopedist.**

Orthoptic (or-thop-TIK)
Referring to normal *binocular vision.*

Orthosis (or-THOE-sis)
A custom-made *orthopedic appliance* (such as a *brace, splint,* or *cast*) used to promote proper body alignment, to stabilize *joints,* or to passively stretch muscle or other *soft tissue.*

Orthotics (or-THOT-iks)
The design and use of an *orthosis.*

Orthotonos/Orthotonus (or-THOT-uh-nuhs)
A severe, continuous *hypertonic* muscle *spasm* causing the body to become rigid and held in a straight line. It can occur for several reasons, including a *tetanus* infection.

OS
The abbreviation for oculus sinister (left eye).

OSEP
The abbreviation for the US federal government's Office of Special Education Programs.

-osis
A suffix meaning condition or process (usually *abnormal*).

oss-, osseo-, ossi-
Prefixes meaning bone or bony.

Osseous (OS-ee-uhs)
Pertaining to bone.

Ossicles (OS-i-kuhlz)
Refer to **Auditory Ossicles.**

ost-, oste-, osteo-
Prefixes meaning bone or bony.

Osteogenesis Imperfecta (os-tee-oe-JEN-uh-sis im-pur-FEK-tuh)
A (usually) *autosomal dominant disorder* characterized by fragile bones that break easily, bluish *sclerae* (the white *membrane* covering most of the back of the eyeball), *hyperextensibility* of *ligaments*, underdeveloped teeth, thin skin, a tendency to bruise easily, recurrent nosebleeds, excess sweating, elevated body temperatures, and possible *hearing loss*. With one *congenital* form of the *disease*, the newborn has many bone defects and, if not *stillborn*, dies in early infancy. If the first bone fractures occur later in infancy, the disease is usually not as severe. With all types of osteogenesis imperfecta, the risk of broken bones decreases as the child gets older. *Intelligence* is not affected.
   Also known as **Fragilitas Ossium.**

Osteopathic Medicine (os-tee-oe-PATH-ik)
A form of medical practice that focuses on the importance of treating the body as an integrated whole, the effects of the body systems on each other, and the role of the *musculoskeletal system* in revealing and influencing health and *disease*. Osteopathy utilizes physical, medicinal, and surgical techniques as well as manipulative therapy for *diagnosing* and treating medical *disorders* and for maintenance of good health. The *physician* practicing osteopathic medicine is called a *Doctor of Osteopathy*, or *DO*.

Osteopenia (os-tee-oe-PEE-nee-uh)
Decreased bone *calcification*, bone density, or bone mass.

Osteotomy (os-tee-OT-uh-mee)
A surgical procedure in which a bone is cut for any purpose, including realigning, shortening, or lengthening it.

Ostium Primum Defect (OS-tee-uhm PRIE-muhm)

An *atrial septal defect* (a type of *heart defect*) in which there is a hole low in the *septum* (the wall separating the right and left *atria* of the *heart*).

> *Compare* **Ostium Secundum Defect** *and* **Sinus Venosus Defect.**
> *Refer to* **Atrial Septal Defect.**

Ostium Secundum Defect (OS-tee-uhm se-KUN-duhm)

An *atrial septal defect* (a type of *heart defect*) in which there is a hole in the central portion of the *septum* (the wall separating the right and left *atria* of the *heart*).

> *Compare* **Ostium Primum Defect** *and* **Sinus Venosus Defect.**
> *Refer to* **Atrial Septal Defect.**

-ostomy

A suffix meaning new opening.

Ostomy (OS-tuh-mee)

A surgically created opening in an organ. *Colostomy* is an example of an ostomy.

ot-, oto-

Prefixes meaning ear.

OT

The abbreviation for occupational therapy or occupational therapist.

Otitis Media (oe-TIE-tis MEE-dee-uh)

An *inflammation* of the *middle ear* usually caused by an upper *respiratory tract* infection that affects the *eustachian tube*. Chronic inflammation results in a collection of fluid that does not drain and becomes infected. Chronic otitis media can cause *hearing impairment*.

> *Also known as* **Ear Infection.**
> *Compare* **Serous Otitis Media.**

Otoacoustic Emissions (OAE) (oe-toe-uh-KOO-stik)

The echoes created by the microscopic outer hair *cells* of the *inner ear* in response to acoustic *stimuli* (amplified clicks). The echoes are used to screen *hearing* in newborns and to evaluate the health of the inner ear.

> *Refer to* **Hearing.**

Otolaryngologist (oe-toe-ler-in-GOL-uh-jist)

A medical doctor who specializes in the *diagnosis* and treatment of *disorders* of the ears, nose, and throat.

> *Also known as an* **Ear, Nose, and Throat (ENT) Specialist.**

Otologist (oe-TOL-uh-jist)

A medical doctor who specializes in *diagnosing* and treating *disorders* of the ear and related structures.

-otomy
A suffix meaning incision.

Otoscope (OE-toe-skope)
An instrument used to examine the *auditory canal* and *tympanic membrane*.

Ototoxicity (oe-toe-toks-IS-i-tee)
Having the property of causing damage to the *auditory nerve* or the ear. For example, certain drugs, such as the *antibiotic drugs* gentamicin sulfate and streptomycin sulfate, can have a *toxic* effect on the organs of *hearing* and *balance* when taken in high doses.

OU
The abbreviation for oculus unitas (both eyes) or oculus uterque (each eye).

Outcome
   Refer to **Annual Goal.**

Outer Ear
   Refer to **Ear** and **External Ear.**

Outtoeing
   Refer to **Toeing Out.**

ov-
A prefix meaning egg.

Ova
Plural of *ovum.*

ovari-, ovario-
A prefix meaning ovary.

Ovaries
Plural of *ovary.*

Ovary
One of a pair of the female *gonads*, or sex *glands*, which forms ova (egg) *cells*, necessary for reproduction. The ovaries are attached to the *uterus* on either side of the pelvic cavity.
   Compare **Testis.**

Overreactive
   Refer to **Hyperresponsive.**

Overresponsive
   Refer to **Hyperresponsive.**

Overstimulation
Refer to Sensory Overload.

Ovum
The egg *cell* (female cell) of reproduction. If the ovum is fertilized by a *sperm* and implants in the *uterus*, the ovum develops into an *embryo*. The plural of ovum is ova.

Oxycephaly (ok-si-SEF-uh-lee)
A *congenital* malformation of the skull caused by premature closure of certain *sutures*. This results in a long, narrow shape to the head, with the top appearing pointed.
> *Also known as* **Acrocephaly, Hypsicephaly,** and **Turricephaly.**
> *Refer to* **Acrocephalopolysyndactyly** *and* **Acrocephalosyndactyly.**

Oxygen (O, O₂)
A gas that is essential for life. Oxygen makes up 21 percent of the earth's atmosphere.

Oxygenate (OK-suh-juh-nayt)
To combine or treat with *oxygen*.
> *Compare* **Deoxygenate.**

Oxygen Hood
A plastic dome that is placed over the infant's head to provide him with a constant flow of warm, moist, *oxygenated* air as he lies in his *incubator*.

Oxygen Saturation (O₂ Sat)
The level of *oxygen* in an individual's bloodstream. An O₂ Sat level of 95 to 100 percent while breathing normal room air is usually maintained by a healthy baby.

Oxygen Tent
> *Refer to* **Tent.**

Oxygen Therapy
Treatment in which *oxygen*-enriched air is supplied to the child who has *hypoxia* (a lack of sufficient oxygen in the body *cells* or blood) or breathing difficulties. Oxygen can be given through a mask worn over the nose and mouth, through a small tube inserted in the nose, through an *oxygen hood* or *tent*, through an *endotracheal tube*, or through a *tracheal tube*.

Oxytocin (ok-see-TOE-sin)
A *hormone* produced by the *pituitary gland* that causes *uterine contractions* and stimulates the flow of milk (the "let down" response) in nursing mothers. Synthetic oxytocin, called Pitocin™, is given to induce uterine contractions.

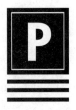

p̄
The abbreviation for after.

p
1. The abbreviation for pulse.
2. Referring to the short arm of a *chromosome*.

p-
Referring to the partial *deletion* of the short arm of a *chromosome*. For example, *5p- syndrome* (*cri du chat syndrome*) is a chromosomal *disorder* that occurs when part of the short arm of chromosome number 5 is deleted.

P
The abbreviation for probability.

Pachygyria (pak-ee-JIE-ree-uh)
A usually *sporadically* occurring *brain* condition in which the *convolutions* (folds) of the surface of the *cerebral hemispheres* are broad and flat (less convolutional than normal). This results in *mental retardation, seizures,* and often *hypertonia.* Some infants with pachygyria are also born with *lissencephaly.*
    Compare **Lissencephaly.**

Palate (PAL-it)
The roof of the mouth. It separates the mouth from the nasal passages.
    Refer to **Hard Palate** *and* **Soft Palate.**

Palatine (PAL-uh-tien)
Relating to the *palate* or the palate bone.

Palliative (PAL-ee-uh-tiv)
Descriptive of treatment that provides relief from some of the *symptoms* of an illness or condition, but not a cure.

Palmar Grasp (PAHL-mer)
Grasp of an object with all four fingers pressing against the palm of the hand

(the thumb is not involved). The palmar grasp usually develops around 4 to 5 months of age.
Refer to Grasp.

Palmar Reflex
Refer to Grasp Reflex.

Palpebral Fissure (PAL-puh-bruhl FISH-uhr)
The opening between the upper and lower eyelids.

Palsy (POL-zee)
A temporary or permanent condition characterized by partial *paralysis*. *Cerebral palsy* is an example.

Pamelor™ (PAM-uh-lor)
Refer to Nortriptyline Hydrochloride.

Pancreas (PAN-kree-uhs)
A *gland* located behind the stomach in the *abdomen*. The pancreas *secretes* digestive *enzymes* and the *hormones insulin* and glucagon.

Pancreatic (pan-kree-AT-ik)
Referring to the *pancreas*.

pancreato-
A prefix meaning *pancreas*.

Pancuronium (pan-kyoo-ROE-nee-uhm)
A *neuromuscular* blocking agent that works as a skeletal *muscle relaxant* and causes temporary *paralysis*. Pavulon™ is the brand name of this drug.

Pancytopenia (pan-sie-toe-PEE-nee-uh)
A pronounced reduction in *red blood cells, white blood cells,* and *platelets.*

P and A
The abbreviation for Protection and Advocacy.

P and PD
The abbreviation for percussion and postural drainage.

Panhypopituitarism (pan-hie-poe-pi-TOO-i-ter-izm)
Poor or absent functioning of the *anterior pituitary gland,* which, when it occurs in young children, can result in *short stature* and low levels of *hormone* functions. In the young child, this condition may be caused by a *brain tumor* or the cause may be unknown.

Panic Disorder
Refer to Anxiety Disorder.

Papule (PAP-yool)
A small (less than one centimeter in diameter) solid raised skin *lesion*.
>   *Compare* **Macule.**

par, para-
Prefixes meaning beside, closely related to, or *abnormal.*

Para (PAR-uh)
A Latin word meaning a woman who has given birth. It applies to a delivery after the stage of viability has been reached whether or not the infant is born alive or dead. A numeral is placed after para to indicate the number of times she has given birth to an infant. For example, *gravida* 2, para 1 describes a woman in her second pregnancy who previously gave birth. (Note: a multiple delivery is considered to be a single parous event.)
>   *Compare* **Gravida.**
>   *Refer to* **Parity.**

Parachute Reflex/Reaction
A protective reaction to a sudden movement of the body. The arms and legs extend in response to the movement to protect the body from falling.
>   *Refer to* **Automatic Reflex.**

Paradoxical Reaction (per-uh-DOKS-i-kuhl)
The opposite reaction than would typically be expected. For example, some drugs worsen rather than alleviate a symptom.

Paraeducator
>   *Refer to* **Paraprofessional.**

Parallel Bars
An ambulation aid that supports the child so she can practice walking. The child uses the bars to support her weight on her arms, allowing her legs to move forward.

Parallel Play
The typical play of the 18- to 24-month-old in which the child plays beside other children, rather than actually interacting with them.

Parallel Speech
Describing the child's experiences for her as they occur. For example, "I am changing your diaper now. A dry diaper sure feels nice!" or "You are bouncing the ball. Uh-oh, it got away! Now you are getting it out of the sand box. No, the ball won't bounce in the sand."

Paralysis (puh-RAL-uh-sis)
Complete or partial loss of muscle movement caused by *brain injury, disease,* or injury to the *nerves* that stimulate the muscles. Paralysis can be a temporary or a permanent condition. Paralysis can make the affected body parts

floppy or stiff (and may cause loss of feeling in those body parts) and can result from many conditions, including a *stroke, cerebral palsy,* and *meningitis.* Paralysis is often described by the areas of the body that are affected, such as *diplegia, hemiplegia, paraplegia,* and *quadriplegia.*

Compare **Paresis.**

Paraphasia (per-uh-FAY-zee-uh)

A form of *aphasia* in which the child is unable to use spoken words correctly. She may transpose letters in a spoken word or substitute one word for another, resulting in jumbled, inaccurate word usage.

Refer to **Aphasia.**

Paraplegia (per-uh-PLEE-jee-uh)

Weakness or *paralysis* of the legs and generally the lower trunk as the result of *disease* or injury to the *nerves* of the *brain* or *spinal cord* that stimulate the muscles. Sometimes the word paraplegia is used to describe *cerebral palsy* in which only the legs are affected.

Refer to **Paralysis** and **Pyramidal Cerebral Palsy.**

Parapodium (per-uh-POE-dee-uhm)

A body *brace* that supports the child's trunk and legs in a standing position. Crutches or a *walker* can be used with a parapodium to help the child walk.

Paraprofessional

A staff member who assists and works under the supervision of an *Early Interventionist* or a *Special Educator.*

Also known as **Paraeducator, Learning Support Assistant, Special Needs Assistant, Special Education Instructional Assistant,** *and* **Shadow.**

Parasite

An *organism* living in or on another organism. The parasite obtains nourishment from the host organism (the organism in which it is living), which is either detrimental to the host or does not contribute to the survival of the host.

Parasympathetic Nervous System

The part of the *autonomic nervous system* that slows *heart rate,* relaxes *sphincters,* and increases the function of the intestinal muscles that push food through the *digestive tract.*

Compare **Sympathetic Nervous System.**

Parathyroid Glands (per-uh-THIE-roid)

Two pairs of *glands* in the region of the *thyroid gland* that *secrete* parathyroid *hormone* and are involved with the *metabolism* of *calcium* and *phosphorus.*

Parenchyma (per-EN-ki-muh)

The functional *tissue* of an organ (as compared to the tissue that forms the framework of the organ or the fibrous outer layer that holds the organ together).

Parenteral Nutrition (puh-REN-tuhr-uhl)
    Refer to **Total Parenteral Nutrition.**

Parent-Professional Partnership
The teaming of parents and teachers (or doctors, *nurses*, therapists, or other professionals) to work together to facilitate the *development* of infants and children with *special needs*.

Paresis (puh-REE-sis or PER-uh-sis)
Muscle weakness or partial *paralysis* caused by *disease* or injury to the *nerves* that stimulate the muscles.
    Compare **Paralysis.**

Parietal Bone (puh-RIE-uh-tuhl)
One of two paired bones that make up part of the side and top of the skull.

Parietal Lobe (puh-RIE-uh-tuhl)
    Refer to **Cerebral Hemisphere.**

Parity (PER-i-tee)
The number of pregnancies a woman has carried to the point of viability.
    Refer to **Para.**

Paroxetine (puh-ROX-eh-teen)
A mood-elevating drug sometimes used in the treatment of depression. Paxil™ is the brand name of this drug.

Paroxysm (PER-uhk-sizm)
1. A sudden, periodic rise, worsening, or occurrence of *symptoms* of a *disease*.
2. A sudden *convulsion* or *spasm*.

Paroxysmal (per-uhk-SIZ-muhl)
Related to, concerning, or occurring in *paroxysms*.

Part B
    Refer to **Individuals with Disabilities Education Act of 1990 (IDEA).**

Part C/Part H
    Refer to **Individuals with Disabilities Education Act of 1990 (IDEA).**

Partial Ankyloglossia
    Refer to **Ankyloglossia.**

Partial Fetal Alcohol Syndrome (PFAS)
A combination of *congenital anomalies* that is caused by *maternal* consumption of alcohol during pregnancy. Characteristics include growth retardation, *central nervous system neurodevelopmental abnormalities*, and some of the characteristic facial features of *fetal alcohol syndrome*.
    Compare **Alcohol-Related Neurodevelopmental Disorder** and **Fetal Alcohol Syndrome (FAS).**
    Refer to **Fetal Alcohol Spectrum Disorder (FASD).**

Partially Sighted

Referring to the child whose *visual acuity* measures better than 20/200 (20/200 is considered *legally blind*), but not more than 20/70 in the corrected, better eye. (20/70 means that the child can only see at 20 feet what can ordinarily be seen at 70 feet.)

Compare **Blindness.**

Partial Seizure

A *seizure* that begins locally or *focally*, affecting a specific part of the *brain*. There are three classes of partial seizures: *simple partial, complex partial*, and partial seizures which become secondarily *generalized*. When the child remains conscious during a partial seizure, this is referred to as a *simple partial seizure*. When consciousness is impaired, it is referred to as a complex partial seizure. When a partial seizure progresses to a *generalized seizure* (a seizure affecting the brain as a whole), it is referred to as a partial seizure which has become secondarily generalized.

Formerly known as **Focal Seizure** and **Local Seizure.**
Compare **Generalized Seizure.**
Refer to **Epilepsy.**

Parturition (par-tyoor-ISH-uhn)

The process of giving birth.

Parvovirus (par-voe-VIE-ruhs)

A group of *viruses* that cause *disease* in humans and animals. One form (human parvovirus B-19) causes *erythema infectiosum,* which is not typically harmful, except to the *fetus* when the mother is infected. When exposed, the fetus is *at-risk* for severe illness or even death.

Passive Range of Motion (PROM)

Guiding the child's movement (such as at an arm or leg *joint*) through the normal *range of motion* without the child's help or effort.

Compare **Active Range of Motion.**
Refer to **Range of Motion.**

Patau Syndrome

Refer to **Trisomy 13.**

Patching

A method for treating certain eye conditions, such as *amblyopia, esotropia,* and *exotropia,* in which the sound eye is covered with a patch to increase the functionality of the other eye.

Patella (pu-TEL-uh)

The kneecap.

Patellar Reflex

A *deep tendon reflex* that can indicate neurological system function. A normal *reflex* is noted when there is a quick upward jerk of the leg at the knee after the *tendon* below the kneecap has been stretched by a tap.

Also known as **Knee Jerk Reflex.**

Patellofemoral Instability (pu-tel-oe-FEM-uh-ruhl)
Instability of the knee cap primarily caused by severe *ligament laxity* and lower leg misalignment (when the bones of the leg turn in or out). This condition is the most common knee problem in children with *Down syndrome*.

Patent (PAT-ent or PAYT-ent)
Open.

Patent Ductus Arteriosus (PDA)
A condition in which the *ductus arteriosus* (the *fetal blood vessel* connecting the *aorta* and the *pulmonary artery* so that blood can bypass the fetal lungs) fails to close at or soon after birth. The patent (open) vessel allows *oxygenated* blood to backflow to the lungs rather than to circulate to the rest of the body, which makes the *heart* overwork. This defect is common in *premature infants* and in newborns with *heart defects*. The ductus often closes on its own, or the drug *indomethacin* may be prescribed. If this treatment is not successful, surgery is done to close the ductus.
> *Refer to* **Ductus Arteriosus.**

path-, patho-
Prefixes meaning *disease*.

Pathogen (PATH-uh-jen)
Any *microorganism* capable of causing *disease*.

Pathogenic (path-uh-JEN-ik)
Capable of causing *disease*.

Pathological (path-uh-LOJ-i-kuhl)
Involving or caused by *disease*.

Pathology (puh-THOI-uh-jee)
The study of the characteristics, causes, and effects of *disease* in the human body.
> *Compare* **Physiology.**

-pathy
A suffix meaning *disease*.

Patterning
Guiding the child's arm or leg through a series of movements without the child's help or effort. Patterning is done to stimulate normal movement patterns. This form of treatment is considered controversial with regard to its benefits.

Pavlik Harness™
A device used to keep the legs apart and the hips back, to treat *dislocated hips*. It consists of a firm *roll* positioned between the child's thighs and a cloth harness worn over the chest.

Pavulon™ (PAYV-yoo-lon)
   Refer to **Pancuronium.**

Paxil™ **(PAKS-il)**
   Refer to **Paroxetine.**

PBS
The abbreviation for Positive Behavior Support.

pc
The abbreviation for the Latin words meaning after a meal.

PCS
The abbreviation for Picture Communication Symbols©.

PCV7
The abbreviation for Pneumococcal Conjugate Vaccine.

PD
The abbreviation for postural drainage.

PDA
The abbreviation for patent ductus arteriosus.

PD and P
The abbreviation for postural drainage and percussion.

PDD
The abbreviation for pervasive developmental disorder.

PDDST-II
The abbreviation for *Pervasive Developmental Disorder Screening Test-II.*

PDD-NOS
The abbreviation for pervasive developmental disorder-not otherwise specified.

PDMS
The abbreviation for Peabody Developmental Motor Scales.

PE
The abbreviation for physical examination.

Peabody Developmental Motor Scales (PDMS) and Activity Cards
A norm-referenced *evaluation* tool used to assess the *fine motor* and *gross motor* skills of children from birth to 7 years old. Activity cards for instructional programming are included. Typically, the PDMS is administered by a professional with a minimum of a bachelor's degree.

Peabody Picture Vocabulary Test - Fourth Edition (PPVT-4)
A norm-referenced *evaluation* tool used to assess the language ability (specifically, the recognition of single words), of people 2½ years or older. Typically, the PPVT-4 is administered by a professional with a minimum of a bachelor's degree.

PECS
The abbreviation for Picture Exchange Communication System.

Pectus Excavatum (PEK-tuhs eks-KAYV-uh-tuhm)
A *congenital* malformation in which the *sternum* (breast bone) is *abnormally* depressed (sunken). This condition may decrease the child's ability to engage in sustained active play and delay recovery from *upper respiratory infections*. It can usually be corrected surgically.

ped/pedia/pedo-
Prefixes meaning child.

PED
The abbreviation for prenatally exposed to drugs.

-pedal/-pedic
Suffixes meaning foot.

Pedaling
A normal movement in the 4- to 6-month-old infant in which the baby, while lying on her back with both hips flexed, extends one leg and then the other, and then flexes both hips again.

Pediatric
Pertaining to children.

Pediatrician
A medical doctor who specializes in the growth and care of infants, children, and adolescents.

Pediculosis (pee-dik-yoo-LOE-sis)
Infestation with *lice*.

PEEP
The abbreviation for positive end expiratory pressure.

Pelizaeus-Merzbacher Disease (PMD)
(pay-leet-SAY-oos MERTS-bah-kur)
An *X-linked recessive demyelinating disorder*. It can result in *hypotonia* and/or fluctuating *muscle tone, ataxia, choreoathetoid movements, dysarthria, nystagmus,* poor *suck reflex, global developmental delay,* and a shortened life span.

Pellagra (puh-LAY-gruh)
A *nutritional disorder* caused by a deficiency of niacin (one of the B-complex *vitamins*). It is characterized by skin, *digestive tract*, and *nervous system* dysfunction and can lead to death.

Pelvic Band
A *band* worn around the waist or *pelvis* to provide extra control for the child using *bilateral* long-legged *braces*.

Pelvis
The bony structure made up of the hipbones, *sacrum* (the fused *vertebrae* that form the back of the pelvis), and the *coccyx* (tailbone). It rests on the legs and supports the *spinal column*.

Pemoline (PEM-oe-len)
A *psychostimulant drug* that had been used in the treatment of certain *behaviors* associated with *autism spectrum disorder* and to treat children with *attention-deficit/hyperactivity disorder*. It is no longer used as frequently because of its association with *liver* damage. Cylert™ is the brand name of this drug.

Pendred Syndrome
An *autosomal recessive disorder* characterized by *congenital bilateral sensorineural hearing impairment,* and associated with *goiter* (enlargement of the *thyroid gland*) in middle childhood. The child usually has *normal intelligence* and physical *development*.

-penia (PEE-nee-uh)
A suffix meaning decrease or deficiency.

Penicillin (pen-i-SIL-in)
Any of a group of *antibiotic drugs* extracted from *cultures* of the mold penicillium or prepared semi-synthetically.

People First Language
The *inclusive* and respectful practice of identifying people with disabilities as people, first and foremost, rather than by *labeling*. For example, saying "A child with Down syndrome," rather than "A Down syndrome child."

pep-
A prefix meaning to digest.

-pepsia
A suffix meaning *digestion*.

Perception
The process of receiving and interpreting *sensory* information that functions as a basis for understanding and learning.
    Compare **Apperception.**

Perceptual Skill
The ability to interpret information gained through the senses.

Percussion (puhr-KUSH-uhn)
A method for examining the organs of the chest and *abdomen* by tapping with the fingers to estimate the condition and size of the organs. (Often, depending on the organ being examined, the examiner does not actually tap the patient's body, but instead taps her own finger, which is placed firmly over the area to be percussed.) The sound made when the organ is tapped as well as the size and borders of the organ that can be felt are all part of the physical examination.
   Compare **Chest Percussion.**

Percussion and Postural Drainage (P and PD)
   Refer to **Chest Percussion** *and* **Postural Drainage.**

Perforated Eardrum
   Refer to **Eardrum Perforation.**

Perfusion (puhr-FYOO-zhuhn)
The movement of blood or fluid through an *artery* to supply an organ or a part of the body with nutrients and *oxygen*. Perfusion also refers to the process of delivering local medication to an organ or part of the body via the blood.

peri-
A prefix meaning around or surrounding.

Perilymph (PER-uh-limf)
A clear fluid in the *inner ear*.

Perilymphatic Fistula (per-uh-lim-FAT-ik FIS-chuh-luh)
A defect within the ear resulting in a leak of *inner ear* fluid that can cause *sensorineural hearing impairment. Hearing* may improve if treatment is received before permanent damage occurs.
   Refer to **Fistula.**

Perinatal (per-uh-NAY-tuhl)
Describing the period from 28 weeks *gestation* to 1 week following delivery.

Perinatologist (per-uh-nay-TOL-uh-jist)
A medical doctor who specializes in *fetal* and *neonatal* care. The doctor has training in *obstetrics* and neonatology.

Perineal (per-uh-NEE-uhl)
Referring to the area between the thighs from the genital organs to the *anus.*

Perineum (per-uh-NEE-uhm)
The part of the body between the thighs from the genital organs to the *anus.*

Periodic Breathing
A pattern of breathing in which the baby stops breathing (has a *respiratory pause*) for at least 3 seconds and not more than 20 seconds. This is followed by a breathing period of 20 seconds or less. Periodic breathing is seen in most *premature infants* and many full-term newborns during their first few days of life. No treatment is necessary unless periodic breathing is associated with recurrent periods of *apnea*.
> *Compare* **Apnea.**

Periodontal Disease (per-ee-oe-DON-tuhl)
Disease of the *gums* and bones that surround the teeth.

Periodontist (per-ee-oe-DON-tist)
A dentist who specializes in treating *disease* of the *tissues* surrounding the teeth.

Perioral (per-ee-OR-uhl)
Surrounding the mouth.

Peripheral
Referring to the parts of an organ distant from the center, such as the *peripheral nervous system* (the *nerves* that branch out from the *central nervous system*).

Peripheral Auditory Disorder
Auditory impairment caused by a problem within the ear.
> *Compare* **Central Auditory Processing Disorder.**
> *Refer to* **Auditory Impairment.**

Peripherally Inserted Central Catheter (Line) (PICC, PIC Line)
A *central line* that is introduced in a *vein* in the arm and inserted far enough so the tip of the *catheter* is positioned in a major vein that leads to the *heart*.
> *Refer to* **Central Line.**

Peripheral Nervous System (PNS)
The *nerves* that branch out from the *central nervous system* and connect the *brain* and the *spinal cord* to the rest of the body.
> *Compare* **Autonomic Nervous System** *and* **Central Nervous System.**

Peripheral Vision
The ability to see objects that are to the sides of straight-ahead vision.

Peritoneal (per-i-tuh-NEE-uhl)
Referring to the *peritoneum*, or *membrane* lining the *abdominal* cavity and covering the organs in it.

Peritoneum (per-i-tuh-NEE-uhm)
The *membrane* lining the *abdominal* cavity and covering the organs in it.

Periventricular Encephalomalacia
(per-uh-ven-TRIK-yuh-luhr en-sef-uh-loe-muh-LAY-shuh)
A condition in which *tissue* around the *ventricles* of the *brain* is damaged due to insufficient blood flow or a lack of *oxygen*. It can cause neurological damage, such as *cerebral palsy*.

Periventricular Hemorrhage (per-uh-ven-TRIK-yuh-luhr HEM-or-ij)
Bleeding in the areas that surround the fluid-filled chambers (*ventricles*) of the *brain*.
> *Refer to* **Intracerebral Hemorrhage.**
> *Compare* **Intraventricular Hemorrhage** *and* **Subarachnoid Hemorrhage.**

Periventricular Leukomalacia (PVL)
(per-i-ven-TRIK-yuh-luhr loo-koe-muh-LAY-shuh)
Brain injury that results from a lack of sufficient *oxygen* and an inadequate blood supply to the *brain*. The *premature infant* is vulnerable to this type of brain injury (with peak *incidence* in babies born between 28 and 32 weeks' *gestation*), largely due to the high incidence of *cardiopulmonary/cardiorespiratory* problems and impaired *cerebrovascular* autoregulation (capable of regulating bloodflow within the *blood vessels* of the brain). The damage caused by periventricular leukomalacia depends on the size of the brain *lesion*, which can range from small affected areas to *multicystic encephalomalacia*. Some premature infants with periventricular leukomalacia initially have *hypotonia* (decreased *muscle tone*) and decreased muscle strength in the lower *extremities*. By around the preterm infant's due date, he becomes increasingly *hypertonic* and usually extremely irritable. A full-term infant can develop PVL due to *heart disease* or infection. Long-term conditions resulting from periventricular leukomalacia include *motor disability* (usually *diplegia* or *quadriplegia*, most often of the lower *limbs*), *cognitive* problems, and *visual impairment*. The resulting conditions relate to where the lesions occurred.

Perlocutionary Stage
A preverbal stage of language development in which the infant's vocal sounds are not yet intentional. This stage typically develops between birth and 6-8 months.
> *Refer to* **Illocutionary Stage** *and* **Locutionary Stage.**

Permanent Teeth
> *Refer to* **Secondary Teeth.**

Peroneal Muscular Atrophy (per-uh-NEE-uhl)
> *Refer to* **Charcot-Marie-Tooth Disease.**

Peroxisomal (puh-roks-i-SOE-muhl)
Pertaining to *peroxisomes*.

Peroxisome (puh-ROKS-i-soem)
A type of *vesicle* (a small fluid-filled sac) that contains *enzymes*. Peroxisomes are primarily found in the *liver* and their absence may indicate *disease*, such as *Zellweger syndrome*.

PERRLA

The abbreviation for pupils equal, round, react to light, and accommodate. It describes a normal condition of the eyes.

Perseveration (pur-sev-ur-AY-shun)

Continuing to repeat a *behavior* or response after it is no longer appropriate. Perseverative movements or speech are seemingly purposeless and may be motivated by a person's inner preoccupations. An example of perseveration is noted when a child of preschool age or older says the same words over and over, even though her words were intelligible the first time uttered and she received acknowledgement that she was understood. (The repetition of sounds, words, or *motor* actions by infants and toddlers younger than preschool age is not considered perseveration.)

Compare Self-Stimulation and Stereotypy.

Persistent Fetal Circulation (PFC)

A condition in which the newborn's blood continues to circulate as it did before birth. In the *fetus*, blood bypasses the lungs through an open *ductus arteriosus*, but at or soon after birth the ductus arteriosus should close, allowing blood to circulate through the infant's lungs to become *oxygenated*. With persistent fetal circulation, the blood continues to bypass the lungs, sending poorly oxygenated blood to the rest of the body.

Also known as Persistent Pulmonary Hypertension.
Compare Circulation and Fetal Circulation.

Persistent Pulmonary Hypertension

Refer to Persistent Fetal Circulation.

Pertussis (per-TUS-is)

An infectious *bacterial disease* that primarily affects children, causing coughing fits. It is spread by airborne droplets and can result in serious illness and lead to death. A vaccine for pertussis is given to immunize against the disease. (This is the "P" part of the *DPT* vaccine.)

Also known as Whooping Cough.

Pervasive Developmental Disorder (PDD)

An umbrella category in the *DSM-IV-TR* to describe any of the following *developmental disabilities*: *autistic disorder*; *Asperger's disorder*; *Childhood disintegrative disorder*; *Rett's disorder*; and *pervasive developmental disorder-not otherwise specified*. Pervasive developmental disorders are characterized by severe and pervasive impairment in *reciprocal* social interaction and *communication* skills, and by the presence of *stereotyped behavior*, interests, and activities. PDD is now commonly referred to as *autism spectrum disorder*.

Refer to Autism Spectrum Disorder.
Compare Pervasive Developmental Disorder-Not Otherwise Specified.

Pervasive Developmental Disorder-Not Otherwise Specified (PDD-NOS)

An *autism spectrum disorder* similar to *autistic disorder*. This *diagnosis* may be given to a child who exhibits some *behaviors* similar to the *symptoms* (signs) associated with *autistic disorder*, but does not meet the exact criteria. That is, she displays fewer than the 6 of 12 symptoms required for a diagnosis of autistic disorder. The *DSM-IV-TR* has recently been amended to state: "This category should be used when there is a severe and pervasive impairment in the development of *reciprocal* social interaction associated with impairment in either verbal and nonverbal communication skills, or with the presence of *stereotyped behavior*, interests, and activities, but the criteria are not met for a specific Pervasive Developmental Disorder..." Thus, the child with PDD-NOS ("NOS" is the abbreviation for "not otherwise specified") generally exhibits fewer or less severe symptoms than the child with autistic disorder. As of yet, there is no clear guideline to differentiate between a diagnosis of PDD-NOS and what some professionals refer to as "high functioning" autistic disorder.

Compare **Autistic Disorder** and **Pervasive Developmental Disorder**.
Refer to **Autism Spectrum Disorder**.

Pervasive Developmental Disorder Screening Test-II (PDDST-II)
A parent-report tool used to screen for an *autism spectrum disorder* in the very young child (as young as 18 months). The PDDST-II was developed by Bryna Siegel, Ph.D.

pes-
A prefix meaning foot.

Pes (peez or pays or pes)
The foot or a foot-like structure.

Pes Cavus (pes KAY-vuhs)
A foot defect in which the arch is excessively high and the tips of the toes turn downward. Pes cavus can occur as a *congenital defect* or result from *nerve* or muscle *disease*.
Also known as **Clawfoot**.

Pes Planus (pes PLAY-nuhs)
A condition in which a child has little or no arch in the foot. Babies are typically born with flat feet, but develop arches in the soles of the feet usually by age 6. A flatfoot which persists may be flexible (it assumes a normal arch when not weight-bearing), for which nothing needs to be done if the child has no *symptoms* of *disease*. When the flatfoot is not flexible, treatment depends on the cause and the symptoms.
Also known as **Flatfeet**.

PET
The abbreviation for positron emission tomography.

Petechiae (pee-TEE-kee-ee)
A pin-point *rash* caused by tiny areas of bleeding under the skin.

Petit Mal Seizure (pet-EE mahl)
Refer to **Absence Seizure** and **Epilepsy**.

Peto (PE-toe)
Refer to **Conductive Education.**

PE Tube
The abbreviation for Pressure Equalization Tube.
Refer to **Ear Tube.**

Pezzer Catheter (pe-ZAY)
Refer to **de Pezzer Catheter.**

Pezzer Tube™
A type of *gastrostomy tube* (a *feeding tube* inserted directly into the stomach through a surgically created opening in the *abdominal* wall).

PFAS
The abbreviation for Partial Fetal Alcohol Syndrome.

PFC
The abbreviation for persistent fetal circulation.

Pfeiffer Syndrome
A rare *genetic disorder* characterized by head, facial, finger, and toe *anomalies*. The head malformations are caused by premature fusion of certain cranial *sutures* resulting in the head appearing short and unusually pointed at the top. Facial features include an unusually high, full forehead; a flattened *midface*; a small nose with a flattened bridge; widely spaced eyes; an underdeveloped upper jaw (which makes the lower jaw look unusually prominent); and/or dental *abnormalities*. Finger and toe anomalies include *syndactyly* of certain fingers and toes; abnormally broad thumbs; and great toes that may bend outward. *Intelligence* is typically normal. The range and severity of characteristics can vary greatly from infant to infant. Pfeiffer syndrome can occur as an *autosomal dominant disorder* or be due to a *sporadic genetic mutation*.
Also known as **Acrocephalosyndactyly, Type V.**

pH
The degree to which a solution is acidic or alkaline. The lower the pH rating, the more acidic the solution. The pH scale expresses values from 0 to 14, with 0 to 6 describing an acidic solution, 7 neutrality, and 8 to 14 an alkaline solution.

Phacomatosis (fak-oe-muh-TOE-sis)
Refer to **Neurocutaneous Disorder.**

phag-, phago-
Prefixes meaning eat.

Phakomatosis (fak-oe-muh-TOE-sis)
Refer to **Neurocutaneous Disorder.**

Phalanges (fay-LAN-jeez)
Plural of phalanx.

Phalanx (FAY-langks)
Any one of the small bones of the fingers or toes. There are three *phalanges* in each finger and toe, except in the thumb and big toe, which each have two.

pharyngo-
A prefix meaning throat.

Pharynx (FER-ingks)
The throat. The pharynx is made up of the *nasopharynx*, the *oropharynx*, and the *laryngopharynx*.

Phenobarbital (fee-noe-BAR-buh-tol)
An *antiepileptic drug*. Luminal™ is the brand name of this drug.

Phenotype (FEE-noe-tiep)
The observable characteristics (the expression of the genes) of an individual, determined by the interactions of *heredity* and the environment.
    Compare **Genotype.**

Phenylalanine (fen-uhl-AL-uh-neen)
An *amino acid* (the basic building block of *proteins*) required by infants and children for normal growth. It is also a dietary requirement for normal protein use.

Phenylketonuria (PKU) (fen-uhl-kee-toe-NOOR-ee-uh)
An *autosomal recessive disorder* in which the inability to break down *phenylalanine* (an *amino acid*) causes a build-up of the amino acid in the body. If the condition is not *diagnosed* soon after birth, the build-up leads to *mental retardation*, progressive neurologic impairment, and seizures. With very early diagnosis, the resulting *symptoms* can be prevented by restricting the infant's intake of phenylalanine (which is found in most *protein* food sources). Newborns are now routinely tested for PKU.
    Refer to **Guthrie Test.**

Phenytoin (FEN-i-toe-in)
An *antiepileptic drug*. Dilantin™ is the brand name of this drug.
    Refer to **Fetal Hydantoin Syndrome (FHS).**

phil-
A prefix meaning affinity for.

-philia
A suffix meaning affinity for.

Philtrum (FIL-truhm)
The grooved area between the upper lip and the nose.

phlebo-
A prefix meaning *vein*.

Phlebogram (FLEB-uh-gram)
> *Refer to* **Venogram.**

Phlegm (FLEM)
A form of *mucus* secreted by the *mucous membranes* lining the *respiratory tract.*
> Compare **Mucus.**

PHN
The abbreviation for Public Health Nurse.

Phobia
> *Refer to* **Anxiety Disorder.**

Phonation (foe-NAY-shuhn)
Voice production. Vocalization is possible when a stream of air passes over the vocal cords, causing them to vibrate.

Phoneme (FOE-neem)
The smallest unit of sound found in speech. *Vowel* and *consonant* sounds are phonemes.

Phonetics (fuh-NET-iks)
The system of speech sounds of a particular language.

Phonics (FON-iks)
The study of speech sounds.

Phonological Development
The development of vocal sound production.

Phonology
The rules followed when combining speech sounds.

Phosphate (FOS-fayt)
A chemical important in living *cells*.

Phosphorus (FOS-fuhr-uhs)
An essential *mineral* element in the diet that is involved in most *metabolic* processes within the body.

Photic Stimulation (FOE-tik)
A technique in which a flashing strobe light is used during an *EEG* (*electroencephalogram*) to stimulate electrical activity. This procedure may be used to determine if a *seizure* can be induced.

Photophobia (foe-tuh-FOE-bee-uh)
Abnormal sensitivity to, and discomfort from, light. It is associated with some eye conditions, including *inflammation* and abrasion to parts of the eye, *congenital glaucoma*, and *albinism*. It may also be one of the *symptoms* of *meningitis*.

Phototherapy
Treatment for *hyperbilirubinemia* (an excess of *bilirubin*, which is the pigment byproduct of the breakdown of *red blood cells*). The infant is placed under *bililights*, which help break down the bilirubin which has accumulated in the skin so it can be *excreted* from the body.

Physical Therapy/Therapist (PT)
Therapeutic treatment designed to prevent or alleviate movement dysfunction through a program tailored to the individual child. The goal of the individualized program may be to develop muscle strength, *range of motion*, coordination, or endurance; to alleviate pain (such as with *contractures*); or to attain new *motor skills*. Physical therapists use a variety of methods of treatment, including therapeutic exercise and the use of physical agents such as heat, cold, and water. Therapeutic exercise for some children may include passive exercise (in which the therapist moves and stretches the child's muscles) or the child may actively participate in learning new ways to acquire and control positions and movement.

Physician
A health care worker who has earned a degree of Doctor of Medicine (*MD*) or of *Doctor of Osteopathy* (*DO*). Physicians are licensed to examine and care for the sick.

Physiological (fizz-ee-uh-LOJ-i-kuhl)
Pertaining to *physiology*.

Physiology (fiz-ee-OL-uh-jee)
The study of essential and characteristic processes and functions of the human body.
> Compare **Pathology**.

Phytanic Acid Storage Disease (fie-TAN-ik)
> *Refer to* **Refsum Disease**.

PI
The abbreviation for present illness.

Piaget, Jean (pee-uh-ZHAY)
A Swiss *psychologist* whose research examined the stages through which infants and children progress as they develop adult patterns of thinking.
> *Refer to* **Sensory-Motor Stage** *and* **Preoperational Stage**.

Pia Mater (PEE-uh MAY-tuhr or PIE-uh MAY-tuhr)

The innermost layer of the *meninges* (the *membranes* surrounding the *brain* and *spinal cord*). The middle layer is the *arachnoid* and the outermost layer is the *dura mater.*

    Refer to **Meninges.**

Pica (PIE-kuh)

A craving to eat non-food substances, such as dirt, hair, or chalk.

PICC/PIC Line

The abbreviation for peripherally inserted central catheter (line).

Picture Communication Symbols© (PCS)

Most widely used (within the U.S.) line drawings of actions, objects, and descriptors used as the basis for pictorial visual language. Developed by Mayer-Johnson LLC.

Picture Exchange Communication System (PECS)

A language training system sometimes used with young children with an *autism spectrum disorder* who do not yet initiate or use speech to communicate. Rather than focusing on teaching the child speech sounds, PECS starts off language instruction by giving the child the opportunity to communicate through the use of picture cards. (The emphasis is on the strength of the child with an autism spectrum disorder in visual processing over verbal processing.) When the child hands the adult a picture card of a desired item or activity, the child is allowed the item or activity to reinforce his attempts at *communication.* Most children with an autism spectrum disorder who use PECS eventually use speech alone or a combination of verbal communication and PECS.

PIE

The abbreviation for pulmonary interstitial emphysema.

Pierre Robin Sequence (pee-YER roe-BA)

A *congenital disorder* characterized by underdevelopment of the lower jaw, *cleft palate*, downward *displacement* or *retraction* of the tongue, and absent *gag reflex* resulting in difficulty in breathing and feeding. Children with this condition may also have defects of the eyes and skeleton, and usually have *normal intelligence.*

Pigeon-Toed

    Refer to **Toeing In.**

Pimozide (PIM-uh-zide)

An *antipsychotic drug* sometimes used to suppress *motor* and verbal *tics.* Orap™ is the brand name of this drug.

Pincer Grasp (PIN-suhr)

Grasp of a small or tiny object using the thumb and index finger of one hand.

    Refer to **Inferior Pincer Grasp** *and* **Neat Pincer Grasp.**

Pineal Body (PIN-ee-uhl)
A tiny *endocrine gland* within the *brain* that *secretes* the *hormone melatonin.*

Pinkeye
> *Refer to* **Conjunctivitis.**

Pinna (PIN-uh)
The *external ear,* consisting of *cartilage* covered by skin. In humans, the pinna plays a very small role in the process of *hearing.*
> *Also known as the* **Auricle.**
> *Refer to* **Ear.**

Pinnae
Plural of *pinna.*

Pinworm
> *Also known as* **Enterobius Vermicularis.**
> *Refer to* **Worms.**

Pitocin™ (pi-TOE-sin)
> *Refer to* **Oxytocin.**

Pituitary Gland (pi-TOO-i-ter-ee)
A tiny *endocrine* (*hormone secreting*) *gland* located at the base of the *brain* that is attached by a stalk to the *hypothalamus.* The hypothalamus stimulates the pituitary gland to secrete hormones which regulate other gland activity. The pituitary gland is important to the growth, *maturation,* and reproduction of the individual.

PKU
The abbreviation for phenylketonuria.

PL
The abbreviation for Public Law.

PL 93-112
> *Refer to* **Section 504 of the Rehabilitation Act of 1973.**

PL 94-142
> *Refer to* **Education for All Handicapped Children Act of 1975.**

PL 99-457
> *Refer to* **Education of the Handicapped Act Amendments of 1986.**

PL 101-336
> *Refer to* **Americans with Disabilities Act (ADA) of 1990.**

PL 101-476
> *Refer to* **Individuals with Disabilities Education Act of 1990 (IDEA).**

PL 105-17
Refer to **Individuals with Disabilities Education Act of 1990.**

PL 108-446
Refer to **Individuals with Disabilities Education Improvement Act of 2004.**

Placement
The selection of the educational program for the child who needs *special education* services.

Placenta (pluh-SEN-tuh)
The organ that supplies the *fetus* with nourishment while in the *uterus*. The placenta also functions to provide the fetus with *oxygen* and to remove the fetus's waste products.
Also known as **Afterbirth.**

Placenta Abruptio (pluh-SEN-tuh uh-BRUP-shee-oe)
Refer to **Abruptio Placenta.**

Placenta Previa (pluh-SEN-tuh PREE-vee-uh)
A condition in which the *placenta* is implanted in the *uterus* near or over the *cervix*. This can result in bleeding during middle or late pregnancy and premature delivery may be unavoidable.

Placing Response
A *primitive reflex* that is triggered when the top of the hand or foot, or the front of the arm or leg (any *extremity*) is touched and the hand/foot/arm/leg responds by placing that extremity on top of the *stimulus*. Normally, a placing response involving the foot and leg is present at birth, and a placing response involving the hand and arm develops at 3 months of age.
Refer to **Primitive Reflex.**

Plagiocephaly (play-jee-oe-SEF-uh-lee)
A *congenital* malformation of the skull in which one side is more developed toward the front and the other side is more developed toward the back. (The maximum length of the head is on a diagonal, not along the *midline*). Premature or irregular closure of certain *sutures* of the *cranium* causes the *asymmetric* shape.

Plantar (PLAN-tuhr)
Referring to the sole of the foot.

Plantar Flexion (PLAN-tuhr FLEX-shuhn)
The position of the foot when the front part is pointing down, such as during the pushing-off action of walking.
Compare **Dorsiflexion.**

Plantar Reflex

A normal response in which a stroke or firm touch to the soles of the feet, from the heel to the base of the toes, causes the toes to flex or curl under. The toes respond in this manner during walking when the foot feels pressure against the floor.

    Refer to **Primitive Reflex.**

-plasia

A suffix meaning growth, formation, or *development*.

Plasma

The clear, fluid portion of blood, excluding the *red* and *white blood cells* and the *platelets*. Plasma differs from *serum* in that plasma still contains clotting factors.

    Compare **Serum.**

Plasticity

Adaptability, flexibility.

-plasty

A suffix meaning shape or repair.

Platelet

One of three types of *blood cells*. The platelet is the smallest cellular element of the blood and is needed for proper clotting.

    Also known as **Thrombocyte.**
    Compare **Red Blood Cell** *and* **White Blood Cell.**

Playful Obstruction

An effective technique to gain a child's attention, to sustain *engagement*, or to expand on the play or interaction in which the adult playfully adds an obstacle to the child's play. For example, the adult can have an action figure jump off the "mountain" in response to the child's repetitive placement of action figures along a table's edge. Playful obstruction can be used when *following the child's lead* during a *floortime* session.

    Refer to **Developmental, Individual-Difference, Relationship-Based (DIR®) Model,** *and* **Following the Child's Lead.**

Play Therapy

A *diagnostic* and treatment method used in child psychotherapy to help children resolve any emotional or psychological conflicts. The child is encouraged to play freely with a selected group of toys as the therapist observes. (The role of the therapist is usually a passive one.) While at play, the child is encouraged to express her thoughts and feelings and to gain understanding of the difference between fantasy (a daydream, or imagined event) and reality.

-plegia

A suffix meaning *paralysis*.

Pleitropia (plie-oe-TROE-pee-uh)
The ability of a single, mutant *gene* to have multiple effects.

Pleura (PLOO-ruh)
A thin two-layered *membrane* that lines the outside of the lungs and the inside of the chest cavity. There is a thin layer of fluid between the two membrane layers.

pleuro-
A prefix meaning rib or *pleura*, or the *membrane* lining the lungs and chest cavity.

Plexus
A network of blood or *lymphatic vessels* and *nerves*.

Plosives
Speech sounds produced when the outgoing breath stream is completely obstructed, such as with /g/ and /k/ (velar plosives) and /b/ and /p/ (*bilabial* plosives).

PMD
The abbreviation for Pelizaeus-Merzbacher disease.

-pnea
A suffix meaning breathing.

pneo-
A prefix meaning breathing or lungs.

pneum-, pneumo-
Prefixes meaning breathing or lungs.

Pneumatogram (noo-MAT-uh-gram)
Refer to **Pneumogram.**

Pneumococcal Conjugate Vaccine (PCV7) (noo-moe-KOK-uhl)
An *immunization* against *pneumococcus*. It is administered by *intramuscular injection*. The child receives doses at 2, 4, 6, and between 12 and 15 months.
Refer to **Pneumococcus.**

Pneumococcus (noo-moe-KOK-uhs)
The *bacterium* which is the most common cause of *bacterial pneumonia*.
Refer to **Pneumococcal Conjugate Vaccine.**

Pneumogram (NOO-moe-gram)
A test to monitor the baby's breathing patterns. Monitoring breathing while the baby sleeps (such as to *diagnose* obstructive sleep *apnea*) is called a sleep study.
Also known as **Pneumatogram.**

Pneumonia (noo-MOE-nee-uh)
An *inflammation* of the lung *tissue*. *Symptoms* include shortness of breath, pain while inhaling, fever, and a sputum-producing cough. Pneumonia is usually caused by either a *viral* or *bacterial* infection, but it can also be caused by other types of *microorganisms*.

Pneumothorax (noo-moe-THOR-aks)
A condition in which air enters and collects between the two layers of the *pleura* (the two-layered *membrane* that lines the outside of the lungs and the inside of the chest cavity). It can be caused by a ruptured lung, a perforation in the chest wall, or as a complication of lung *disease* such as *asthma*. The *premature infant* who requires high *ventilator* pressures is vulnerable to the bursting of the *alveoli* (air sacs) in her lungs, which causes pneumothorax.

PNS
The abbrevation for peripheral nervous system.

PO/po
The abbreviation for the Latin words meaning by mouth.

POE Position
The abbreviation for prone on elbows (lying on the stomach with weight on the forearms).

PO Feeding
The abbreviation for the Latin words meaning by mouth (oral feeding).

-poiesis
A suffix meaning make or produce.

Polio
The informal word for *poliomyelitis*.

Poliomyelitis (poe-lee-oe-mie-uhl-IE-tuhs)
A *viral* infection that can affect the *central nervous system*, specifically the *gray matter* (nervous *tissue*) of the *spinal cord*, causing *paralysis*. Infants and young children are given a vaccine to immunize them against the *disease*.
>   *Also known as* **Polio.**
>   *Refer to* **Inactivated Poliovirus Vaccine of Enhanced Potency (IPV-E).**

Poliovirus (poe-lee-oe-VIE-ruhs)
The *viral organism* that causes *poliomyelitis*.
>   *Refer to* **Poliomyelitis.**

poly-
A prefix meaning much or many.

Polycythemia (pol-ee-sie-THEE-mee-uh)
A condition in which there is an *abnormally* high number of *red blood cells*. It can result from another *disorder* such as lung or *heart disease*, or from *hypoxia*

(a lack of sufficient *oxygen* in the body *cells* or blood), and can cause impaired blood *circulation*. Polycythemia most commonly occurs when a newborn receives more blood than normal from the *placenta*.

Polydactyly (pol-ee-DAK-ti-lee)
A *congenital anomaly* that results in one or more extra fingers or toes. They may look like the other *digits* or they may be incompletely formed.
> Compare **Adactyly.**

Polyhydramnios (pol-ee-hie-DRAM-nee-os)
> *Refer to* **Hydramnios.**

Poly-Vi-Flor™
A multivitamin containing *fluoride* (a *mineral* used to prevent tooth decay) and *iron*.

Poly-Vi-Sol™
A multivitamin containing *iron*.

Pommel (POM-uhl)
A piece of *adaptive* equipment that is placed between the legs to keep them apart, such as while sitting in a *wheelchair*.

Pons (ponz)
The middle part of the *brainstem*.
> *Refer to* **Brain.**

Pope Night Splint™
A *splint* that is typically worn while the child sleeps to help prevent heel cord (*Achilles tendon*) tightness and *contracture*.

Popliteal (pop-LIT-ee-uhl)
Referring to the back surface of the knee.

Porencephaly (por-en-SEF-uh-lee)
A *cyst* that develops within the *brain* and connects the *ventricles* with the subarachnoid space (the space inside the *arachnoid membranes* that surround the brain). It may develop either *prenatally* due to a *congenital anomaly*, or in early infancy as a result of poor blood supply (which may be the result of a birth *trauma*). *Motor* and/or *sensory* function may be impaired, depending on the size and location of the cyst, and *hydrocephalus* may result. Some children have *normal intelligence*.
> Compare **Schizencephaly.**

Portage Project
One of the early model programs for providing home-based *early intervention* services in which parents are trained to teach their children. It was initially funded by the United States Department of Education's Office of Special Education and Rehabilitative Services (formerly known as the Bureau of Educa-

tion for the Handicapped) in 1969. The program includes *assessment*, curriculum planning, and a family focus.

Port Wine Stain
A flat, purple-red birthmark. It is usually found on the head or neck and usually persists throughout life.
> *Also known as* **Nevus Flammeus.**
> *Refer to* **Hemangioma.**

Positioning
Placing a child's body in correct alignment to facilitate optimal *posture* and performance. Special equipment, such as an *adaptive* seat, may be required for the child to maintain proper positioning.

Positive Behavior Support (PBS)
Strategies used to teach new skills and make changes in a child's environment so that events or circumstances that trigger unwanted behaviors are removed. First, *Functional Behavior Analysis* (FBA) is used to determine the purpose of a child's undesirable behavior, then an individualized intervention plan that is positive, proactive, and functional can be developed and implemented.

Positive End Expiratory Pressure (PEEP) (ik-SPIE-ruh-tor-ee)
The constant pressure provided by a *ventilator* to help keep the baby's lungs from collapsing.

Positive Reinforcement
> *Refer to* **Reinforcement.**

Positive Support Reflex
A normal *reflex* in infants from birth to 6 to 8 weeks of age and then again from approximately 3 months to 10 months of age. The infant extends her legs and hips when held upright with the balls of her feet touching the floor, supporting some of her weight. It is not desirable for this reflex to continue beyond 10 months of age because the increased *muscle tone* in the legs makes learning to walk difficult.
> *Refer to* **Primitive Reflex.**

Positron Emission Tomography (PET) (POZ-i-tron tuh-MOG-ruh-fee)
A *diagnostic* imaging technique used to study the *metabolic* and chemical activity of *tissue*, especially that of the *brain*, *heart*, and *blood vessels*. PET scanning visualizes the organ, producing 3-dimensional color images.

post-
A prefix meaning behind or after.

Posterior
Behind.
> *Also known as* **Dorsal.**
> *Compare* **Anterior.**

Posterior Rhizotomy
> *Refer to* **Dorsal Rhizotomy.**

Postictal (poest-IK-tuhl)
Referring to the recovery period just after a *seizure* during which the child is usually sleepy.
> *Refer to* **Epilepsy.**

Postpartum
After delivery (childbirth).
> *Compare* **Antepartum** and **Prenatal.**

Post Traumatic Stress Disorder
> *Refer to* **Anxiety Disorder.**

Postural Drainage (PD)
A technique which allows *mucus* to drain from the lungs in which the baby is tilted with the head positioned below the lungs. This can be accomplished by placing the infant in different positions on a bed in which the foot of the bed is raised higher than the head of the bed, and is usually accompanied by *chest percussion.*
> *Refer to* **Chest Percussion.**

Postural Drainage and Percussion (PD and P)
> *Refer to* **Chest Percussion** and **Postural Drainage.**

Postural Reaction/Reflex
> *Refer to* **Automatic Reflex.**

Posture/Posturing
Positioning of the body.

Potassium (K)
A *mineral* needed by the body for *nerve* and muscle functioning, for regulation of the body's water and acid-base balance, and to assist with maintaining the *heart's* normal rhythm.

Potter Syndrome
A *congenital disorder* characterized by absence of both *kidneys*. Other characteristics that may be present include poor lung development, a flat nose, a small lower jaw, low-set and malformed ears, *epicanthal folds* (vertical skin folds at the inner corner of the eyes), and *clubbed* hands and feet (broadening and thickening of the *soft tissues* of the ends of the fingers and toes). Potter Syndrome is thought to result from an insufficient amount of *amniotic fluid* around the *fetus.*

Potts Shunt™
A surgically created *heart* connection that enables blood to bypass the malformed *pulmonary valve.*

PPVT-4
The abbreviation for Peabody Picture Vocabulary Test-Fourth Edition.

pr
The abbreviation for the Latin words meaning by *rectum*.

Prader-Willi Syndrome (PRAH-duhr WIL-ee)
A *congenital disorder* characterized by almond-shaped eyes, *strabismus,* low forehead, small lower jaw, *abnormalities* of the hands and fingers, *hypogonadism* (abnormally low activity of the *gonads*), slow height growth, early *hypotonia* (decreased *muscle tone*), *cognitive* impairment (frequently *mental retardation*), and *failure to thrive* in early infancy, with obesity beginning between 1 and 3 years of age. Prader-Willi syndrome is caused by an alteration of the chromosomal material on *chromosome* 15.

Pragmatics
The understanding of how and why language is used. Pragmatics involves understanding the context in which language is expressed and the intent of what is expressed. Elements of pragmatics include facial expressions, the appropriate use of space and distance in interpersonal situations, and conversational skills such as taking turns, knowing how to make requests, and clarifying misunderstandings. Usually, infants develop an early understanding of pragmatics even before they are able to speak. For example, an infant who tosses her spoon to the floor and waits in anticipation for her parent to retrieve it and continue the game is expressing something different than an infant who tosses her spoon to the floor and squirms to get out of her high chair.

Praxis (PRAK-sis)
The ability to plan and perform movements.
        Refer to **Dyspraxia.**

pre-
A prefix meaning before or in front of.

Precipitate/Precipitous Delivery
The sudden, uncontrolled delivery of an infant.

Precise Finger Opposition
        Refer to **Opposition Movement** *and* **Neat Pincer Grasp.**

Precursor
A skill that precedes and indicates the emergence of a related skill.

Prednisone (PRED-ni-soen)
A *corticosteroid* drug used to treat *inflammation* associated with different *disorders* including severe *asthma*.

Pre-eclampsia (pree-ee-KLAMP-see-uh)
A serious complication of the second half of pregnancy in which the woman develops high *blood pressure* and *edema*, and has *protein* in the urine. Pre-eclampsia must be treated to prevent *eclampsia*, which can be fatal.
> *Previously known as* **Toxemia of Pregnancy.**
> *Compare* **Eclampsia.**

Pregestamil™
A predigested *protein* formula (the protein is broken down), fed to infants with *malabsorption* problems, such as *celiac disease* or *cystic fibrosis*.

Prehension
The act of *grasping* or holding.
> *Refer to* **Grasp.**

Prelingual
Describing the vocalizations an infant produces prior to the development of speech (verbal) skills, such as *cooing* and *babbling*.

Prelingual Deafness
Loss of *hearing* occurring before the development of speech and language skills. Prelingual deafness may be *congenital* or *adventitious*.
> *Refer to* **Deafness.**

Premature Infant
A baby born before 37 weeks' *gestation*. (Babies born at 35-36 weeks' gestation are considered mildly premature. Babies born between 30-34 weeks' gestation are considered moderately premature. Babies born between 26-29 weeks' gestation are categorized as extremely premature. Babies born earlier than 26 weeks' gestation are categorized as *micropremies*.) The cause of premature delivery cannot always be determined, but often it is caused by *maternal* conditions such as bleeding, high *blood pressure*, or infection, or by *fetal* conditions such as a multiple pregnancy or *hydramnios* (excessive *amniotic fluid*). Babies have different problems depending on the reasons for and the amount of prematurity. These complications may include a *low birth weight, respiratory distress syndrome, apnea, bradycardia, patent ductus arteriosus*, feeding difficulties, *necrotizing enterocolitis, jaundice*, infection, *seizures*, and *brain damage*. As of 2003, approximately 1 in 8 babies in the United States is born prematurely.
> *Also known as a* **Premie/Preemie.**
> *Compare* **Micropremie/Micropreemie** *and* **Term Infant.**
> *Refer to* **Gestation.**

Premie/Preemie (PREE-mee)
> *Refer to* **Premature Infant.**

Prenatal/Prenatally (pree-NAY-tuhl/pree-NAY-tuhl-lee)
Before birth.
> *Compare* **Postpartum.**

Prenatal Diagnosis
The determination of a baby's illness or *developmental disability* before birth.

Prenatally Exposed to Drugs (PED)
Referring to an infant who was exposed to drugs as a *fetus* due to *maternal* substance abuse. The effects of drug exposure can range from slight to severe, in part due to the many variables associated with substance abuse. These variables include the type and/or combination of drugs taken; the amount, frequency, and route of use; the *gestational* period in which the fetus was exposed to drugs; the *genetic* make-up of the fetus and *prenatal* care received; and the environment in which the newborn lives. Infants prenatally exposed to drugs often have a withdrawal period. They suffer damage to the *central nervous system* and display *behaviors* that reflect this damage. These behaviors might include poor impulse control, being easily distracted or stimulated, delayed language skills, difficulty with following directions, and difficulty with developing appropriate *attachments* to others. Infants prenatally exposed to drugs are sometimes referred to as "drug babies."

> *Also known as* **Drug Baby, Infant of a Substance Abusing Mother, and Infant of a Chemically-Dependent Mother.**
> *Refer to* **Neuro-Neonatal Abstinence Syndrome, Alcohol Related Neurodevelopmental Disorder,** *and* **Fetal Alcohol Syndrome.**

Preoperational Stage
The second stage of Jean *Piaget's* theory of *cognitive* development in which the 2- to 7-year-old child acquires a symbolic system to represent her world, based on her own *perceptions*. Much of her play involves imitation, symbolic play, drawing, and use of language.

> *Compare* **Sensory-Motor Stage.**

Presentation
> *Refer to* **Fetal Presentation.**

Pressure Equalization Tube (PE Tube)
> *Refer to* **Ear Tube.**

Pre-Term Infant
> *Refer to* **Premature Infant** *and* **Assessment of Pre-Term Infant Behavior.**

Primary Caregiver/Caretaker
The adult who provides care for, and is best known and depended upon by the young child. The primary caregiver is usually the mother but may be another adult who provides quality love and attention to the child.

Primary Circular Reactions
According to Jean *Piaget's* theory of *cognitive* development, primary circular reactions describes the infant's repetition of an action involving her body that initially occurred as an accident. After the first accidental occurrence, the 1- to 4-month-old attempts and eventually succeeds at repeating the action

(such as getting her fist to her mouth). Primary circular reactions is a substage of the *sensory-motor stage.*
>   Compare **Secondary Circular Reactions.**
>   *Refer to* **Sensory-Motor Stage.**

Primary Epilepsy
>   *Refer to* **Idiopathic Epilepsy** *and* **Epilepsy.**

Primary Seizure
>   *Refer to* **Idiopathic Epilepsy** *and* **Epilepsy.**

Primary Teeth
The first teeth, which are shed and replaced by permanent (*secondary*) *teeth.* There are 20 primary teeth, 10 in each jaw. The primary teeth usually begin to appear around 6 months of age.
>   *Also known as* **Baby Teeth** *and* **Deciduous Teeth.**
>   Compare **Secondary Teeth.**

Primidone (PRIM-i-doen)
An *antiepileptic drug.* Mysoline™ is the brand name of this drug.

Primigravida (prie-mi-GRAV-i-duh or pri-mi-GRAV-i-duh)
A woman pregnant for the first time. Also known as gravida 1.
>   *Refer to* **Gravida.**

Primitive Reflex
A *reflex* response to a *stimulus* such as touch or movement that is normal in infants. The word "primitive" refers to the fact that these are involuntary survival responses with which infants are born. As the newborn moves through her first year of life, reflexive (involuntary) movement is replaced by (integrated into) voluntary movement. The absence of a primitive reflex at the age at which it should be present, or presence beyond the age at which it should disappear, can interfere with normal *motor* function and may be an indication of neurological damage. The *asymmetrical tonic neck reflex* (*ATNR*), the *grasp reflex*, and the *suck reflex* are examples of primitive reflexes.
>   Compare **Automatic Reflex.**

p.r.n.
The abbreviation for pro re nata, meaning as needed or when necessary.

pro-
A prefix meaning before or prior to.

Problem Solving
Experimenting with different methods and/or materials to reach a goal. Standing on a stack of books to obtain a toy that is out of reach is an example of problem solving.

Process-Oriented Measure
A type of *assessment* tool used to evaluate the child's problem-solving techniques. The process involved in task completion is the focus.

procto-
A prefix meaning *anus* or *rectum*.

Proctoscopy (prok-TOS-koe-pee)
Refer to **Rectoscopy.**

Prodrome (PROE-droem)
An early *sign* or *symptom* that may be a first indication of a developing illness or condition, such as a *rash* that precedes an infectious *disease*. For example, prodromal labor is a condition in which a pregnant woman experiences sometimes painful but unproductive (no dilation of the *cervix*) *uterine contractions* that indicate actual *labor* is impending.

Profound Mental Retardation
Refer to **Intelligence.**

Progeria (proe-JEE-ree-uh)
A *congenital* condition of premature old age, characterized by graying hair, baldness, loss of fat, a wizened face, sagging skin, and small stature. The cause of this extremely rare condition is unknown. It is usually fatal before 20 years of age.
Also known as **Hutchinson-Gelford Syndrome.**

Progesterone (proe-JES-tuhr-oen)
A female sex *hormone* essential to pregnancy and the menstrual cycle.

Prognathism (PROG-nuh-thizm)
A condition in which one or both jaws project further out than the forehead.

Prognosis (Px)
An estimate of the course and outcome of a *disease*, including the chance of recovery.

Project TEACCH
Refer to **TEACCH.**

Prolapse (PROE-laps or proe-LAPS)
A condition in which an organ has fallen or slid from its normal position in the body. An example of a prolapsed organ is *rectal prolapse*, in which *bowel tissue* has pushed down through the *anus*.

Prolonged Regard
The newborn's ability to look at someone or something for 4 to 5 seconds.

Prompt

Input that encourages the child to perform a movement or activity. A prompt may be verbal, *gestural*, physical (such as a touch or manually guiding the child), or a demonstration. An example of prompting is tapping beneath one's chin as a visual reminder to the child to close her mouth to prevent drooling.

> *Also known as* **Cue.**
> *Refer to* **Fading.**

Prompt Dependence

Relying on a prompt to elicit demonstration of a skill or to stop an unwanted behavior. For example, a child has become prompt dependent if she only requests a piece of fruit when prompted with, "Do you want to eat an apple or banana?"

Prompt Fading

> *Refer to* **Fading.**

Pronation

Turning of the hand or foot so the palm faces downward or the sole faces outward.

> *Compare* **Supination.**

Prone

Lying with the face down, on the stomach.

> *Compare* **Supine.**

Prone Board

A padded board to which the front side of the child's body is strapped so she is positioned in properly aligned standing. This piece of equipment allows the child to bear some of her own weight (leaning at an angle, such as against a table), and to engage in table activities while developing *head control.*

> *Also known as a* **Prone Stander.**

Prone On Elbows (POE Position)

Lying on the stomach with weight on the elbows.

Prone Pivoting

Moving in a circular pattern (as opposed to forward and backward movement) while lying on the stomach. The infant's arm and leg movements pivot her before she is able to *crawl.*

Prone Stander

> *Refer to* **Prone Board.**

Pronominal Reversal (proe-NOM-uh-nuhl)

Switching (reversing) first and second person pronouns during speech, such as a child saying, "You want a cookie" when she actually means, "I want a cookie." Pronominal reversal may occur in a child with an *autism spectrum disorder* or certain *language disorders.*

Prophylactic Therapy (proe-fi-LAK-tik)
Treatment to prevent *disease,* including use of drugs, equipment, or procedures. Using drugs to prevent *seizures* is an example of prophylactic therapy.

Propionic Acidemia (proe-pee-ON-ik as-i-DEE-mee-uh)
A rare *autosomal recessive metabolic disorder* caused by the body's inability to metabolize 3 *amino acids.* A low *protein* diet (restriction of the 3 amino acids) may help. The defect is characterized by lethargy, vomiting, and *coma,* and can result in *mental retardation,* physical *developmental delay,* and death.

Proprioception (proe-pree-oe-SEP-shuhn)
The body's conscious or unconscious awareness of its position, movement, *posture,* and *balance* in relation to the surrounding environment. *Nerve* sensors (proprioceptors) within the *inner ear,* muscles, *tendons,* and *joints* provide information about the body's position in space.

Proptosis (prop-TOE-sis)
An *abnormal* protrusion of a body organ, usually referring to the eye.

Propulsid™ (proe-PUL-sid)
    Refer to **Cisapride.**

Pro Sobee™
A milk-free *protein* formula for infants sensitive to milk.

Prosodic Pattern/Prosody (pruh-SOD-ik/PROS-uh-dee)
The stress and intonation aspects of speech production. For example, the same sentence can convey more than one meaning depending on how and which words are stressed: "We're having a baby!" (excitement) versus "We're having a baby?" (surprise).

Prostaglandin (PROS-tuh-gland-in)
A *fatty acid* substance found in body *tissues* that functions in many ways within the body, including to stimulate *uterine contractions* and to widen or constrict certain *blood vessels.*

Prosthesis (PROS-thee-sis or pros-THEE-sis)
An artificial replacement for a missing body part, such as a leg, arm, or eye. Prostheses may be designed to restore normal function of the missing body part, or for cosmetic enhancement.

Protection and Advocacy (P and A)
A federally mandated system of non-governmental state agencies established to protect the rights of, and advocate for, people with *developmental disabilities.* Examples of services the staff of P and A agencies may provide include legal intervention; administration; negotiation with schools or agencies on behalf of a student; and education to the public about the rights of children with developmental disabilities.

Protective Extension
A response to a sudden body movement that upsets *balance*, in which the arm(s) and/or leg(s) *extend* to try to protect oneself from a fall. An example of protective extension is the *parachute reflex*. Another example is extending one arm to the side while sitting on the floor to avoid falling all the way over when one's balance is lost.
    *Refer to **Automatic Reflex** and **Extension**.*

Protein (PROE-teen or PROE-tee-in)
An *organic* compound that is made up of linked *amino acids* and is necessary for life. Protein is a part of many body *tissues* and is an essential component of a balanced diet.

Protein Binding
The process by which *proteins* in the blood attach to and carry medications and other chemicals through the bloodstream. This is a major factor determining distribution of various molecules (the smallest portion into which a substance can be divided and still retain its properties) to different organs of the body.

Protodeclarative Pointing
Pointing to an object or action for the purpose of guiding someone else's attention to the same thing. Protodeclarative pointing is a form of *shared attention and meaning* and is a skill that typically develops in toddlers. Initially (around 12 months of age), the toddler points to indicate that she wants something. Around 18 months, the child points to objects on request. By 24 months, the toddler points for the purpose of *joint attention* to an object or activity. Delay in the development of protodeclarative pointing is often a *sign* of an *autism spectrum disorder*.

Protraction
To move the shoulder or hip forward from its natural resting position, such as reaching forward toward something just out of reach with the arm extended at shoulder level.

Proventil™ (proe-VEN-til)
    *Refer to **Albuterol**.*

Proximal (PROK-suh-muhl)
Referring to the body parts that are closest to the point of attachment to, or to the center part of, the body. For example, the elbow is proximal to the shoulder while the fingers are *distal* to the shoulder. The development of movement skills follows a pattern of proximal to distal development, meaning that skills involving proximal body parts (such as the elbow) are acquired before skills involving distal body parts (such as the fingers).
    *Compare **Distal**.*

Prozac™ (PROE-zak)
    *Refer to **Fluoxetine Hydrochloride**.*

pseudo-
A prefix meaning false.

Pseudohypertrophic Muscular Dystrophy (soo-doe-hie-puhr-TROE-fik)
Refer to Duchenne Muscular Dystrophy.

Pseudomonas (soo-doe-MOE-nas or soo-DOM-uh-nas)
A type of *bacteria* often found in *urinary tract* infections and in wounds.

Psychiatric (sie-kee-AT-rik)
Pertaining to mental, emotional, and *behavioral disorders*.

Psychiatrist (sie-KIE-uh-trist)
A *physician* who specializes in *diagnosing* and treating mental illness. The psychiatrist can prescribe medications (unlike the *psychologist*, who is not a medical doctor).
*Compare **Psychologist**.*

psycho-
A prefix meaning mind.

Psychologist (sie-KOL-uh-jist)
A professional who specializes in the study of human *behavior* and the function of the *brain*, including *intelligence*. There are several types of psychologists, including clinical psychologists, who test and counsel children with emotional or *behavioral disorders*; school psychologists, who give *standardized tests* and make recommendations regarding school *placement* for the child with *special needs*; and developmental psychologists, who assess the child's intellectual *development*.
*Compare **Psychiatrist**.*

Psychomotor (sie-kuh-MOE-tuhr)
An educational term meaning voluntary *motor* activity. Sitting up and *bladder* control are examples of psychomotor skills.

Psychomotor Seizure
*Refer to **Complex Partial Seizure**, **Partial Seizure**, and **Epilepsy**.*

Psychosis/Psychotic (sie-KOE-sis/sie-KOT-ik)
A severe mental *disorder* that alters the child's understanding of reality and ability to participate normally with others. The child may exhibit personality changes, loss of *affect*, disturbed thought processes, depression, confusion, a decrease in language skills, aggression, agitation, delusions, or hallucinations. (Individual *symptoms* can occur with disorders other than psychoses, as well.) *Schizophrenia* is an example of a psychosis.
*Refer to **Antipsychotic Drug**.*

Psychostimulant Drug (sie-koe-STIM-yuh-luhnt)
A medication prescribed to elevate mood or to treat depression.

Psychotropic Drug (sie-koe-TROP-ik)
A drug used in the treatment of mental illness. Psychotropic drugs are some-times used in the treatment of certain *autistic-like behaviors*.

PT
The abbreviation for physical therapy or physical therapist.

pt
The abbreviation for patient.

pto-
A prefix meaning fall.

-ptosis
A suffix meaning *prolapse* or drooping of an organ or body part.

Ptosis (TOE-sis)
A drooping down of an organ or body part, usually referring to the drooping of the upper eyelid. Ptosis of the eye can occur *congenitally* or be caused by in-jury or *disease* to the muscle or *nerve* supply to the eye.

Pubis (PYOO-bis)
The most *anterior* bone in the *pelvis*.

Public Law 93-112
> *Refer to Section 504 of the Rehabilitation Act of 1973.*

Public Law 94-142
> *Refer to Education for All Handicapped Children Act of 1975.*

Public Law 99-457
> *Refer to Education of the Handicapped Act Amendments of 1986.*

Public Law 101-336
> *Refer to Americans with Disabilities Act (ADA) of 1990.*

Public Law 101-476
> *Refer to Individuals with Disabilities Education Act of 1990 (IDEA).*

Public Law 105-17
> *Refer to Individuals with Disabilities Education Act of 1990 (IDEA).*

Public Law 108-446
> *Refer to Individuals with Disabilities Education Improvement Act of 2004.*

pulmo-
A prefix meaning lung.

Pulmonary (PUL-muh-ner-ee)
Referring to the lungs.

Pulmonary Artery
Either the right pulmonary artery or the left pulmonary artery that delivers blood from the right side of the *heart* to the lungs to be *oxygenated*.
　　Compare **Systemic Circulation.**

Pulmonary Function Test
A set of several tests to assess lung function, including determination of the volume of air that moves in and out of the lungs, the ability of the lungs to exchange *oxygen* and *carbon dioxide,* and the degree of airway obstruction.

Pulmonary Hypertension
High *blood pressure* in the *vessels* supplying blood to the lungs caused by inadequate blood flow through the lungs. High blood pressure occurs when the *heart* must pump harder to maintain proper blood flow and results in enlargement of the heart muscle. The underlying problem of inadequate blood flow can be caused by a decreased supply of *oxygen* to the lungs or other lung *disease*.

Pulmonary Interstitial Emphysema (PIE)
(PUL-muh-ner-ee in-tuhr-STISH-uhl em-fuh-SEE-muh)
A condition in which air bubbles leak from the lungs into the *tissue* of the lungs. It can be caused by high pressure to the lungs associated with use of a *ventilator*. Pulmonary interstitial emphysema usually improves after *respirator* pressure is decreased.

Pulmonary Stenosis (PUL-muh-ner-ee sti-NOE-sis)
An obstruction of the outflow from the right ventricle of the *heart*, which causes the heart to pump harder to move blood to the lungs. Pulmonary stenosis is usually a *congenital* condition, and may be caused by narrowing of the *pulmonary valve*, the *pulmonary artery*, or part of the right ventricle, but obstruction can develop after birth. In severe cases, the obstruction (narrowing) can be improved through surgery.

Pulmonary Valve
One of the four *valves* in the *heart* that open and close with each heartbeat to control the flow of blood. Blood exits each chamber of the heart through one of the valves. The pulmonary valve is located between the *pulmonary artery* and the right ventricle. The three cusps (small flaps) of the pulmonary valve close during each heartbeat to prevent blood from flowing back into the right ventricle.
　　Compare **Aortic Valve, Mitral Valve,** *and* **Tricuspid Valve.**

Pulmonary Vein
One of four *blood vessels* that return *oxygenated* blood from the lungs to the left *atrium* of the *heart*.

Pulse
The expansion and *contraction* of an *artery* caused by the pumping of blood through it, by the *heart*. Each pulse beat reflects a beat of the heart.

Pupil (PYOO-puhl)
The opening in the center of the *iris* of the eye through which light enters. The iris constricts to change the size of the pupil. The pupil becomes smaller, or constricted, in bright lighting to decrease the amount of light entering the eye, and becomes larger, or dilates, in dim lighting to admit more light.
Refer to ***Eye.***

Puppy Position
The *prone* position with weight on the forearms and the head up.

Purulent (PUR-yoo-lent)
Containing or producing *pus*.

Pus
A creamy substance indicating the site of *inflammation*. Pus contains dead *white blood cells* and cellular debris.

PVL
The abbreviation for periventricular leukomalacia.

Px
The medical abbreviation for prognosis.

pyelo-
A prefix meaning *kidney* or *pelvis*.

Pyelogram (PIE-uh-loe-gram)
Refer to ***Intravenous Pyelogram.***

Pyloric Stenosis (pie-LOR-ik sti-NOE-sis)
A relative narrowing of the pyloric *orifice* (the opening between the stomach and the *duodenum*), where food passes from the stomach into the *small intestine*. The narrowing is caused by a thickening of the pyloric muscle, which obstructs the passage of food from the stomach. This results in persistent vomiting, *constipation*, and failure to gain (or loss of) weight. Pyloric stenosis is sometimes improved with medication, but often surgery is required to correct the narrowing.

pyo-
A prefix meaning *pus*.

Pyramidal Cerebral Palsy (pi-RAM-i-duhl)
Cerebral palsy that results from damage to the part of the *brain* that controls the initiation of voluntary movement or to the *nerve* pathways that transmit

these *motor* impulses from the brain to the *spinal cord*. Pyramidal cerebral palsy is characterized by *spasticity* (stiffness) in certain muscle groups. It is the most common type of cerebral palsy and can take the form of *monoplegia, diplegia, hemiplegia, paraplegia, quadriplegia,* or *double hemiplegia* depending on the location of *brain damage*.

> *Also known as* **Spastic Cerebral Palsy.**
> *Compare* **Extrapyramidal Cerebral Palsy.**
> *Refer to* **Cerebral Palsy.**

Pyramidal Tract

The *nerve* pathways that transmit impulses for initiating voluntary movement from the *brain* to the *spinal cord*.

> *Compare* **Extrapyramidal Tract.**

Pyrexia (pie-REK-see-uh)

Fever.

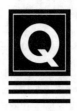

q
1. The abbreviation for every.
2. Referring to the long arm of a *chromosome*.

q-
Referring to the partial *deletion* of the long arm of a *chromosome*. For example, *13q- syndrome* occurs when part of the long arm of a number 13 chromosome is deleted.

qd
The abbreviation for every day.

qh
The abbreviation for every hour.

qid
The abbreviation for four times a day.

qns
The abbreviation for quantity not sufficient.

qod
The abbreviation for every other day.

qq
The abbreviation for each or every.

qs
The abbreviation for quantity sufficient.

Quadriceps (KWOD-ri-seps)
The large muscle on the front of the thigh. The quadriceps is made up of four sections which function to extend the leg at the knee.

Quadriparesis (kwod-ruh-puh-REE-sis)
*Refer to **Quadriplegia**.*

Quadriplegia (kwod-ruh-PLEE-jee-uh)

Paralysis in both arms and both legs, and often the head or face and the trunk, caused by *disease* or injury to the *nerves* of the *brain* or *spinal cord* that stimulate the muscles. (The word *quadriparesis* may be used to describe *motor* weakness or partial paralysis in both arms, both legs, and often the head or face and the trunk.) Sometimes the word quadriplegia is used to describe *cerebral palsy* in which the legs, arms, face, and trunk are affected, with the legs and feet (and often the face) most affected.

Refer to **Paralysis, Pyramidal Cerebral Palsy,** *and* **Spastic Quadriplegia.**

Quadruped (KWOD-roo-ped)

Referring to an "all fours" (hands and knees) position.

Qualitative Developmental Assessment

An *evaluation* of the quality, rather than the quantity, of a child's *cognitive* skills.

Quetiapine Fumarate (cue-TIE-ah-peen FYOO-muh-rayt)

An *antipsychotic drug.* Seroquel™ is the brand name of this drug.

qwk

The abbreviation for every week.

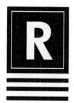

R
The abbreviation for respiration or response.

Radial (RAY-dee-uhl)
Referring to the thumb side of the forearm and the hand.

Radial Digital Grasp
Grasp of an object using the middle and index fingers, and the thumb (without the use of the palm of the hand). The radial digital grasp usually develops between 7 and 9 months of age.
　　Refer to **Grasp.**

Radial Palmar Grasp
Grasp of an object using the thumb, index and middle fingers, and the palm of the hand. The radial palmar grasp usually develops between 4½ and 6 months of age.
　　Refer to **Grasp.**

Radiation Therapy (ray-dee-AY-shuhn)
Treatment of *disease* caused by *tumor* growth by using *x-rays* or *gamma rays* (*gamma radiation*).
　　Also known as **Radiotherapy.**

Radiotherapy (ray-dee-oe-THER-uh-pee)
　　Refer to **Radiation Therapy.**

Radius (RAY-dee-uhs)
The long bone on the thumb side of the forearm, extending from the elbow to the wrist. The radius is the smaller of the two forearm bones. (The other bone is the *ulna*.)

Rale
An *abnormal* breathing sound heard through a stethoscope placed on the chest. Breathing is heard as a crackling sound when air passes through *bronchial tubes* congested with fluid.

Range of Motion (ROM)
The amount of motion in a *joint* from endpoint to endpoint (or extreme to extreme). This reflects the total distance through which a joint can be moved in natural directions. An example of the effects of a limited range of motion is seen in children with *pyramidal cerebral palsy*.
> *Refer to* **Active Range of Motion** *and* **Passive Range of Motion.**

Rash
A skin eruption. A rash can be a *sign* of a childhood *disease*, a skin *disorder*, an *infection,* or an *allergic* reaction.

Raw Score
The number of test items "passed."

RBC
The abbreviation for red blood cell.

RDS
The abbreviation for respiratory distress syndrome.

RE
The abbreviation for right extremity.

Reabsorption (ree-uhb-SORP-shuhn)
The process by which a substance is absorbed again, such as when *calcium* from bone is moved back into the blood.
> *Compare* **Absorption** *and* **Malabsorption.**

Reactive Attachment Disorder of Infancy or Early Childhood
A *disorder* that can develop in infants or young children prior to 5 years of age that is caused by emotional or physical *neglect* or abuse, or by lack of *attachment* to a *primary caregiver*. The *symptoms* of this disorder include inhibited types of *behaviors* such as failure to respond to or initiate social interactions, or disinhibited types of behaviors such as indiscriminate sociability with strangers. For Reactive Attachment Disorder of Infancy or Early Childhood to be *diagnosed*, the child's disturbance must not be due solely to *mental retardation* or attributed to a *pervasive developmental disorder*. Some affected infants experience *failure to thrive* and *developmental delays*. When adequate stable care is provided, the infant can improve.

Receptive Aphasia
> *Refer to* **Aphasia.**

Receptive-Expressive Emergent Language Scale – Third Edition (REEL-3)
A screening tool used to assess the verbal abilities of young children. A parent interview format is used.

Receptive Language
The ability to understand what is being expressed, including verbal and *nonverbal communication*, such as *sign language*.
> *Compare* **Expressive Language.**

Recessive Gene

A *gene* (unit of *heredity*) capable of producing an effect in the *organism* (such as the human body), only when it is transmitted to the offspring by both parents.
*Compare **Dominant Gene**.*
*Refer to **Autosomal Recessive Disorder** and **Gene**.*

Reciprocal Movement (ri-SIP-ruh-kuhl)

Alternating movements of the arms and legs, such as the movement involved in walking or in *creeping* on the hands and knees. With creeping, the right arm and left leg move forward more or less simultaneously, then the left arm and right leg move forward at the same time. Both sides of the body are involved in reciprocal movement.
*Compare **Non-Reciprocal Gait**.*

Reciprocating Gait Orthosis (RGO)

An *orthotic* device that assists with reciprocal walking. This *brace* provides support at the chest, hips, knees, ankles, and feet, and through the use of attached cables, allows the child to swing one leg forward at a time in a reciprocal motion.
*Refer to **Orthosis**.*

Reciprocity/Reciprocal

A mutual exchange of gestures, sounds, play, attention, or conversation between two or more people. Children with *autism spectrum disorders* have difficulty engaging in social and emotional reciprocity.

Recklinghausen Disease (REK-ling-hou-zen)

*Refer to **Neurofibromatosis**.*

Rectal

Pertaining to the *rectum*.

Rectal Administration

Administration of a drug via the *rectum*. *Absorption* is much faster than by *intramuscular injection* or by mouth and is very useful when an *IV* cannot be used.

Rectal Prolapse

*Refer to **Prolapse**.*

Rectal Temperature

The body's temperature reading when the thermometer is placed in the *rectum*. It runs approximately ½ to 1 degree higher than the *oral temperature* and is considered most accurate.
*Compare **Axillary Temperature, Oral Temperature**, and **Tympanic Membrane Temperature**.*

recto-

A prefix meaning *rectum*.

Rectoscopy (rek-TOS-kuh-pee)
A *diagnostic* technique for examining the *rectum* and *anus* in which a long, narrow, flexible tube is inserted into the rectum so the inside *tissues* can be seen. Tissue samples can also be obtained during this procedure.
Also known as **Proctoscopy.**

Rectum
The lowest part of the *large intestine* just before the anal canal and *anus*. The rectum moves *fecal matter* toward the anus for elimination from the body.

Red Blood Cell (RBC)
One of three types of *blood cells*. RBCs contain *hemoglobin*, which picks up *oxygen* from the lungs and carries it to body *tissues*.
Also known as **Erythrocyte.**
Compare **Platelet** *and* **White Blood Cell.**

REEL-3
The abbreviation for Receptive-Expressive Emergent Language Scale – Third Edition.

Reflex/Reflexive
An involuntary and unlearned response to a *stimulus* that occurs without thinking. Removing the hand when something hot is touched and the *patellar* ("knee jerk") *reflex* are examples of reflexes. Some reflexes (*primitive reflexes*) are normally only present in infants and disappear with normal *motor development*. When primitive reflexes persist beyond infancy, it may signify a *pathological* condition.
Refer to **Primitive Reflex** *and* **Automatic Reflex.**

Reflex Arc
A simple muscle action started by a *nerve* message that involves one muscle and one nerve pathway to and from the *spinal cord*. The *reflex* that is checked by tapping the knee with a rubber mallet is an example of a spinal reflex arc.

Reflux
A backward flow. An example is *gastroesophageal reflux.*
Refer to **Gastroesophageal Reflux.**

Refraction
1. The bending of light rays as they pass into a medium of different density. Refraction is part of the process of vision, which allows images to be focused on the *retina*.
2. The examination of the eye to determine if there is a refractive eye defect, such as *myopia*, and if there is a need for prescription eyeglasses.

Refractive Error
An eye defect that causes decreased *visual acuity*. Examples of refractive errors include *myopia* (*nearsightedness*, or blurred vision of distant objects), in

which the *lens* focuses distant objects in front of the *retina* because the eyeball is too long, and *hyperopia* (blurred vision of close objects), in which the lens focuses close objects behind the retina because the eyeball is too short.
Refer to **Refraction.**

Refractory Epilepsy
Seizures that don't respond to *antiepileptic drugs* and medical management.

Refsum Disease (REF-soom)
An *autosomal recessive neurologic disease* caused by the inability to *metabolize* phytanic acid (a *fatty acid* normally found in trace amounts), resulting in an accumulation of the acid. The disease may be detected in early childhood or not until middle age. *Symptoms* include night *blindness*, vision loss, *nerve inflammation, heart disease,* and *ataxia.* Refsum disease generally progresses slowly, with periods of waxing and waning of symptoms. Dietary management can relieve some of the symptoms of the disease.
Also known as **Phytanic Acid Storage Disease.**

Regard
To look or gaze.

Registered Nurse (RN)
A professional *nurse* who has completed the educational requirements (usually a bachelor's degree) and passed the necessary examination. RNs are licensed and registered by the state.
Compare **Licensed Practical Nurse** *and* **Licensed Vocational Nurse.**

Reglan™ (REG-lan)
Refer to **Metoclopramide Hydrochloride.**

Regression
Reverting to a more immature form of *behavior* or decreased skill level. For example, the young child who resumes sucking her thumb after a substantial period (months or years) of no thumb-sucking. Regression is usually felt to be an unconscious protective mechanism.

Regulation
Refer to **Self-Regulation** *and* **Sensory Regulation.**

Regulatory-Sensory Processing
The ability to receive *sensory* information (such as what the child touches, sees, hears, or senses about body position) and then accurately interpret it.
Refer to **Self-Regulation.**

Regulatory-Sensory Processing Disorder (RSPD)
One of a group of *disorders* in which the primary challenge to the child involves her *sensory*, visuospatial, auditory, and language processing, or *motor planning* and sequencing capacities. *Symptoms* can include inattention, overreac-

tivity, or sensory-seeking. RSPD is one of the five main categories of primary *diagnoses* (Axis 1) listed in the *Interdisciplinary Council on Developmental and Learning Disorders' Diagnostic Manual for Infancy and Early Childhood.*

> *Refer to* **Diagnostic Manual for Infancy and Early Childhood** *and* **Regulatory-Sensory Processing.**

Regurgitate (ree-GUR-ji-tayt)
To flow backwards, as when swallowed food or liquid flows back into the mouth from the stomach. Regurgitation also refers to blood flow back through a defective *heart valve.*

Rehabilitate
To provide an individual with treatment, education, and/or training designed to help her attain or restore her potential for normal living, including learning the skills necessary for *activities of daily living,* working, and engaging in social or leisure activities.

Rehabilitation Act of 1973 (PL 93-112)
A federal law that helps protect the rights of individuals with *disabilities.*

> *Refer to* **Section 504 of the Rehabilitation Act of 1973 (PL 93-112).**

Reinforcement
A *behavior modification* technique used to increase the likelihood of a desired response or *behavior.* Positive reinforcement is accomplished by immediately strengthening or rewarding a desirable behavior. The reward can be a social reinforcer, such as praise or a hug, or it can be material, such as a sticker or cookie. Negative reinforcement is accomplished by removing the usual unpleasant consequence of the child's behavior (such as yelling "No!") and, instead, ignoring the behavior. (It could be that the child is seeking the attention she gets for her undesirable behavior and so the adult's response actually reinforces, or encourages, the behavior.) For example, if the child typically hears "No!" every time she throws her cup on the floor, negative reinforcement would be to ignore her behavior, thereby depriving her of the satisfaction of the adult's attention. As might be expected, positive reinforcement is generally more effective than negative reinforcement.

Reinforcer
> *Refer to* **Reinforcement.**

Related Services
Services that enable a child to take advantage of *special education.* Related services include such things as *speech-language, occupational,* and *physical therapies,* and transportation, and are required under the *Individuals with Disabilities Education Improvement Act of 2004.*

> *Also known as* **Support Services.**

Reliability
The consistency of the results of a particular test instrument.

Remission
1. A decrease in the severity of the *symptoms* of a *disease*.
2. The period of time in which symptoms of a disease improve.

ren-, reno-
Prefixes meaning *kidney*.

Renal (REE-nuhl)
Pertaining to the *kidney*.

Renal Failure
Reduced function of the *kidney*. The kidney's ability to filter waste products from the blood and *excrete* them in the urine, to control the body's water and salt balance, and to regulate the *blood pressure* is diminished. Renal failure can be an *acute* or *chronic* condition. Acute renal failure is usually a temporary condition, and, once the underlying cause is treated, full kidney function returns. There are several causes of acute renal failure, including fluid and *electrolyte* depletion, *hemorrhage*, a *tumor* of the *bladder*, *nephritis* (*inflammation* of the kidney), *arterial* or *venous* obstruction, and severe injury, such as a burn. Chronic renal failure may result from any cause of significant *renal* dysfunction, such as *congestive heart failure*, infection, *hypercalcemia*, or obstruction, and it leads to *uremia*. If chronic renal failure is caused by a progressive and untreatable *disorder*, it usually progresses to complete loss of kidney function.
    *Also known as **Kidney Failure**.*

Representation
The use of a symbol to stand for an actual object or activity. An example of representation is understanding that a picture of a dog is a symbol for an actual dog.
    *Also known as **Symbolic Representation**.*

Rescue Breathing
    *Refer to **Resuscitation**.*

Reservoir
A place or body cavity that serves as a storage structure for fluids. An example is the *vitreous chamber*, which is the part of the cavity of the eyeball behind the *lens*.

Resident
A *physician* in his or her second or third year of postgraduate training at a hospital.

Residential Program
An educational or other treatment program that provides room and board for its clients.

Residual Hearing
The level at which the child can hear after impairment or injury, without *amplification*.
    *Refer to **Auditory Impairment**.*

Residual Vision
The level of vision in a child with *visual impairment*.

Resource Specialist
A teacher who provides *special education* instruction to children who are taught by regular classroom teachers for the majority of the school day.

Respiration (res-puh-RAY-shuhn)
Breathing. The process of inhaling and exhaling by which *oxygen* is delivered to the lungs and *carbon dioxide* is eliminated.

Respiration Rate (RR)
The rate of breathing. It is typically from 30-50 breaths per minutes for newborns, 20-30 breaths per minutes for toddlers, 18-24 breaths per minute for preschoolers, and decreases to 15-20 breaths per minute by puberty.

Respirator
>Refer to **Ventilator.**

Respiratory (RES-purh-uh-tor-ee)
Pertaining to *respiration*.

Respiratory Acidosis
An excess of acid in the blood and body *tissues* that occurs when the body is not able to remove *carbon dioxide* from the lungs due to illness, such as *respiratory distress syndrome* of the *premature infant* or *bronchitis*. It may also occur due to an obstruction in the *respiratory tract*. This condition can lead to disruption of the chemical processes within the body.
>Compare **Metabolic Acidosis.**

Respiratory Distress Syndrome (RDS)
A lung *disorder* that results in breathing difficulties and an insufficient level of *oxygen* in the blood. RDS is common in *premature infants* because the infant is born too early to have produced enough *surfactant*, which is the agent needed to keep the lungs' air sacs open for breathing.
>Also known as **Hyaline Membrane Disease.**

Respiratory Failure
Inadequate gas exchange (low *oxygen*, high *carbon dioxide*) by the *respiratory system*. This condition can lead to brain and heart malfunction resulting in deteriorating consciousness or unconsciousness and *abnormal* heart rhythms (*arrhythmias*), which can lead to death.

Respiratory Suctioning
>Refer to **Suctioning.**

Respiratory Syncytial Virus (RSV) (sin-SI-shuhl)
A type of *virus* that causes acute *respiratory disease* (such as *pneumonia*) in children.

Respiratory System
*Refer to **Respiratory Tract.***

Respiratory Therapist
A specialist who uses various techniques to preserve or improve the breathing abilities of children with breathing problems, such as infants who are *ventilator*-dependent or children with other types of lung *disease*.

Respiratory Tract
The organs and structures involved in the process of breathing. The respiratory tract also warms air entering the body and assists in speech function.
*Also known as **Respiratory System.***

Respite Care (RES-pit)
Skilled caregiving service that can be provided to the parent of a child who is disabled or seriously ill. Respite care allows parents time away from home for several hours or overnight to rest or attend to other needs. Respite care is provided in the family's home or in the home of a care-provider. The duties of the respite worker usually include feeding, hygiene care, and companionship for the child.

Restraint
A device used to prevent a child from moving in such a way that could injure her. A restraint might be used when the child who has *seizures*, or is unable to sit without support, is placed in a chair.

Resuscitation (ri-sus-i-TAY-shuhn)
*Also known as **Rescue Breathing.***
*Refer to **Artificial Respiration, Cardiopulmonary Resuscitation,** and **Mouth-to-Mouth.***

Retardation
A slowing of, as in physical growth or mental maturation.
*Refer to **Mental Retardation.***

reti-, reticulo-
A prefix meaning network.

Retina (RET-i-nuh)
The *membrane* lining the back of the inside of the eyeball on which images from the *cornea* and *lens* of the eye are focused and transmitted to the *brain* for vision.
*Refer to **Eye.***

Retinitis Pigmentosa (ret-in-IE-tis pig-men-TOE-suh)
A *disorder* in which there is *degeneration* in the *retinas* of both eyes (with corresponding areas of *abnormal* pigment accumulation) that leads to varying degrees of *visual impairment*. Retinitis pigmentosa usually occurs due to *genetic* factors.

Retinoblastoma (ret-i-noe-blas-TOE-muh)
A *malignant congenital tumor* of the *retina* of the eye that affects the infant's vision. Retinoblastoma sometimes occurs due to *genetic* factors. Treatment involves removal of the *diseased* eye, followed by *radiation therapy* and *chemotherapy*.

Retinoic Acid
A drug used for treating severe acne that has been associated with *brain* malformation and other significant *anomalies* of children whose mothers used it during pregnancy. Accutane™ is the brand name of this drug.

Retinopathy of Prematurity (ROP) (ret-in-OP-uh-thee)
An eye *disorder* that can develop in the *premature infant*. (Retinopathy occurs primarily, but not exclusively, in premature babies.) The *etiology* is not quite clear, but there is an increased *incidence* in infants who are given high levels of *oxygen* for long periods of time to treat *respiratory distress*. There is also an association between ROP and the bright lights of the *neonatal intensive care unit*, *hypoxia*, *shock*, *asphyxia*, and *vitamin* E deficiency. Most ROP gradually resolves, but some children develop other visual problems later in life. Generally, the lower the infant's *birth weight*, the more severe the *disease*. A small percentage of children have progressive disease, and, in the most severe cases eventually have *retinal* detachment and/or *blindness*. The stages of ROP are scored from 1 through 4, with 4 describing the most severe level of the disease.
    Refer to **Retrolental Fibroplasia.**

Retraction
1. An *abnormal* sinking in of the chest that occurs when the infant is making great efforts to breathe.
2. A drawing back of a body part (usually referring to the hips or shoulders), to a point behind its normal resting position.

retro-
A prefix meaning backward or located behind.

Retrolental Fibroplasia (RLF) (ret-roe-LEN-tuhl fie-broe-PLAY-zee-uh)
The severe stages of *retinopathy of prematurity,* which involve scarring of the *retinal vessels* and can result in retinal detachment and *blindness*.
    Refer to **Retinopathy of Prematurity.**

Retrusion (ri-TROO-shun)
A condition in which a body part, such as the teeth, is displaced backward or is being forced backward.

Rett's Disorder
A very rare *autism spectrum disorder* occurring in approximately 1 of 15,000 births that almost exclusively affects girls. Children with Rett's disorder demonstrate typical *development* in early infancy, then move through 4 stages of the *disorder* in which skills are lost (especially in the social, language, and *gross motor* areas, and in purposeful use of the hands); interest in people and

things in the environment decreases; hand-wringing and *seizures* may begin; irritablility and insomnia may develop; and health, eating, and *motor* coordination concerns may arise. A *diagnosis* of Rett's disorder is made when a child frequently demonstrates all of the following *symptoms*: 1) apparently normal *prenatal* and *perinatal* development; 2) apparently normal *psychomotor* development through the first 5 months after birth; 3) normal *head circumference* at birth; 4) deceleration of head growth between ages 5 and 48 months; 5) loss of previously acquired purposeful hand skills between ages 5 and 30 months with subsequent development of *stereotyped* hand movements (such as hand-wringing); 6) loss of social *engagement* early in the course (although often social interaction develops again later); 7) appearance of poorly coordinated *gait* or trunk movements; 8) severely impaired *expressive* and *receptive* *language* development with severe psychomotor retardation.

Refer to **Autism Spectrum Disorder.**

Reye Syndrome (RAY)
A rare *disorder* characterized by *brain* and *liver* damage that develops suddenly after a flu or chickenpox (*viral*) infection, often after a child has been treated with *aspirin* (*salicylate*). Depending on the severity of the *central nervous system* involvement, Reye syndrome can be a life-threatening condition. (Thirty percent of children who develop Reye syndrome do not survive.)

RGO
The abbreviation for reciprocating gait orthosis.

Rheumatic Fever (roo-MAT-ik)
A *disease* in which there is *tissue inflammation*, especially of the larger *joints* of the body. It may develop after infection with certain strains of *streptococcal* *bacteria*. Rheumatic fever is characterized by the sudden occurrence of fever and pain and stiffness of the joints; small, solid nodules (masses) under the skin; *involuntary movements* that affect the *gait*, arm movements, and speech; *erythema* (an inflammation of the skin resulting in redness); and occasionally *heart* damage of varying degrees.

Rheumatic Heart Disease
Heart disease caused by *rheumatic fever*. Damage to the *heart* is usually related to the *valves* and causes *heart murmurs*.

Rh Factor
A type of *protein* that is present on the *red blood cells* of people who have Rh positive blood. The Rh factor is an *inherited* trait. The Rh factor is important in blood transfusion (Rh negative recipients cannot receive Rh positive blood) and in pregnant women who are Rh negative with an Rh positive *fetus*.

Refer to **Rh Incompatibility.**

rhin-
A prefix meaning nose.

Rh Incompatibility
A condition that occurs when a woman with Rh negative blood is pregnant with an infant with Rh positive blood (an *inherited* trait from the baby's father). Some of the baby's Rh positive blood may enter the mother's *circulation* at the time of birth or *miscarriage*, causing the mother to develop *antibodies* against Rh positive blood. In subsequent pregnancies with an Rh positive *fetus*, the antibodies are passed through the *placenta* to the fetus, destroying the fetus's *red blood cells*. Injections can and should be given to prevent Rh *disease* in future pregnancies. Rh incompatibility can also occur if a woman with Rh negative blood mistakenly receives a transfusion of Rh positive blood.
> *Refer to* **Rh Factor.**

Rhinitis (rie-NIE-tis)
Inflammation of the *mucous membranes* of the nose, usually accompanied by a "runny" nose (nasal discharge).

rhino-
A prefix meaning nose.

Rhinorrhea (rie-noe-REE-uh)
The discharge of *mucus* from the nose.

Rhizotomy (rie-ZOT-uh-mee)
> *Refer to* **Dorsal Rhizotomy.**

Riboflavin (rie-boe-FLAY-vin)
Vitamin B2, a component of the B vitamin complex. Riboflavin deficiency causes skin changes, and problems with vision and growth.

Rickets
A condition caused by *vitamin* D deficiency. It is characterized by *abnormalities* in the shape and structure of bones, delayed closure of the *fontanelles* (the two soft spots on the top of the infant's head), body pain or tenderness, sweating of the head, and an enlarged *liver* and *spleen*. Rickets is treated with vitamin D, sunlight, and adequate diet.

Ride-On Toy
A wheeled toy on which the child can sit and move about, using her feet on the floor to propel herself forward.

Righting Reaction
An automatic movement response to bring or restore the head and body to an upright position. Righting reactions are normal responses. An example of a righting reaction is the automatic response of holding the head upright even if the body is tilted.
> *Refer to* **Automatic Reflex.**

Rigid Cerebral Palsy
A form of *extrapyramidal cerebral palsy* characterized by extremely high *muscle tone*. Rigid cerebral palsy is caused by damage to the *nerve* pathways that

transmit impulses for controlling movement and maintaining *posture* from the *brain* to the *spinal cord*.
>   *Refer to* **Extrapyramidal Cerebral Palsy.**

Rigidity

1. Extremely high *muscle tone* in any position, combined with very limited movement.
2. Inflexibility of *behavior* or needing things to happen in a very specific way in order for them to "feel right" to the child.

Riley-Day Syndrome

An *autosomal dominant disorder*, most commonly seen in Ashkenazi Jews, characterized by *autonomic nervous system* problems including difficulty with swallowing, excessive salivation and sweating, unstable temperature and *blood pressure*, *taste* deficiency, insensitivity to pain, and skin blotching; *dysarthria*; lack of *motor* coordination; emotional instability; *seizures* in about 50 percent of affected children; ulceration of the *cornea* (due to lack of tearing); and, often, recurring *aspiration pneumonia*. Approximately 50 percent of individuals with Riley-Day syndrome do not survive beyond 20 years of age.
>   *Also known as* **Dysautonomia, Familial Autonomic Dysfunction, and Familial Dysautonomia.**

Ring Chromosome

A *chromosome* that forms a circular shape due to fusion of the two ends. Ring chromosome *anomalies* often result in growth and *mental retardation*.

Ring Sit

Sitting on the buttocks with the knees bent and the bottoms of the feet together.

Ringworm

>   *Refer to* **Tinea Capitis.**

Risperdol™ (RIS-pur-dol)

>   *Refer to* **Risperidone.**

Risperidone (ris-PUR-i-don)

An *antipsychotic drug*. Risperdol™ is the brand name of this drug.

Ritalin™ (RIT-uh-lin)

>   *Refer to* **Methylphenidate Hydrochloride.**

Ritualistic Behavior

Seemingly purposeless *behavior* that a child always engages in when in a particular situation. For example, on entering a room, a child may always have to turn the lights off and on twice.

Rivotril™

>   *Refer to* **Clonazepam.**

RLE
The abbreviation for right lower extremity.

RLF
The abbreviation for retrolental fibroplasia.

RN
The abbreviation for Registered Nurse.

Roberts Syndrome
An *autosomal recessive disorder* characterized by imperfect development of the long bones of the *limbs* (resulting in short arms and legs), *cleft palate,* lip, eye and other *anomalies,* and, often, *mental retardation.*

Robinow-Silverman-Smith Syndrome
Refer to Robinow Syndrome.

Robinow-Silverman Syndrome
Refer to Robinow Syndrome.

Robinow Syndrome (ROB-i-nou)
A rare *congenital disorder* characterized by *short stature,* shortened forearms, facial features similar to a young *fetus,* spinal *anomaly* in which half of an individual *vertebra* is missing, underdeveloped *genitalia,* a prominent forehead, widely-spaced eyes, shorter fingers, occasional speech delay, and, usually, *normal intelligence.* Robinow syndrome is most often an *autosomal dominant disorder,* but *recessive* and *sporadic* cases have been reported. Both boys and girls are affected.
   *Also known as **Robinow-Silverman Syndrome, Robinow-Silverman-Smith Syndrome,** and **Fetal Face Syndrome.***

Rocker-Bottom Foot
Refer to Congenital Rocker-Bottom Foot.

Rolandic Epilepsy
Refer to Benign Rolandic Epilepsy.

Rolfing (ROL-fing)
Refer to Structural Integration.

Roll
A cylindrical piece of equipment (often made of foam) on which the infant with *special needs* is placed to help develop muscle strength and control, *balance* and protective reactions, the ability to assume and maintain new positions, and/or weight-bearing and weight-shifting skills. The infant may be placed over the roll on his *abdomen,* he may be placed on the roll in a straddle position, or he may be placed on the roll in a sitting position with the legs together.
   *Also known as **Bolster** and **Therapy Roll.***

Rollator™
An adjustable *walker* that only has wheels on the front two legs.

ROM
The abbreviation for range of motion.

Room Air
The regular air we breathe. Room air is 21 percent *oxygen* by volume.

Rooting Reflex
A normal response in infants up to 4 months of age in which, when the baby's cheek is stroked, the head turns to the same side as the stroked cheek and the baby begins to suck. The rooting reflex is present until approximately 12 months of age in the sleeping baby.
    Refer to **Primitive Reflex.**

ROP
The abbreviation for retinopathy of prematurity.

Roseola (roe-zee-OE-luh or roe-ZEE-oe-luh)
1. A *viral* infection that mainly affects children between 6 months and 2 years of age. Roseola causes a high spiking fever that lasts for usually 3 but up to 5 days, and is followed by a *rash* over most of the body. The rash usually appears after the fever disappears.
2. Any rose-colored rash.

Rossetti Infant-Toddler Language Scale™
A *criterion-referenced* instrument designed to assess the preverbal and verbal language skills of the birth to 36-month-old. The Rossetti Infant-Toddler Language Scale is a measure of *communication* and interaction and it assesses the following areas of *development*: interaction-attachment, *pragmatics, gesture,* play, language comprehension, and language expression. It was developed by Louis Rossetti, Ph.D.

Rotary Chewing
Normal *chewing* in which there is rotary jaw movement, rather than an up-and-down biting motion. The tongue moves food within the mouth from side to side and front to back. Rotary chewing develops between 18 and 24 months of age.
    Refer to **Chewing.**

Rotation Movement
A turning or twisting movement between two body parts. Examples of rotation include the head turning from side to side, or the trunk twisting. Rotation is one of the four basic kinds of movement by the *joints* of the body.
    Compare **Angular Movement, Circumduction Movement,** *and* **Gliding Movement.**

Roussy-Levy Syndrome (roo-SEE lay-VEE)
A slowly progressive *familial disorder* characterized by muscle wasting, especially of the calves and the hands; *scoliosis*; and *ataxia* (an inability to coordinate muscles in voluntary movement).

RR
The abbreviation for respiration rate.

-rrhagia
A suffix meaning excessive discharge.

-rrhaphy
A suffix meaning *suture* or sew.

-rrhea
A suffix meaning flowing.

-rrhexia
A suffix meaning break or rupture.

RSPD
The abbreviation for regulatory-sensory processing disorder.

RSV
The abbreviation for respiratory syncytial virus.

Rubella (roo-BEL-luh)
A mild, *contagious viral* infection *symptomized* by *rash*, fever, enlarged *lymph nodes,* and *respiratory* symptoms. Rubella is only serious in the pregnant woman who is infected during the first 4 months of pregnancy, when the *virus* can cause *fetal abnormalities* including *mental retardation, heart disease, deafness,* and eye *disorders.* The rubella vaccination provides *immunity* to the virus.
> Also known as **Three-Day Measles** and **German Measles.**
> Compare **Measles.**
> Refer to **Congenital Rubella** and **Measles, Mumps, and Rubella Vaccine.**

Rubenstein-Taybi Syndrome (ROO-bin-stien-TAY-bee)
A *congenital disorder* characterized by *short stature*; *anomalies* of the *vertebrae* and *sternum*; small head; facial anomalies including *ptosis* (drooping of the upper eyelid), slanting eyes, *exophthalmos* (*abnormal* protrusion of the eyeball), *epicanthal folds* (a vertical skin fold at the inner corner of the eyes), *strabismus* (a condition in which the eyes do not work together), a thin beaked nose, high arched *palate,* and underdeveloped upper jaw; low-set and/or malformed ears; occasional *cardiac* anomaly; broad thumbs and great toes; *undescended testes*; and *mental retardation.*

Rubeola
> Refer to **Measles.**

RUE
The abbreviation for right upper extremity.

Rx
The abbreviation for prescription.

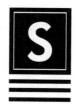

s
The abbreviation for without.

Sabin Vaccine (SAY-bin)
Refer to Oral Polio Vaccine.

Sacral (SAK-ruhl or SAY-kruhl)
Pertaining to the *sacrum*.

Sacrum (SAK-ruhm or SAY-kruhm)
The five fused *vertebrae* of the lower back that form the back part of the *pelvis*. The sacrum is triangular in shape and is located between the two hip bones.

Saethre-Chotzen Syndrome (SAY-truh-KOT-zuhn)
An *autosomal dominant disorder* characterized by a *congenital* malformation of the skull caused by premature closure of certain *sutures* (resulting in a head that appears pointed at the top); mildly webbed or fused fingers and/or toes; an *abnormally* wide space between the eyes; drooping upper eyelids; and, sometimes, *mental retardation*.
Also known as Acrocephalosyndactyly, Type III.

Sakati-Nyhan Syndrome (sah-KAH-tee-NIE-han)
An *autosomal dominant disorder* characterized by a *congenital* malformation of the skull caused by premature closure of certain *sutures* (resulting in a head that appears pointed at the top); webbed or fused fingers and/or toes; extra fingers and/or toes; underdeveloped *tibias*; and malformed, displaced *fibulas*. *Intelligence* is usually normal.
Also known as Acrocephalopolysyndactyly, Type III.

Salicylate (sal-i-SIL-ayt or sal-IS-il-ayt)
A white substance used to make *aspirin*.

Saline Solution (SAY-leen or SAY-lien)
A solution containing salt (sodium chloride).

Salk Vaccine
*Refer to **Inactivated Poliovirus Vaccine of Enhanced Potency (IPV-E).***

salpingo-
A prefix meaning fallopian tube.

Sanfilippo Syndrome (san-fi-LIP-oe)
An *autosomal recessive mucopolysaccharidosis disorder* characterized by *coarse facial features, hirsutism* (excessive body hair), mildly stiff *joints,* normal growth for 1 to 3 years followed by slowed growth, and *mental retardation* by 1½ to 3 years of age. The child with this *disorder* tends to have *severe mental retardation,* and to deteriorate in *motor,* speech, and *social skills.*
*Also known as **Mucopolysaccharidosis III or MPS III.***

sarc-
A prefix meaning similar to or resembling flesh.

SBFE
The abbreviation for Stanford-Binet Intelligence Scale - Fourth Edition.
*Refer to **Stanford-Binet Intelligence Scale – Fifth Edition (SBIS – V).***

SBIS – V
The abbreviation for Stanford-Binet Intelligence Scale - Fifth Edition.

Scalp IV
The placement of an *intravenous* needle in a *vein* in the scalp. The scalp is often chosen as the location for *IV* placement in an infant because the scalp has an abundance of surface veins and because an IV placed there does not restrict the baby's arm and leg movements.

Scaphocephalism (skaf-oe-SEF-uh-lizm)
*Refer to **Scaphocephaly.***

Scaphocephaly (skaf-oe-SEF-uh-lee)
A condition in which the child's head is shaped *abnormally* long and narrow. Scaphocephaly is a form of *craniosynostosis* and is sometimes associated with *mental retardation.*
*Also known as **Scaphocephalism.***

Scaphoid Bone (SKAF-oid)
*Refer to **Navicular Bone.***

Scaphoid Pad
*Refer to **Arch Insole Pad.***

Scapula (SKAP-yuh-luh)
The shoulder blade.

Scarlet Fever
A *contagious* childhood *disease* characterized by a widespread red *rash*, sore throat, and fever. It is caused by a type of *streptococcal (strep throat) bacteria* that can be treated with *antibiotic drugs*.

Scattered Scores
Scores on an *assessment* that range between high scores and low scores. Achieving high scores in some *developmental* areas and low scores in other areas shows an uneven quality to the child's development and may indicate that the child is *at-risk* or *developmentally delayed*.

Scheie Syndrome (SHAY)
An *autosomal recessive mucopolysaccharidosis disorder* characterized by a broad mouth with full lips that develops between 5 and 8 years of age, opacity of the *corneas* of the eyes, *retinitis pigmentosa*, *joint* limitation, mild deformities of the bones, including broad and short hands and feet, *cardiac* defect, a short neck, and *normal intelligence*.
Also known as **Mucopolysaccharidosis V** *or* **MPS V**.

Schizencephaly (skiz-en-SEF-uh-lee)
A (usually) *sporadically* occurring condition in which the baby is born with elongated *clefts* (openings) in the *cerebral hemispheres* of the *brain*. Schizencephaly can result in *mental retardation, spasticity, hemiparesis, hypotonia, microcephaly, epilepsy,* or a combination of *symptoms*, depending on the location of the clefts. The level of severity depends upon the size and number of clefts.
Also known as **Schizencephalic Porencephaly**.
Compare **Porencephaly**.

Schizophrenia (skit-suh-FREE-nee-uh or skit-suh-FREN-ee-uh)
Any of a group of mental illnesses in which the individual displays characteristic *psychotic symptoms* (such as delusions, hallucinations, and *flat affect*) and functions at a lower level than before the onset of the disturbance (or, in the case of children and adolescents, fails to achieve the *social skills* expected of their age group). The individual with schizophrenia usually withdraws and displays thoughts and feelings that do not relate to each other in a normal way. Schizophrenia usually appears during adolescence or early adulthood. Investigators have found both *genetic* and non-genetic causes associated with schizophrenia.

School Psychologist
Refer to **Psychologist**.

Schwa (shwah)
The *vowel* sound produced when the lips and tongue are relaxed (the /uh/ sound).

Scissoring
Bringing the extended legs together so they are tightly crossed at the knees. Scissoring can occur if there is extreme tightness of the *adductor* muscles in the inner thighs. The child with *pyramidal cerebral palsy* may scissor his legs.

Sclera (SKLER-uh)
The tough, dense white *membrane* starting at the edges of the *cornea* and covering most of the back of the eyeball.

Sclerae (SKLER-ay)
Plural of *sclera*.

sclero-
A prefix meaning hardening.

Sclerosis (skluh-ROE-sis)
A condition in which there is hardening of body *tissue*. The cause is not always understood but it can be caused by chronic *inflammation* or by plaque formation (raised areas). *Atherosclerosis* (thickening of the inside walls of the *arteries*) and *multiple sclerosis* (a progressive *central nervous system disease* that affects adults and may result in *paralysis*) are examples.

Scoliosis (skoe-lee-OE-sis)
A C-shaped or S-shaped *lateral* (sideways) *curvature of the spine*. Scoliosis can occur as a result of *poliomyelitis* or other *neuromuscular disease*, of *paralysis* of spinal muscles, of one leg being shorter than the other, or due to a *congenital abnormality* of the *vertebrae*. Often the cause of scoliosis is unknown.
> Compare **Kyphosis** and **Lordosis**.
> Refer to **Congenital Scoliosis**.

Scooter Board
A *mobility aid* that holds the child in proper alignment to allow him to move about and explore his environment. The child lies on his *abdomen* on a board with casters and uses his hands to propel forward. Adaptations may be necessary depending on the child's *muscle tone*, *head control*, tendency to scissor his legs, etc.

Screening Test
1. Any test designed to minimize *false negatives* (to not miss any patient with a particular condition).
2. An *evaluation* tool designed to identify children who are *at-risk* for having or developing a *developmental disability*. The *Denver Developmental Screening Test (Denver II)* is an example of a screening test.
> Compare **Criterion-Referenced Test** and **Norm-Referenced Test**.

Screening Tests for Young Children and Retardates
> Refer to **STYCAR**.

Script
> Refer to **Auditory Script** and **Textual Script**.

Script-Fading
> Refer to **Auditory Script**.

Seborrheic Dermatitis (seb-oe-REE-ik dur-muh-TIE-tis)
A common skin condition affecting the scalp and face. It consists of thick, yellow scales and *erythema* (*inflammation* of the skin resulting in redness) on the scalp, and occasionally the face, neck, chest, or the infant's diaper area. The cause is unknown.
> *Also known as* **Cradle Cap** *(in infants).*

Seckel Syndrome
An *autosomal recessive disorder* characterized by *short stature* (*prenatal* onset of growth deficiency), *microcephaly* (an *abnormally* small head size), *strabismus* (a condition in which the eyes do not work together), prominent beaked nose, low-set and/or malformed ears, *simian crease* (a single crease across the palm of the hand), absent thumb, *clinodactyly* (an incurved fifth finger), *hip dislocation*, and moderate to *severe mental retardation*.

Secondary Circular Reactions
According to Jean *Piaget's* theory of *cognitive* development, the infant's repeating of an action involving an object that initially occurred as an accident. After the first accidental occurrence, the 4- to 8-month-old attempts and succeeds at repeating the action (such as batting a toy that makes noise). Secondary circular reactions is a substage of the *sensory-motor stage*.
> *Compare* **Primary Circular Reactions.**
> *Refer to* **Sensory-Motor Stage.**

Secondary Epilepsy
> *Refer to* **Symptomatic Epilepsy** *and* **Epilepsy.**

Secondary Seizure
> *Refer to* **Symptomatic Epilepsy** *and* **Epilepsy.**

Secondary Teeth
The permanent teeth that begin to replace the *primary teeth* (*baby teeth*) starting around 6 years of age. There are 32 secondary teeth, 16 in each jaw.
> *Also known as* **Permanent Teeth.**
> *Compare* **Primary Teeth.**

Secrete/Secretion (si-KREET/si-KREE-shuhn)
To release *cell* products for use in the body.
> *Compare* **Excrete.**
> *Refer to* **Gland.**

Secretin (si-KREE-tin)
A naturally occurring *hormone* that aids in *digestion*. Some people have theorized that a deficiency in secretin plays a role in causing *symptoms* of *autism spectrum disorders*.

-sect
A suffix meaning cut or divide.

Section 504 of the Rehabilitation Act of 1973 (PL 93-112)

A federal law that helps protect the rights of students with *disabilities*. It requires states to provide education programs for eligible students with disabilities that are equal to those for students without disabilities. Students eligible for a program under Section 504 include any child who a) has a physical or mental impairment that limits one or more major life activities; b) has record of such an impairment; or c) is regarded as having such an impairment. A major life activity under Section 504 includes breathing, *hearing*, learning, seeing, speaking, walking, caring for oneself, performing manual tasks, and working. At age 3 years, a child may be eligible for Section 504 services, even if they do not qualify for the *Individuals with Disabilities Education Improvement Act of 2004.*

SEE

The abbreviation for Signed Exact English.

Segmental Rolling

Rolling, in which the body moves sequentially; i.e., the head moves first, then the shoulders, then the hips.

Seizure (SEE-zhur)

Involuntary movement or changes in consciousness or *behavior* brought on by *abnormal* and excessive bursts of electrical activity in the *brain*.

>*Refer to* **Convulsion** *and* **Epilepsy.**

Seizure Disorder

>*Refer to* **Epilepsy.**

Seizure Threshold

The amount of *abnormal* and excessive bursts of electrical activity in the *brain* necessary to cause a *seizure*. A child who experiences spontaneous seizures due to a *seizure disorder* is said to have a "low seizure threshold."

Selective Dorsal Rhizotomy

>*Refer to* **Dorsal Rhizotomy.**

Selective Mutism

A *disorder* characterized by failure to speak in specific social situations (in which there is an expectation to speak, such as at school), despite the ability to speak in other situations.

>*Formerly known as* **Elective Mutism.**
>*Compare* **Mutism.**

Selective Posterior Rhizotomy

>*Refer to* **Dorsal Rhizotomy.**

Selective Serotonin Reuptake Inhibitor (SSRI)
(si-LEK-tiv ser-uh-TOE-nin ree-UP-tayk in-HIB-i-tuhr)
Any of several *antidepressant drugs* that prevent (inhibit) the *reabsorption* (reuptake) of the *neurotransmitter serotonin* produced in the *brain*. Preventing serotonin from being reabsorbed quickly increases the amount of serotonin available in the brain. SSRIs selectively act on serotonin and have zero to little effect on other brain chemicals. SSRIs are sometimes used to treat *behavioral rigidity* and *ritualistic behaviors* associated with *autism spectrum disorders* and *obsessive-compulsive disorder*.

Self-Comforting Behavior
Activity in which the baby engages to comfort himself, such as sucking on his fist or fingers.

Self-Help
The developmental area that involves skills that enable the child to care for his own needs, such as feeding, bathing, and dressing himself.
*Refer to **Activities of Daily Living** and **Adaptive Behavior/Skill**.*

Self-Injurious Behavior (SIB) (SELF-in-JOOR-ee-uhs)
Repetitive *abnormal behaviors* that are harmful to oneself, such as *head banging* or scratching or biting oneself.
*Compare **Self-Stimulation**.*

Self-Regulation
The ability to organize and respond to internal *stimuli*, as well as environmental demands. Self-regulation includes the control of body temperature, *heart rate*, *respiratory rate*, voluntary body movements, and arousal level.

Self-Stimulation
Persistent, repetitive *abnormal behaviors* such as watching the fingers wiggle or rocking side to side, that interfere with the child's ability to "sit still" and focus or to participate in meaningful activity. It may also be considered self-stimulation if the child plays with a toy, but without purpose, such as only spinning the wheels on a toy truck rather than exploring it in other ways as well. The child may engage in self-stimulatory behavior (often referred to as "stimming") if he cannot readily participate with people and objects in his environment. Self-stimulation is most common in children who have *mental retardation*, an *autism spectrum disorder*, or a *psychosis*.
*Compare **Perseveration**, **Self-Injurious Behavior**, and **Stereotypic Behavior**.*

Semantics
The study of the meaning of language, specifically the understanding of the relationship between words (not just of the meaning of individual words). An example of semantics is the understanding that "kick the ball" is different than "throw the ball." The child must not only be able to identify the ball, but also understand how to act upon it.

semi-
A prefix meaning half.

Semicircular Canal
One of the three bony, fluid-filled passages of the *inner ear*. The semicircular canals are involved in detecting motion for the sense of *balance*.

Sensorimotor (sen-suh-ree-MOE-tuhr)
Referring to *input* from the senses, in conjunction with purposeful *motor* responses. For example, catching a ball is a sensorimotor activity because both vision and raising the arms to the right place and at the right time are required.

Sensorimotor Integration
The ability to receive *input* from the various individual senses, organize them into a meaningful whole, and produce a purposeful *motor* response. For example, when running, leaning forward as the ground slopes upward. (This response may not be on a conscious level.)

Sensorineural Hearing Impairment (sen-suh-ree-NOOR-uhl)
Auditory impairment that results from permanent damage to the *inner ear* or to the *auditory nerve*, which transmits sound *stimuli* (in the form of electrical impulses) to the *brain*. Sensorineural hearing impairment can occur *congenitally* or be *acquired*. If senorineural hearing impairment is acquired (such as from a *tumor* of the auditory nerve) and if the child receives treatment before permanent damage, his *hearing* may improve.
>	*Compare* **Conductive Hearing Impairment** *and* **Mixed Hearing Impairment.**
>	*Refer to* **Auditory Impairment.**

Sensory
1. Pertaining to sensation.
2. Relating to the body's *sensory nerve* network.

Sensory Defensiveness
The fight or flight responses of a child reacting to a *sensory* experience that most children would consider common or tolerable. The child experiences the *sensory stimulation* as unpleasant, uncomfortable, or intolerable. For example, a child with auditory defensiveness may be terrified of loud noises and therefore avoid activities such as birthday parties or amusement parks that may be noisy.
>	*Refer to* **Oral Tactile Defensiveness** *and* **Tactile Defensiveness.**

Sensory Diet
A "kit" of materials or activities (usually designed by an *occupational therapist*) for a child and his family that provides individualized *sensory input* or movement suggestions for that child to utilize throughout the day. The kit should be organized according to the child's specific needs and should be available for home/school/other use. Appropriate materials and activities often provide *proprioceptive* input (pressure/sensations provided to *joints* and

muscles) and/or *vestibular* input (sensations related to *balance* and movement in space). Kit materials may include a squishy rubber ball to play with during circle time, whistles/bubbles to play with before meal time, or finding hidden treasures in playdough to warm up fingers prior to *fine motor* exercises. Kit activities may include performing *jumping* activities prior to seated tasks, rolling up (with face exposed) in heavy blanket prior to difficult *cognitive* tasks, and sitting on a large therapy ball during tabletop tasks. These tools and techniques are intended to enable the child with *sensory integration* difficulties to stay focused, *on-task*, and ready to learn.

Sensory Dysfunction
Refer to Sensory Integration Dysfunction.

Sensory Impairment
A problem with receiving information through one or more of the senses (sight, *hearing*, touch, etc.). For example, *deafness* is a sensory impairment.

Sensory Integration (SI)
A child's ability to receive, interpret, organize, and respond to *sensory* information (experienced through the 7 senses including touch, movement, sight, sound, smell, *proprioception*, and *vestibular*) and then use that information to complete physical actions in response to environmental demands. Sensory integration refers to the entire sequence of events from the initial sensory *stimulus* to the final environmental interaction. For example, listening to and following simple directions involves sensory integration.
Refer to Sensory Integration Dysfunction and Sensory Processing.

Sensory Integration Dysfunction (DSI)
A *neurological disorder* characterized by an inability to receive, interpret, organize, and respond to *sensory* information and have an appropriate reaction. Children with DSI have difficulty tolerating, detecting, or processing *sensory stimulation* and may respond in an oversensitive (*hyperresponsive*) or undersensitive (*hyporesponsive*) manner. For example, a child who is *hyperresponsive* may feel true discomfort from loud sounds, firm hugs, or the way new or stiff clothing feels against his skin. A child who is *hyporesponsive* may crave the sensations that constant movement and rougher play bring. A child with DSI can appear clumsy due to the challenges he experiences with *motor planning*. The cause of DSI is unclear, but there is an association with *traumatic* or premature birth (the environmental *stimulation* and painful procedures of the *neonatal intensive care unit* may have bombarded the newborn's underdeveloped sensory systems) and with *hereditary* factors. Some research also suggests that unidentified environmental *toxins* may cause DSI. While many people experience degrees of under- or overresponsiveness to sensory stimulation, a diagnosis of DSI is not made unless the child's ability to participate in typical daily activities is disrupted. Although children with DSI typically have *normal intelligence*, it should be noted that DSI is seen in the majority of children with *learning disabilities*, and that there is an association with some *developmental disabilities*, such as *autism spectrum disorder* and attention-

deficit/hyperactivity disorder. Occupational therapy is often recommended to help the child learn to regulate his attention and activity levels, to better tolerate sensory stimulation, and to increase motor planning skills.

> *Also known as* **Dysfunction in Sensory Integration.**
> *Refer to* **Sensory Diet, Sensory Integration, Sensory Integration Therapy,** *and* **DSI.**

Sensory Integration Therapy

A therapy technique used to help a child integrate (receive, interpret, organize, and respond to) sensations from his body and from the environment. The goal is to help the child with *hypo-* or *hyperresponsiveness, motor planning* difficulties, decreased *attending* skills, or inadequate body awareness to process, organize, and respond to *sensory* information. Sensory integration therapy often involves activities and movement that provides the child with *vestibular, proprioceptive,* and *tactile stimulation.* It may include massage; use of vibration; and play activities that involve swinging, rocking, *bouncing,* spinning, *crawling/creeping* through tunnels or over mats, *jumping* on a mat or trampoline, and playing on inclines or *scooter boards.* Encouraging the child to touch or play with different textures and mediums, such as fabrics, sand, water, paint, or playdough may be a part of sensory integration therapy. Sensory integration therapy was developed by A. Jean Ayres, Ph.D., OTR.

> *Refer to* **Sensory Integration Dysfunction** *and* **Sensory Diet.**

Sensory Modulation

A child's ability to regulate and organize his *behavioral* reactions to incoming *sensory input.* A child's level of modulation is dependent upon his ability to demonstrate graded and *developmentally* appropriate responses to input.

> *Also known as* **Sensory Regulation.**
> *Refer to* **Self-Regulation.**

Sensory-Motor Stage

The first stage of Jean *Piaget's* theory of *cognitive* development in which the birth to 2-year-old child learns about objects and events in the environment and how to respond to and manipulate them. As the child progresses through the sensory-motor stage, he refines his *reflexive* (involuntary) movements and his actions become more purposeful. It is during this stage that the child understands *object permanence.*

> *Compare* **Preoperational Stage.**

Sensory Nerve

A nerve that conducts *sensory* impulses from the *peripheral nervous system* to the *central nervous system.*

> *Refer to* **Peripheral Nervous System.**

Sensory Overload

The condition that occurs when one or more of the senses have been overstimulated beyond the child's level of tolerance. The *sensory input* is overwhelming, and the child may respond by becoming *hyperresponsive* (i.e., over-excited and unable to *attend* to an activity or to speech), or by withdrawing. The child who is overstimulated also has a difficult time being comforted and utilizing sensory information. Sensory overload may occur as the result of too much noise, light, or movement, even in amounts that might be considered by others as ordinary and tolerable.

    *Also known as **Overstimulation**.*

Sensory Processing

A child's ability to receive, interpret, organize, and respond to *sensory input* affecting the *central nervous system*. Sensory processing is commonly observed as a child's *behavior* when he experiences a sensation by touching it, seeing it, *hearing* it, smelling it, tasting it, or feeling it (*vestibular/proprioception*).

    *Refer to **Sensory Integration**.*

Sensory Regulation

    *Refer to **Sensory Modulation**.*

Sensory Seizure

A type of *partial seizure* that produces dizziness or disturbances in vision, *hearing, taste*, smell, or other senses. For example, the child may hear sounds or see images that are not actually present.

    *Refer to **Partial Seizure** and **Epilepsy**.*

Sensory Stimulation

Any arousal of one or more of the senses. For example, a play activity that includes touching strips of shiny cellophane, listening to them crinkle, and watching while a bright light is shone on them against a contrasting background might be a fun and stimulating activity for the child with *low vision*.

seps-

A prefix meaning decay.

Sepsis (SEP-sis)

A *bacterial* infection.

Septal Defect

A hole in the *septum* (wall) that divides the right and left *atria* or the right and left *ventricles* of the *heart*.

    *Also known as a **Hole in the Heart**.*

    *Refer to **Atrial Septal Defect** and **Ventricular Septal Defect**.*

-septic

A suffix meaning infection.

Septic

Related to *sepsis* (a *bacterial* infection).

septo-

A prefix meaning fence.

Septra™

A trademark for a drug made of two *antibacterial drugs* (*Sulfamethoxazole* and *Trimethoprim*) to treat certain *bacterial* infections such as *urinary tract, respiratory,* or *middle ear infections*.

Septum

A dividing wall in the body, such as in the chambers of the *heart* or in the nose dividing the nostrils.

Sequela (see-KWEE-luh)

A condition that follows as a consequence of *disease,* injury, or *disorder*. An example of a sequela is *bronchitis,* which can be a complication of the *common cold*.

Serology (see-ROL-uh-jee)

The medical science involved with studying blood *serum*.

Seroquel™ (SER-oe-kwel)

Refer to **Quetiapine Fumarate.**

Serotonin (ser-uh-TOE-nin)

A naturally-occurring substance found in *platelets* and in *cells* of the *brain* and intestine. It functions as a vasoconstrictor (it causes *constriction* of *blood vessels*), as an agent to cause the smooth muscle of the intestines to contract, and as a *neurotransmitter* in the *central nervous system* (regulating such things as sleep, mood, body temperature, and pain *perception*).

Refer to **Selective Serotonin Reuptake Inhibitor (SSRI).**

Serous (SIR-uhs)

Pertaining to, producing, or containing *serum* (a thin, watery fluid).

Refer to **Serum.**

Serous Otitis Media (SIR-uhs oe-TIE-tis MEE-dee-uh)

An acute or chronic ear condition in which fluid collects in the *middle ear* causing *inflammation,* but not an infection. The condition usually is painless. It can cause some degree of temporary *conductive hearing impairment,* or cause permanent hearing loss if, over time, untreated serous otitis media damages the bones of the middle ear.

Compare **Otitis Media.**

SERs

The abbreviation for somatosensory-evoked responses.

Sertraline Hydrochloride (SIR-truh-leen hie-droe-KLOR-ied)

A *selective serotonin reuptake inhibitor* (*SSRI*). It is prescribed as an *antidepressant drug* and to treat *obsessive-compulsive disorder*. Zoloft™ is the brand name of this drug.

Refer to **Selective Serotonin Reuptake Inhibitor (SSRI).**

Serum (SIR-uhm)

1. The clear, sticky, fluid part of blood that remains after clotting and removal of the *blood cells.*
2. Any thin, watery fluid that has been separated from its more solid elements.
3. A *vaccine* made from the serum of a patient with a particular *disease* and used to protect someone else from the same disease.
    Compare **Plasma.**

Serum Hepatitis

Refer to **Hepatitis B Virus.**

Service Coordinator

The person who, under the *Individuals with Disabilities Education Improvement Act of 2004,* is responsible for coordinating performance *evaluations* and the development of the *Individualized Family Service Plan*; identifying, coordinating and monitoring service delivery; informing the family of the availability of advocacy services; coordinating with medical and health providers; and facilitating the development of *transition planning*. The service coordinator was formerly known as the case manager.

Severe Mental Retardation

Refer to **Intelligence.**

Sex Chromosome

One of a pair of *chromosomes* that determines gender. It may carry *genes* that transmit *sex-linked* traits and *disorders*. In humans, the normal chromosome combination for females is *XX* and the normal chromosome combination for males is *XY*.

Sex-Linked Disorder

Any *disease* or *abnormal* condition that is caused by a defect in the *sex chromosomes* or in the *genes* of the sex chromosomes. Sex-linked disorder is often used interchangeably with X-linked disorder since no known *disorders* are associated with genes of the Y chromosome (the other sex chromosome). *Turner syndrome* is an example of a sex-linked disorder.

Sexual Abuse

Acts of sexual molestation or exploitation of a minor. Signs of suspected sexual abuse in children include: *sexually transmitted diseases*; evidence of injury to the genital or anal areas; vaginal discharge or blood in the diaper or underwear; frequent *urinary* or *yeast* infections; unusual sexual *behavior*, acting out, or knowledge; and sudden change in behavior or emotions such as moodiness, fear, *regression*, or withdrawal. (Signs of force or penetration are not the only indicators of sexual abuse.)
    Refer to **Child Abuse and Neglect** and **Mandated Reporter.**

Sexually Transmitted Disease (STD)

A *contagious disease* transmitted through sexual contact. STDs can also be transmitted other ways, such as through blood contact (as with drug users who share needles). An infant can be infected with an STD *prenatally* or during delivery as he passes through the birth canal and comes in contact with his infected mother's *tissues* or bodily fluids.

> *Formerly known as **Venereal Disease (VD)**.*

SGA
The abbreviation for small for gestational age.

Shadow
> *Refer to **Paraprofessional**.*

Shaken Baby Syndrome
A group of *symptoms* that, occurring together, characterizes injury sustained by the infant who has been shaken (not necessarily with much force). The infant will have bleeding in his *brain* and also in the *retinas* of his eyes. Abusing an infant this way is likely to result in both mental and *motor* damage, and often death.

Shaping
A method of teaching a new skill or *behavior* by reinforcing responses that most closely approximate the desired goal. The goal is broken down into small steps, and as each step is mastered, it is rewarded. For example, if the goal is for the child to make eye contact with the person speaking to him, he would be rewarded (reinforced) initially for directing his face toward the speaker. Then after this skill is demonstrated consistently, it can be shaped into the even more appropriate response of making eye contact briefly, then shaped into the skill of holding eye contact for a designated period of time, etc., until the desired goal is attained.

Shared Attention and Meaning
The interaction between two people, such as a child and his parent, when they are playing and both are focused on the same object or idea.

> *Also known as **Joint Attention**.*

Sheridan Tests for Young Children and Retardates
> *Refer to **STYCAR**.*

Shock
Reduced blood flow to vital organs that leads to low *blood pressure*, collapse, pale skin, sweating, and a fast *pulse* and rate of breathing. Untreated shock may result in unconsciousness or death. Shock may occur for many reasons, including failure of the *heart* to pump normally, severe *hypoxia* (a lack of sufficient *oxygen* in the body *cells* or blood), decreased blood volume, infection, severe injury, severe bleeding or burns, persistent vomiting or diarrhea, or poisoning.

Short Stature
Abnormal underdevelopment of the body. Body height is below the level obtained at that age by 70 percent of the population. Short stature can result from hormonal or *nutritional* deficiencies or from *intrauterine growth retardation*.

> *Also known as **Dwarfism**.*

Shoulder Presentation

The birth (delivery) of a baby in which the shoulder is the part of the body that first appears in the mother's *pelvis*.

Refer to **Fetal Presentation.**

Shprintzen Syndrome (SHPRINT-suhn)

Refer to **Velocardiofacial Syndrome.**

Shunt

A surgical procedure in which a *catheter* (tube) is placed to divert an accumulation of fluid. For example, with increased fluid pressure in the *brain*, a catheter is placed through the skull to drain excess *cerebrospinal fluid* from the ventricles of the brain. The fluid may be drained into the *abdominal* cavity (through a *ventriculoperitoneal shunt*) or into the right *atrium* of the *heart* (through a *ventriculoatrial shunt*), where it is absorbed. Draining the excess fluid relieves the pressure on the brain caused by the fluid. If the pressure is not relieved, *hydrocephalus* or *brain damage* may occur.

Refer to **Hydrocephalus.**

Shunt Revision

A surgical procedure to replace a *shunt* that is malfunctioning.

SI

The abbreviation for sensory integration.

sial-

A prefix meaning saliva.

SIB

The abbreviation for self-injurious behavior.

Sickle Cell Anemia

An *autosomal recessive hemoglobin abnormality* characterized by the presence of crescent- or sickle-shaped *red blood cells*. It is a serious *disease,* which can render the child vulnerable to *bacterial* infections (because the *spleen* functions poorly), painful crises (periods of obstructed *capillary* blood flow and inadequate *oxygen* supply that are *symptomized* by fever and pain in the *joints* and *abdomen*), and *aplastic anemia*. Sickle cell anemia occurs primarily in African-Americans and is an incurable disease.

SID

The abbreviation for Sensory Integration Dysfunction. However, "*DSI*" is used rather than "SID" in order to distinguish it from *SIDS (Sudden Infant Death Syndrome)*.

Refer to **Sensory Integration Dysfunction.**

Side Effect

A reaction to medication or therapy that occurs in addition to the desired effect. A side effect is usually, but not necessarily, an adverse effect. For example, drowsiness may be a side effect of *phenobarbital*, which is prescribed to control *seizures*.

Side Lyer
A piece of *adaptive equipment* that supports the child's body so he can bear weight on his side and bring his hands together at *midline* to play.

Side Sitting
Sitting with both knees bent and to one side of the body.

SIDS
The abbreviation for Sudden Infant Death Syndrome.

Sigmoid Colon
The last four sections of the *colon*, which extend to the *rectum*.

Sigmoidoscopy (sig-moi-DOS-koe-pee)
A procedure for examining the *rectum* and the *sigmoid colon* in which a lighted viewing tube is inserted through the rectum.

Sign (Sx)
An indication of a *disease* or a *disorder* that is noticed by a *physician*.
> Compare **Symptom.**
> Refer to **Soft Sign.**

Signed Exact English (SEE)
A form of *sign language* (in English) in which each word expressed is represented with a hand sign. For words that do not have a sign, *fingerspelling* is used.
> Refer to **American Sign Language.**

Sign Language
One of several methods for communicating in which hand signs are used to express thoughts and feelings. *American Sign Language* and *Signed Exact English* are examples of forms of sign language.

Simian Crease (SIM-ee-uhn)
A single crease across the palm of the hand. This is a common feature of *Down syndrome* and other syndromes.

Simple Partial Seizure
A type of *partial seizure* confined to one area of the *brain,* which causes involuntary jerking of the muscle groups controlled by that brain region. During this type of seizure, the child remains conscious (unless the seizure spreads to involve the whole brain, in which case the seizure is described as secondarily *generalized*).
> Compare **Complex Partial Seizure.**
> Refer to **Partial Seizure** and **Epilepsy.**

Single Gene Disorder
One of many *genetic disorders* caused by a change (*mutation*) in one or both copies of a specific *gene* pair. Some single gene disorders develop frequently from a new mutation (such as *neurofibromatosis*) and other single gene disorders result primarily in a person with a family *history* for the condition (such as *fragile X syndrome*).
> *Compare* **Cytogenetic Syndrome.**
> *Refer to* **Gene.**

Sinus (SIE-nuhs)
A cavity or hollow space.

Sinus Venosus Defect (SIE-nuhs vee-NOE-suhs)
An *atrial septal defect* (a type of *heart defect*) in which the upper portion of the *atrium* fails to develop.
> *Compare* **Ostium Primum Defect** *and* **Ostium Secundum Defect.**
> *Refer to* **Atrial Septal Defect.**

Situated Learning
Learning embedded in everyday *natural environments*, for example, during bath time, at the grocery store, or with a play group.

Sjogren-Larsson Syndrome (SHOE-gren LAHR-suhn)
An *autosomal recessive disorder* characterized by *spasticity* (especially in the lower *extremities*), dry and scaly skin, brittle and sparse hair, *short stature*, and *mental retardation*.

Skin Graft
A procedure in which a piece of skin is transferred to an area where skin has been lost through burns, injury, or surgical removal of *diseased tissue*.

Skinner, B.F.
> *Refer to* **Mand** *and* **Tact.**

Skin Tag
A small flap of skin that may occur spontaneously or as the result of a wound that is not healing properly.
> *Also known as* **Cutaneous Papilloma.**

Skull
The bony structure of the head. The skull is comprised of the *cranium*, which consists of 8 bones and is responsible for containing and protecting the *brain*, and the facial skeleton, which consists of 14 bones.

Sleep Study
> *Refer to* **Pneumogram.**

SLO Syndrome
The abbreviation for Smith-Lemli-Optiz syndrome.

SLP
The abbreviation for Speech-Language Pathologist.

Sly Syndrome
An *autosomal recessive disorder* of *carbohydrate metabolism* (it is a *mucopolysaccharidosis*) with several clinical forms. All forms are characterized by *short stature* and *abnormalities* of the skeletal system, but other characteristics may include enlarged *liver* and *spleen*, *heart murmurs*, and *mental retardation*. (In milder forms of Sly syndrome, the child may have *normal intelligence*.)
Also known as **Mucopolysaccharidosis VII or MPS VII.**

Small For Dates
Refer to **Small For Gestational Age.**

Small For Gestational Age (SGA)
A newborn whose weight is low (below the tenth percentile) for his *gestational age*. This indicates that the baby has a low *birth weight* due to growth retardation while *in utero* (compared to the simple *premature infant* who has a low birth weight due to a shortened length of time in utero).
Also known as **Small For Dates.**
Compare **Appropriate for Gestational Age** *and* **Large for Gestational Age.**
Refer to **Intrauterine Growth Retardation** *and to the* **CDC Growth Charts** *in the Appendix.*

Small Intestine
The longest part of the *digestive tract*, extending from the stomach to the *large intestine*. The small intestine is approximately 21 feet long and is made up of three sections: the *duodenum*, the *jejunum*, and the *ileum*. Most *absorption* of nutrients takes place here.
Refer to **Bowel** *and* **Large Intestine.**

Smith-Lemli-Opitz Syndrome (SLO Syndrome)
An *autosomal recessive disorder* characterized by poor growth, *microcephaly* (an *abnormally* small head size), low-set or slanted ears, short nose with upturned nostrils, small jaw, arched *palate*, *ptosis* (drooping) of the eyelids, *epicanthal folds* (a vertical skin fold at the inner corner of the eyes), *strabismus* (a condition in which the eyes do not work together), *simian crease* (a single crease across the palm of the hand), fusion of second and third toes, *metatarsus adductus* (inward turning of the *forefoot*), short thumbs and toes, genital abnormalities, feeding problems, *failure to thrive*, irritability, and *mental retardation*.

Smith-Magenis Syndrome (SMS)
A *chromosome disorder* caused by a *microdeletion* on chromosome 17 (at 17p11.2—on the *proximal* short arm of chromosome 17). It is characterized by *brachycephaly*; a flat *midface*; a prominent forehead and deep set eyes; a broad nasal bridge; an upper lip shaped like a "cupid's bow"; a prominent jaw; *short stature*; short, broad hands; visual problems; ear *anomalies*; and a deep, hoarse voice. Medical concerns are often present as well, and can include *peripheral*

neuropathy (with *symptoms* of decreased sensitivity to pain or temperature, decreased *deep tendon reflexes*, and *scoliosis*), *heart defects*, *seizures*, *auditory impairment*, and *kidney* anomalies. Children with Smith-Magenis syndrome typically function in the mild range of *mental retardation*; have delayed speech acquisition; and exhibit *behaviors* such as *self-injurious behavior*, sleep problems, aggression, *impulsivity*, and *hyperactivity*. Smith-Magenis syndrome is considered a rare disorder, however under- or *misdiagnosis* may make it more prevalent than the research indicates (affecting 1 person in 25,000).

SMO
The abbreviation for supra malleolar orthosis.

SMS
The abbreviation for Smith-Magenis syndrome.

Social/Emotional
The *developmental* area that involves the development of self-concept and the skills that enable the child to function in a group and to interact appropriately with others. Smiling at one's mirror image, playing a circle game with other children, and comforting someone who is crying by offering a hug are examples of social/emotional skills.

Social Maturity
The ability to function in a socially responsible manner appropriate to the child's age. An example is the ability of the 3-year-old to cooperatively join other children in forming a circle so that the group can play a circle game.

Social Security Administration (SSA)
The US federal agency that administers both *Supplemental Security Income* (*SSI*) and *Social Security Disability Insurance* (*SSDI*).

Social Security Disability Insurance (SSDI)
A federally funded *disability* insurance program. This money has been paid into the Social Security System through payroll deductions on earnings. Disabled workers are entitled to these benefits. People who become disabled before the age of 22 years may collect SSDI under a parent's account, if the parent is retired, disabled, or deceased. The applicant's financial need is not an eligibility consideration.

Social Skills
Abilities involving the development of a child's self-concept (such as his ability to distinguish himself as separate from his parent) and his interactive skills (i.e., his ability to lift his arms to indicate that he wants to be picked up.)

Social Worker
A professional who helps individuals manage within society. The social worker may function as a counselor or *service coordinator*, as well as help to secure services, such as counseling, financial assistance, *respite care*, or crisis intervention.

Sodium (Na)
A *mineral* needed in small amounts for the body's health.

Sodium Bicarbonate (NaHCO₃)
A substance that helps neutralize excess acid in the blood.
> *Also known as* **Bicarbonate.**

Soft Palate
The movable structure made of muscular fibers and *mucous membrane* that is attached to the back edge of the *hard palate* (the bony front part of the roof of the mouth). The soft palate rises during sucking and swallowing to close off the nose and *sinuses* from the mouth and throat. The soft palate is also involved in the production of speech sounds such as the /g/ and /k/ sounds.
> *Compare* **Hard Palate.**
> *Refer to* **Palate.**

Soft Sign
Any of several neurological *signs* (indicators of *disease* or *disorder* that are noticeable by a *physician* or a qualified *physical therapist*) that, collectively, suggest the presence of damage to the *central nervous system*. Soft signs include a disturbance of *balance* or *proprioception*, visual *motor* difficulties, a lack of *motor control* or coordination, *associated reactions*, or *nystagmus*. Soft neurological signs can be difficult to detect or interpret because they are so mild or slight.

Soft Tissue
Tissue that surrounds bones and *joints*, including *ligaments, tendons*, and muscles.

Soft Tissue Release
A surgical procedure (or a manual therapy, i.e., massage technique called *myofascial release*) on the muscles, *tendons*, or *ligaments* to correct deformities or improve *positioning* and movement.

soma-, somat-
Prefixes meaning body.

Somatic (soe-MAT-ik)
A word that means related to the body.

Somatic Growth Measurements
> *Refer to* **Body Measurements.**

Somatosensory (soe-muh-toe-SEN-suh-ree)
Pertaining to the parts of the *central* and *peripheral nervous systems* that receive and process information about pain and touch, including temperature; pressure; *joint* position; and muscle length, degree of stretch, *tension*, and *contraction*.

Somatosensory-Evoked Responses (SERs)
> *Refer to* **Evoked Potential Studies.**

-some
A suffix meaning body.

Somophyllin-CRT™ (som-AH-fi-lin)
*Refer to **Theophylline**.*

Sonogram (SOE-noe-gram)
A 2-dimensional image produced by *ultrasound*.

Sonography (soe-NOG-ruh-fee)
*Refer to **Ultrasound Scanning**.*

Sotos Syndrome (SO-toes)
A *disorder* of unknown cause characterized by advanced height, weight, and bone age at birth; large hands and feet; facial *anomalies* including a large skull, a prominent forehead, a receding hairline, wide-set eyes, downslanting *palpebral fissures*, a large jaw with a pointed chin, an upturned nose, and teeth present at birth (in over 50 percent of affected children); *motor* delays; and *mental retardation*. Children with Sotos syndrome experience rapid growth during the first 4-5 years of life, but typically only reach heights in the normal range.
*Also known as **Cerebral Gigantism**.*

Spasm
A sudden, involuntary muscle *contraction*.

Spastic
*Refer to **Spasticity**.*

Spastic Cerebral Palsy
*Refer to **Pyramidal Cerebral Palsy**.*

Spastic Diplegia (die-PLEE-jee-uh)
*Refer to **Pyramidal Cerebral Palsy**.*

Spasticity (spa-STIS-i-tee)
A type of muscle *hypertonicity* with increased resistance to muscle stretch and, usually, increased *deep tendon reflexes* and muscle weakness. Spasticity results in difficulty performing movements.
*Refer to **Antispastic Drug**.*

Spastic Quadriplegia (kwod-ruh-PLEE-jee-uh)
A form of *cerebral palsy* with *spasticity* in all four *extremities*.
*Refer to **Cerebral Palsy** and **Pyramidal Cerebral Palsy**.*

Spatial Relationships (SPAY-shuhl)
The understanding of the relationship between the position of an object and the infant's own body or another object. For example, when the infant plays at placing objects in and removing them from a container, he is experimenting with the spatial relationship between objects and his own hand.

Special Education
Specialized instruction tailor-made to fit the unique learning strengths and needs of the individual student with *disabilities*, from age 3 through 21 years. A major goal of special education is to teach the skills and knowledge the child needs to be as independent as possible. Consequently, special education programs do not just focus on academics, but also include special therapeutic and other *related services* to help the child overcome difficulties in all areas of *development*. Special education and related services may be provided in a variety of educational settings, but are required by *IDEA 2004* to be delivered in the *least restrictive environment*.
*Refer to **Individualized Education Program**.*

Special Education Instructional Assistant
*Refer to **Paraprofessional**.*

Special Needs
Referring to the needs of the child who requires special services to assist with his acquisition of skills in one or more *developmental* areas: *cognition, communication* (language), *gross motor, fine motor* (perceptual), social, and *self-help* (*adaptive*). The needs are generated by the child's *disability*.
*Refer to **Early Intervention**.*

Special Needs Assistant
*Refer to **Paraprofessional**.*

Speech and Language Pathologist
*Refer to **Speech-Language Pathologist**.*

Speech Disorder
A condition that affects the ability to speak. Speech disorders include *articulation* problems, such as sound substitutions (saying "wan" instead of "ran"); rate and rhythm problems, such as *stuttering*; and voice production (or resonance) *disorders*, such as a voice that is too soft or *hypernasal*. Speech disorders are often associated with another disorder, such as *cerebral palsy*, but can occur on their own.
*Compare **Language Disorder**.*

Speech Generating Device
*Refer to **Voice Output Communication Aid**.*

Speech-Language Pathologist (SLP)
A therapist who works to improve the child's speech and language skills, as well as to improve *oral motor* abilities, such as feeding. Speech-language pathologists are required to have a master's degree in speech *pathology* and either a teaching credential to work in a school district setting or a state license to work in private practice or other agencies. (A therapist without this level of training is not a speech-language pathologist.)
*Also known as **Speech and Language Pathologist**.*

Speechreading

A form of *communication* for the child with *auditory impairment* in which the child uses visual *input* (watching the speaker's mouth, facial movements, and *gestures*) to help him understand what he cannot hear.

> *Also known as* **Lipreading.**

Speech Therapist

> *Refer to* **Speech-Language Pathologist.**

Sperm

The male sex *cell.* An *embryo* can only develop if a sperm fertilizes an *ovum* (egg).

> *Also known as* **Spermatozoa.**

sperma-

A prefix meaning seed, or relating to *sperm.*

Spermatozoa

> *Refer to* **Sperm.**

Sphenoid Bone (SFEE-noid)

The bone that makes up the front portion of the base of the skull and parts of the *orbits* (the bony sockets that contain the eyes) and nose.

Sphincter (SFINGK-tuhr)

A ring-like muscle around a natural body opening, such as the anal sphincter.

Sphingolipid (sfing-goe-LIP-id)

A *lipid* (fat) substance found in *nervous system tissue*, including the *brain.*

Sphingolipidosis (sfing-goe-lip-id-OE-sis)

One of a group of *hereditary disorders* of *lipid* (fat) *metabolism* in which a specific *enzyme* used in the breakdown of a specific lipid is missing, resulting in fat accumulation in body *tissue. Tay-Sachs disease* is an example of a sphingolipidosis. .

> *Also known as* **Sphingomyelin Lipidosis.**

Sphingomyelin (sfing-goe-MIE-uh-lin)

A *sphingolipid* (a *lipid*, or fat, substance) that contains *phosphorus* and is found in *nervous system tissue* and in the lipids in the blood. It is also a component in *surfactant* (a substance formed in the lungs that is needed to keep the air sacs in the lungs open).

Sphingomyelin Lipidosis (sfing-goe-MIE-uh-lin lip-id-OE-sis)

> *Refer to* **Sphingolipidosis.**

Spike-and-Wave Abnormality

A *brain wave abnormality*, as seen on an *EEG* (*electroencephalogram*), that is associated with a susceptibility to having *seizures.*

Spina Bifida (SPIE-nuh BIF-uh-duh)

A *congenital neural tube defect* in which part of the *spinal column* (one or more *vertebrae*) fails to close completely, exposing the *membranes* covering the *spinal cord* or the membranes and the spinal cord. Sometimes the membranes and cord protrude out through the back of the *spine*. The severity of damage depends on the degree and the placement of the exposure, and can range from no apparent damage to *paralysis* below the level of the protrusion and severe *brain damage*. Spina bifida is often associated with *hydrocephalus*. Other conditions that may be associated with spina bifida include *Arnold-Chiari Malformation*; *curvature of the spine* (*scoliosis* and *kyphosis*); foot *anomalies*, including *clubfoot* and *congenital rocker-bottom foot*; and problems with the *heart*, *kidneys*, intestines, *bladder*, and rectal and anal *sphincters*. The exact cause is not known; it is a multi-factorial *disorder* and it is believed that there are many contributing factors. Adequate daily intake of *folic acid* prior to conception and during early pregnancy has been found to decrease the risk of *fetal* neural tube defects. There are 4 forms of spina bifida: *spina bifida occulta, meningocele, myelocele*, and *encephalocele*. (Encephalocele is actually a cranial defect in which the *brain, meninges*, or both protrude through an opening in the skull.)

Spina Bifida Occulta

A *congenital anomaly* defect in which a minimal amount of *spinal cord tissue* is exposed due to the *spinal column* failing to form completely. This form of *spina bifida* may not be detected without an x-ray, but is often suspected because of a dimple or tuft of hair on the skin that lies over the defective *vertebrae*.
>   *Refer to* **Spina Bifida.**

Spinal Cerebellar Degeneration
(SPIE-nuhl ser-uh-BEL-uhr di-jen-uh-RAY-shuhn)
>   *Refer to* **Friedreich's Ataxia.**

Spinal Column

The 33 *vertebrae* that form the *spine* and the spongy disks that separate the vertebrae. The spinal column extends from the base of the skull to the *pelvis* and supports the trunk and head. It is within the spinal column that the *spinal cord* is located.
>   *Also known as* **Vertebral Column.**
>   *Refer to* **Vertebra.**

Spinal Cord

The *nerve tissue* located within the canal of the *spinal column* that runs from the base of the *brain* to the lower back area. The spinal cord passes *sensory* information to the brain and passes on *motor* signals from the brain. The spinal cord is also responsible for certain *reflex* actions that do not require brain involvement. The brain and the spinal cord form the *central nervous system*.

Spinal Fusion

A surgical procedure (*arthrodesis*) to join an unstable part of the *spine* (to reduce movement between two *vertebrae*). This may result in some loss of mobility.

Spinal Muscular Atrophy

A *genetic disorder* in which the muscles do not receive impulses from the *spinal cord* due to a wasting of *motor neurons* (*nerve cells* that convey impulses, which initiate muscle *contraction*) of the spinal cord. This results in severe wasting of muscle, which can render the child unable to walk. There are several forms of this *disease*, including *Werdnig-Hoffmann Disease* (Infantile Spinal Muscular Atrophy) and *Kugelberg-Welander Disease (*Juvenile Spinal Muscular Atrophy). Some forms of spinal muscular atrophy are fatal.

Spinal Tap

*Refer to **Lumbar Puncture.***

Spine

*Refer to **Spinal Column.***

Spironolactone (spie-roe-noe-LAK-toen)

A *diuretic* (a drug that helps remove excess water from the body). Aldactone™ is the brand name of this drug.

Spleen

The organ located in the upper left part of the *abdomen* beneath the *diaphragm*. The spleen produces *blood cells* in the *fetus* and, after birth, functions to destroy old blood *cells* and to help fight infection.

Splenomegaly (splee-noe-MEG-uh-lee)

An enlarged *spleen* that can result from many *diseases*, including certain types of *anemia, infectious mononucleosis, thalassemia, leukemia,* and *tumors* in the spleen.

Splint

A device used to stretch *soft tissues*, prevent movement, or hold a *limb* in a position that makes movement easier. An example of a splint is an *opponens splint*, which may be prescribed for the child with *cerebral palsy* to hold the thumb in correct alignment.

Splinter Skill

A skill that is striking because it is so much more advanced than other areas of a child's *development*. Splinter skills are frequently demonstrated by children with *autism spectrum disorders* and often involve visual-spatial skills. For example, a 30-month-old may be able to complete complex puzzles, but not demonstrate age-appropriate *cognitive* skills, such as identifying body parts or following simple directions.

spondyl-

A prefix meaning *vertebra*.

Spontaneous Abortion

*Refer to **Miscarriage.***

Sporadic
Occurring only occasionally, at apparently random intervals.

Squamous (SKWAY-muhs)
Scaly.

Squint
*Refer to **Strabismus.***

S-R
The abbreviation for stimulus-response.

SSA
The abbreviation for Social Security Administration.

SSDI
The abbreviation for Social Security Disability Insurance.

SSI
The abbreviation for Supplemental Security Income.

SSRI
The abbreviation for Selective Serotonin Reuptake Inhibitor.

Stammering
*Refer to **Stuttering.***

Standard Deviation
A measurement of the degree to which a given test score differs from the *mean* (average) score. For example, on the *Bayley Scales of Infant and Toddler Development™ – Third Edition,* the majority of children score within 15 points above to 16 points below the mean score of 100, so 1 standard deviation is considered to be 15 points. That is, a *score* of 85 is considered to be 1 standard deviation below the mean.

Standardization
The process of testing a sample population to establish general evaluative criteria (the average scores or standards against which the child is evaluated). For example, a test may be standardized to children of a specific age who have *auditory impairments*.

Standardized Test
A test that has set standards on which the child is evaluated, in addition to set administration and scoring procedures. The standardized test yields a score that may be used to compare the child's performance with those of others in his age group. *Norm-referenced tests* are standardized tests, as are some *criterion-referenced* tests.

Standard Score

A test score based on the normal distribution curve (the "bell curve"). In tests scored with standard scores, 100 is usually considered exactly average, with scores from 85 to 115 considered to be in the average range.
    Compare *Age-Equivalent Score.*

Stanford-Binet Intelligence Scale - Fifth Edition (SBIS - V)
(STAN-fuhrd bi-NAY)

A *standardized test* used to evaluate the *intelligence* (reasoning, knowledge, memory, visual-spatial processing) of children 2 years of age to adulthood.

Stanford-Binet Intelligence Scale - Fourth Edition (SBFE)

    Refer to Stanford-Binet Intelligence Scale – Fifth Edition (SBIS – V).

Stapes (STAY-peez)

One of the three small bones of the *middle ear*. (The other two bones are the *malleus* and the *incus*.)
    Also known as the Stirrup.
    Refer to Ear.

Staph

The abbreviation for *staphylococcus*.

Staphylococcus (staf-il-oe-KOK-uhs)

An infection-causing *bacterium*.

Startle Reflex

A startle reaction normal in infants up to 4 months of age. The startle reflex is observed when the infant reacts to a sudden loud noise by bringing his arms and legs in close to his body.
    Compare *Moro Reflex/Response.*
    Refer to Primitive Reflex.

State

A condition or status. For example, a newborn experiences several states of alertness or *arousal levels*.
    Refer to Arousal Level.

Static Splint

A device that supports body parts, such as the wrist and hand, in correct alignment.
    Compare *Dynamic Splint.*

Status Epilepticus (STAY-tuhs ep-i-LEP-ti-kuhs)

A single or series of *convulsive seizures* throughout which the child remains unconscious. If the seizures are not stopped, *brain damage* will result. (Untreated, they will last more than 30 minutes, even up to 1 hour.) Status epilepticus may be caused by the sudden withdrawal of seizure medication, erratic administering of medication, *low blood sugar*, a *brain tumor*, infection, head injury, or poisoning. Status epilepticus is a life-threatening condition and patients may have permanent neurologic *sequelae* (resulting damage).

STD
The abbreviation for sexually transmitted disease.

Steady State
A term that describes the drug level in the blood once it has reached a level around which it is fairly stable. Daily doses of medication maintain this level.

Stelazine™ (STEL-uh-zeen)
Refer to **Trifluoperazine Hydrochloride.**

sten-
A prefix meaning narrow.

Stenosis (sti-NOE-sis)
Constriction or narrowing of an opening or passageway in the body, such as a *blood vessel*. An example is *aortic stenosis*.

Stepping Reflex
A normal response that occurs in newborns up to 2 months of age, and then again at 6 months of age, when the baby is held upright with the soles of the feet touching a firm surface. It causes the baby to simulate walking movements with each leg moving forward as weight is placed on the other leg.
Also known as **Walking Reflex.**
Refer to **Primitive Reflex.**

Stereotypic/Stereotyped Behavior (ster-ee-oe-TIP-ik)
Persistent repetitive actions or vocalizations that appear to have no meaning or logical motivation. *Hand flapping* and rocking back and forth are examples.
Also known as **Stereotypy.**
Compare **Perseveration** *and* **Self-Stimulation.**

Stereotypy (ster-ee-O-tuh-pee or STER-ee-uh-tie-pee or ster-ee-oe-TIE-pee)
Refer to **Stereotypic Behavior.**

Sternum (STUR-nuhm)
The breastbone.

Steroids (STIR-oids)
A group of chemical substances including natural and synthetic compounds. They may be prescribed to replace natural *corticosteroid hormone* (one of the hormones produced by the *adrenal glands*) or to treat inflammatory *disorders*. These are corticosteroid drugs. Another type of steroid works in a manner similar to male sex hormones. These are called *anabolic steroids*. Anabolic steroids are any of a group of synthetic derivatives of testosterone. They are used

primarily to repair and build *tissue* and to promote body growth. They are also used to treat some types of *anemia* and *leukemia*.

Stickler Syndrome

An *autosomal dominant disorder* characterized by progressive vision problems (severe *nearsightedness* and, often, *retinal* detachment that can lead to *blindness*); *joint abnormalities* (prominent and *hyperextensible* joints that can become painful and stiff if overused); facial *anomalies*, including a small jaw, an underdeveloped *midface*, flat nasal bridge, prominent eyes, *epicanthal folds*, and a short nose with nostrils tipped forward (some of these facial anomalies can become milder as the child develops); *cleft palate*; *sensorineural hearing impairment*; and *short stature*. With proper medical treatment (especially to prevent retinal detachment), children with Stickler syndrome can have a normal lifespan.

Stiffness

Refer to **Hypertonia.**

Stigma (STIG-muh)

A physical mark or *sign* that serves to identify a *disease* or condition, such as a limp or unusual *gait,* which may be a manifestation of an individual's *disability.*

Stillbirth/Stillborn

An infant who dies *in utero* and is born dead. In many cases, the cause of stillbirth is unknown, but seriously malformed infants (such as infants with *anencephaly*) account for a significant number of stillbirths. Other causes include *maternal disease* (such as *cytomegalovirus* or high *blood pressure*), *fetal oxygen* deprivation, and *Rh incompatibility*.

Stimming

Refer to **Self-Stimulation.**

Stimulant Drug

A drug that increases *nerve* activity in the *brain.* A stimulant is a *psychotropic drug* and is sometimes used to control *hyperactivity* in children. An example of a stimulant drug is caffeine.

Stimuli

Plural of *stimulus.*

Stimulus/Stimulation

A physical object or an environmental event that may affect an individual's *behavior* or elicit a response. Some *stimuli* are internal (such as earache pain), while others are external (such as a smile from a loved one).

Stirrup

Refer to **Stapes.**

STNR
The abbreviation for symmetrical tonic neck reflex.

Stoma (STOE-muh)
A surgically created opening from an internal organ (such as the *colon*) to the surface of the body. For example, a stoma is created at the site of a *colostomy* to allow *feces* to be passed from the body when it cannot be passed through all of the colon or through the colon and *rectum*.

Stomach
The organ located in the left upper part of the *abdomen* that is connected to the *esophagus* and *small intestine*. The stomach is the main organ of enzymatic *digestion* and also functions to receive food.

Stomach Tube
A *gastrostomy tube*.
> *Refer to* **Gastrostomy.**

stomato-
A prefix meaning mouth.

Stop
A *consonant* sound that is made when the flow of air is stopped as it passes through the mouth. Usually the tongue (and sometimes the lips) is what stops the air stream, such as when producing the /t/, /d/, /p/, and /b/ sounds.

STORCH Infections
A group of *congenital infections*, each responsible for causing illness, handicapping conditions, or death: *Syphilis*, *Toxoplasmosis*, Other Infections (such as *HIV* and *hepatitis B*), *Rubella*, *Cytomegalic Inclusion Disease*, and *Herpes*.
> *Also known as* **TORCH-S.**

Stork Bite
> *Refer to* **Telangiectatic Nevus.**

Strabismus (struh-BIZ-muhs)
A condition in which the eyes do not work together, in that one eye deviates (wanders) from its position, relative to the other eye. Strabismus may be convergent (deviate inward, also known as *esotropia*, or *cross-eye*), or divergent (deviate outward, also known as *exotropia*, or *wall-eye*). It may result from an inability of the muscles to align the eyes, from a defect such as a *cataract*, or from a *visual acuity* problem.
> *Also known as* **Squint.**

Strawberry Mark
A raised red birthmark. Strawberry marks nearly always resolve spontaneously.
> *Also known as a* **Capillary Hemangioma.**
> *Refer to* **Hemangioma.**

Strep Throat

A throat infection caused by *streptococcal bacteria*. Strep throat is spread by airborne droplets and usually causes a sore throat, fever, enlarged *lymph nodes* in the neck, and general discomfort. Strep throat is treated with *antibiotic drugs*.

Streptococcal (strep-tuh-KOK-uhl)

Pertaining to any of the types of *streptococcus*.

Streptococcus (strep-toe-KOK-uhs)

An infection-causing *bacterium*.

Streptomycin Sulfate (strep-toe-MIE-sin SUL-fayt))

An *antibiotic drug* used to treat infections.

Stress Test

1. A test to record the *fetus's heart rate* patterns in response to the stress of *uterine contractions*. The drug *oxytocin* is usually given to induce the contractions, which are monitored by a device worn around the mother's *abdomen*. A stress test is done during certain types of high risk pregnancies, but should not be used with women who have a *history* of premature *labor*.
2. A test to measure a body system's response to carefully controlled stress, such as the *heart's* response to monitored exercise.

Stricture (STRIK-chur)

A narrowing of a tube, *duct*, hollow organ, or other passage within the body. A stricture may be a *congenital* condition, or it may be the result of another condition, such as the growth of a *tumor, inflammation*, damage to the passage that results in scar *tissue*, or *spasm* of the muscles in the passage wall. For example, a stricture may develop in the *esophagus* or in a *ureter*.

Stridor (STRIE-dor)

An *abnormal*, high-pitched breath sound, caused by a blockage in the throat or *larynx*. Stridor may occur due to *croup*, growth of a *tumor* in the larynx, *laryngomalacia* (softening of the *tissues* of the larynx), or a foreign object that has been inhaled.

Stroke

Sudden onset of damage to part of the *brain* that can occur if the area does not receive its blood supply or if there is bleeding within or over the surface of the brain. Stroke does not always result in other problems, but problems that may occur range from a *seizure*, or a language *disability* and/or *motor* impairment, or even death.

    *Also known as **Cerebrovascular Accident** or **Brain Attack**.*

Structural Integration

A therapeutic treatment to improve body function developed by Ida Rolf. Using this treatment, the *fascia* (the fibrous *connective tissue* in the body that surrounds and supports organs and separates muscle) is manipulated and stretched with applied pressure. This is done to realign the segments of the body (head, torso, *pelvis*, legs, and feet), thereby increasing ease of movement and decreasing fatigue. Structural integration should only be done by a certified practitioner, as some of the techniques may be injurious to infants and children with *disabilities*.

    Also known as **Rolfing.**

Structure

1. An organ, a body part, or a complete *organism*.
2. The parts and their arrangement in forming a whole.

Sturge-Weber Syndrome

A *congenital neurological disorder* characterized by a *port wine stain* (a flat, purple-red birthmark), commonly on one side of the face, and a *hemangioma* (a usually harmless *tumor* caused by an *abnormal* distribution of *blood vessels*) of the *brain*. The brain hemangioma may result in a lack of brain growth and development (progressive *mental retardation*), *seizures*, and *motor* impairment caused by *hemiparesis*. Other features include *exophthalmos* (abnormal protrusion of the eyeballs), *optic atrophy* (wasting of the *optic nerve* fibers that leads to *visual impairment*), *glaucoma*, and malformation of blood vessels.

    Also known as **Encephalofacial Angiomatosis** *and* **Encephalotrigeminal Angiomatosis.**

Stuttering

A *speech disorder*, usually beginning by 8 years of age and sometimes continuing into adulthood, in which the person's speech has many hesitations, repetitions of syllables or words, and prolonged sounds. Stuttering may be associated with certain *learning disabilities* or with *mental retardation*, but it also occurs in children who have no other *disability*. Stuttering most commonly occurs in children between 2 and 4 years of age, as a temporary condition.

    Also known as **Stammering.**

STYCAR

Tests for assessing vision and *hearing* in infants as young as 6 months old and overall *development* in children who have *developmental delays* up until 5 years of age. Although the test is often referred to as the STYCAR, the actual test name is Screening (or Sheridan) Tests for Young Children and Retardates.

sub-

A prefix meaning under.

Subacute Necrotizing Encephalomyelopathy

(sub-uh-KYOOT NEK-roe-tie-zing en-sef-uh-loe-mie-el-OP-uh-thee)

    Refer to **Leigh Disease.**

Subacute Necrotizing Encephalopathy

(sub-uh-KYOOT NEK-roe-tie-zing en-sef-uh-LOP-uh-thee)

    Refer to **Leigh Disease.**

Subacute Sclerosing Panencephalitis
(sub-uh-KYOOT sklir-OE-zing pan-uhn-sef-uh-LIE-tis)
A rare childhood *disorder* that develops 6 to 8 years after a child 2 years old or younger becomes infected with the *measles virus*. (It has also been reported as a result of *rubella*.) The child recovers from the illness but later (usually by age 10) develops *inflammation* of *brain tissue, seizures, ataxia, spasticity,* muscle jerking, vision problems, impaired *cognition*, personality changes, and *dementia*. The *disease* is usually fatal.

Subarachnoid Hemorrhage (sub-uh-RAK-noid HEM-uhr-ij)
Bleeding in the subarachnoid space (the space inside the *arachnoid membranes* that surround the *brain*).
> *Compare* **Intracerebral Hemorrhage, Intraventricular Hemorrhage,** *and* **Periventricular Hemorrhage.**

Subclinical
Denoting the presence of *disease* without *symptoms* or *signs* (disease that cannot be noted clinically), either because the disease is mild or because the disease is in an early stage.

Subcutaneous (sub-kyoo-TAY-nee-uhs)
Beneath the skin.

Subdural (sub-DYOO-ruhl)
Pertaining to the space between the outermost and middle layers of the *meninges*.
> *Refer to* **Meninges.**

Subdural Hematoma (sub-DYOO-ruhl hee-muh-TOE-muh)
A condition in which blood accumulates between the outermost and middle layers of the *meninges* (the *membranes* surrounding the *brain* and *spinal cord*). It is usually caused by an injury.

Subependymal Hemorrhage (sub-ep-EN-di-muhl HEM-uhr-ij)
> *Refer to* **Intraventricular Hemorrhage.**

Subglottic (sub-GLOT-ik)
Referring to beneath the *glottis* (the vocal cords and the slit-like opening between them).

Subglottic Stenosis (sti-NOE-sis)
A narrowing of the area beneath the *glottis* (the vocal cords and the slit-like opening between them). It can be a *congenital* condition, but more commonly is the result of *endotracheal intubation*.

Subluxation (sub-luks-AY-shuhn)
A partial *dislocation* of the two bones of a *joint*. The bone surfaces are displaced to the degree that they are only partly in contact.
> *Compare* **Dislocation.**

Subluxed Hip
A partially *dislocated hip*.
> *Refer to* **Subluxation.**

Subthreshold
Not meeting full criteria (guidelines) for a *diagnosis*.

Suck Reflex
A normal response in infants up to 12 months in which the baby starts sucking when something is placed in his mouth. Sucking is sometimes noticed during sleep, also.
> *Refer to* **Primitive Reflex.**

Sucrose (SOO-kroes)
Sugar derived mainly from sugar cane and sugar beets.

Suctioning
A procedure to rid the body of unwanted or excess fluid, often referring to a procedure to remove excess *mucus* from the *respiratory tract*. Suctioning may be done with a syringe and hollow needle, a bulb syringe, or with one end of a narrow tube inserted into the respiratory tract and the other end attached to a machine that suctions out fluid.
> *Also known as* **Respiratory Suctioning.**

Sudden Infant Death Syndrome (SIDS)
The unexpected and sudden death of an infant who had appeared to be healthy. SIDS occurs during sleep (this is why it is also known as *crib death*), and is the most common cause of death in children between 1 month and 1 year of age. Peak *incidence* occurs between 2 and 4 months. The cause of SIDS is still unknown. A number of hypotheses have been offered, such as a *heart rate* or breathing problem, or a disruption of proper brain activation mechanisms, but nothing has been proven and post-mortem examination fails to demonstrate the cause of death. Research has shown, however, that the incidence of SIDS decreases when infants are positioned to sleep on their backs or sides, rather than on their *abdomens* ("back to sleep"), on a firm sleeping surface free of pillows, toys, or cushions, which can interfere with breathing or cause *suffocation*. Sleeping on their backs might also prevent infants from inhaling their exhaled breath or increase their ability to awaken themselves should they experience *apnea* in their sleep. A recent study also indicated that use of a pacifier is associated with a reduction of SIDS.
> *Also known as* **Crib Death.**

Suffocation
> *Refer to* **Asphyxia.**

Sulci (SUL-kie)
Plural of *sulcus*.

Sulcus (SUL-kus)
1. A shallow groove. An example of a sulcus is one of the grooves that separates the *gyri* (*convolutions*) of the surface of the *cerebral hemispheres* of the *brain*.
2. Singular of *sulci*.
>   Compare **Fissure**.

Sulfamethoxazole (sul-fuh-meth-OKS-uh-zoel)
An *antibacterial drug*.
>   *Refer to* **Septra**™.

Sulfatide Lipidosis (SUL-fuh-tied lip-i-DOE-sis)
>   *Refer to* **Metachromatic Leukodystrophy**.

Sulfisoxazole (sul-fi-SOK-suh-zoel)
An *antibacterial drug* used to treat *conjunctivitis* and *urinary tract* infections. Gantrisin™ is the brand name of this drug.

Sun-setting Sign
A condition, or *sign*, associated with *hydrocephalus* in which it appears that the baby's eyes only look downward, showing more of the white (rather than the colored) part of the eye than is typical.

super-
A prefix meaning above or extreme.

Superior
Situated above.

Superior Vena Cava (VEE-nuh KAY-vuh)
>   *Refer to* **Vena Cava**.

Supination (soo-pin-AY-shuhn)
Turning the forearm so the palm faces upward.
>   Compare **Pronation**.

Supine (SOO-pien)
Lying on the back.
>   Compare **Prone**.

Supplemental Security Income (SSI)
A US federally funded public assistance program for people who are 65 or older or people of any age who are *blind* or have a *disability*. The individual's income is an eligibility consideration. (SSI is based on financial need, not on past earnings.)

Support Services
>   *Refer to* **Related Services**.

Support Trust
A trust that requires that funds be expended to pay for the beneficiary's expenses of living, such as housing, food, and transportation.

Suppository
A bullet-shaped mixture of a drug and an easily-melted material (such as cocoa butter) that is placed in the *rectum* or vagina when the drug cannot be administered orally, or if the drug is for treating rectal or vaginal *disorders*. A suppository is a useful means of administering medication to infants and young children.

supra-
A prefix meaning above or extreme.

Supra Malleolar Orthosis (SMO)
(SOO-pruh muh-LEE-uh-lar or-THOE-sis)
A *brace* that provides support to the ankle *joint* and the foot.
> *Refer to* **Orthosis.**

Surfactant (sur-FAK-tuhnt)
A substance formed in the lungs that is needed to keep the *alveoli* (air sacs) in the lungs open. Without surfactant, the alveoli would collapse at the end of each exhalation and stick together. A *fetus* born before 36 weeks *gestation* usually has not produced enough surfactant and often develops *respiratory distress syndrome.*

Surgeon
A medical doctor who performs operations that involve cutting body *tissue* for the treatment of *disease*, deformity, or injury.

Suture (SOO-chur)
1. The border (joint) of the bones of the skull.
2. A surgical stitch.

Swayback
> *Refer to* **Lordosis.**

Sweat Test
A test to measure the concentration of *sodium* and chloride in the child's sweat to *diagnose cystic fibrosis.*

Swimming Position
A position that the 4- to 6-month-old may assume while lying on his stomach in which he extends and lifts his arms and legs, and supports most of his weight on his *abdomen.*

Switch
> *Refer to* **Adaptive Switch.**

Switch Interface
A connector piece that allows an *adaptive switch* to activate software on a computer.

Swivel Walker
A type of *walker* consisting of a supportive body *brace* secured to a base that has two foot plates that rise and swivel forward.

Sx
The abbreviation for symptom or sign.

Symbolic Representation
Refer to **Representation.**

Symmetrical (si-MET-ri-kuhl)
Referring to parts of the body that are equal in size or shape, or are similar in arrangement or movement patterns.
Compare **Asymmetrical.**

Symmetrical Movements
Moving corresponding parts of the body, such as both arms, at the same time and in the same movement pattern.

Symmetrical Tonic Neck Reflex (STNR)
A *reflex*, normal (and faint) in infants from about 2 to 6 months of age, in which the infant's arms flex and the legs extend when the neck is flexed (when the head moves forward) and the infant's arms extend and the legs flex when the neck is extended (when the head falls back).
Compare **Asymmetrical Tonic Neck Reflex.**

Sympathetic Nervous System
The part of the *autonomic nervous system* that increases *heart rate*, constricts *blood vessels*, and raises *blood pressure*.
Compare **Parasympathetic Nervous System.**

Symptom (Sx)
An indication of a *disease* or *disorder* that is noticed by the patient. For example, a sore throat may be a symptom of an *upper respiratory infection*.
Compare **Sign.**

Symptomatic
Pertaining to a *symptom* or a condition that is indicative or characteristic of a particular *disease* or *disorder*. For example, *emesis* (vomiting) is symptomatic of *abdominal* disorders.
Compare **Asymptomatic.**

Symptomatic Epilepsy

Epilepsy that has an identifiable cause, such as an infection, a *tumor*, a reaction to a *toxin*, or a *metabolic* disturbance.

> *Also known as* **Secondary Epilepsy.**
> *Refer to* **Epilepsy.**

Symptomatic Seizure

> *Also known as* **Secondary Seizure.**
> *Refer to* **Symptomatic Epilepsy** *and* **Epilepsy.**

syn-

A prefix meaning with or together.

Synapse (SIN-aps)

A junctional region between two *nerve cells* (*neurons*), forming the place across which a *nerve impulse* is transmitted from one *neuron* to another by chemical neurotransmitting substances.

> *Refer to* **Neurotransmitter.**

Syncopal (SIN-kuh-puhl or SING-kuh-puhl)

Referring to a short period of unconsciousness (fainting).

Syncope (SIN-kuh-pee or SING-kuh-pee)

Fainting or a short period of unconsciousness caused by poor blood supply to the *brain*. It can be mistaken for a seizure.

Syndactyly (sin-DAK-tuh-lee)

A *congenital anomaly* in which there is partial or complete *webbing* or fusion of fingers or toes.

> *Refer to* **Acrocephalopolysyndactyly** *and* **Acrocephalosyndactyly.**

Syndrome

A group of *signs* and *symptoms*, or *genetic* traits, that, occurring together, are characteristic of (describe) a particular *disease* or *disorder*. A child *diagnosed* with a given syndrome may or may not exhibit all the signs or symptoms.

Synergy (SIN-uhr-jee)

The action of two drugs or body structures which, working together, can achieve an effect that is greater than the simple addition of the two actions. An example is two muscles which must work together to produce a certain movement.

Syntax

The rules that govern the way in which words are arranged to form meaningful sentences or phrases. For example, "He ran outside" compared to, "Outside ran he."

Synthroid™ (SIN-throid)

> *Refer to* **Levothyroxine Sodium.**

Syphilis (SIF-uh-lis)
Refer to **Congenital Syphilis.**

Systemic (sis-TEM-ik)
Of, or relating to, the whole body rather than a specific area or part of it.

Systemic Circulation
The blood circulation of the body, excluding the lungs.
Compare **Pulmonary Artery.**
Refer to **Circulation/Circulatory System.**

Systole (SIS-tuh-lee)
The muscular *contraction* phase of the *heart*. (The heart rests in between *contractions*.) During systole, blood is pumped out of the heart to the rest of the body. The systole is what is felt when the *pulse* is taken and is the first sound of the heartbeat.
Compare **Diastole.**
Refer to **Blood Pressure.**

Systolic Murmur (sis-TOL-ik)
A type of *heart murmur* that occurs during *heart contraction*. This type of murmur is commonly harmless and does not necessarily indicate *heart disease*.

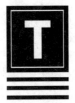

t
The abbreviation for time.

T
The abbreviation for temperature.

T & A
The abbreviation for tonsillectomy and adenoidectomy.

tachy-
A prefix meaning fast.

Tachycardia (tak-ee-KAR-dee-uh)
A condition in which the *heart rate* is excessively rapid (although the rhythm of the *heart's contractions* is normal). For an infant, tachycardia is a heart rate over 180 to 200 beats per minute. (A healthy newborn heart rate is over 100 beats per minute.) Tachycardia occurs when infants are upset or excited, but can also be an indication of infection, *heart disease*, or breathing problems. An increased heart rate may also be a *side effect* of certain drugs or fever. (For an adult, tachycardia is a resting heart rate of more than 100 beats per minute.)

Tachypnea (tak-ip-NEE-uh)
An *abnormally* rapid rate of breathing. An infant whose breathing rate is over 60 breaths per minute is experiencing tachypnea. (A newborn baby breathes at an approximate rate of 40 breaths per minute.) Tachypnea occurs when the infant is upset or excited, but can also be an indication of *respiratory* distress, *heart disease*, or infection. (For an adult, tachypnea is a breathing rate of more than 20 breaths per minute.)

Tact
The name of something, such as when a child is shown a picture of a ball and is asked, "What is this?" and she responds (names it), "ball." (Tact is derived from "contacting the environment," and is a concept developed by American *psychologist*, B.F. Skinner as he studied the functions of how people use language to communicate.)

Tactile (TAK-til)
Pertaining to touch.

Tactile Defensiveness
An *abnormal* sensitivity to touch, indicated by an infant's avoidance or rejection of touching and handling. The infant who has tactile defensiveness may resist touching or being touched by something that is wet, that is an unusual texture, or that is of an unfamiliar temperature or pressure. For example, a child may perceive the unexpected, mild bump from someone while standing in line, as rough and aggressive. Tactile defensiveness may be the result of having difficulty with processing and *discriminating tactile stimulation*.

Tactile Discrimination
The ability to perceive the differences between various *stimuli* to the skin, either when touching objects or when being touched by someone or something.

Tailor Sitting
Sitting with the buttocks on the floor with the legs bent and feet crossed at the ankles.

TAL
The abbreviation for tendo-achilles lengthening.
>   *Refer to* **Achilles Tendon Lengthening.**

Talipes (TAL-i-peez)
Any deformity of the foot involving the *talus* (the foot bone that connects with the *tibia* and *fibula* to form the ankle).
>   *Refer to* **Clubfoot.**

Talipes Equinovalgus (TAL-i-peez ee-kwie-noe-VAL-guhs)
A form of *clubfoot* in which the foot is bent downward and the heel is elevated and turned outward (away from the *midline* of the body).
>   *Refer to* **Clubfoot.**

Talipes Equinovarus (TAL-i-peez ee-kwie-noe-VER-uhs)
A foot deformity (the most common form of *clubfoot*) in which the foot is twisted in an *abnormal* position of *plantar flexion, adduction,* and *inversion* (the foot is bent downward and inward, with the heel turned inward as well). Talipes equinovarus should be treated as soon as possible after birth in order to restore the foot to the normal position.
>   *Refer to* **Clubfoot.**

Talus (TAY-luhs)
The foot bone that connects with the *tibia* and *fibula* (the bones of the lower leg) to form the ankle.

Tandem Walking
Walking forward in a straight line with the heel of one foot touching the toe of the opposite foot (heel-to-toe walking).

Tantrum

A normal *behavior* exhibited especially by children under 3 years of age that is typically caused by the child's inability to tolerate frustration. To some adults, yelling or crying angrily constitutes a tantrum. To others, lying on the floor kicking and screaming for a long period of time is a tantrum. Most adults find it difficult to deal with a child who is having a tantrum. An important first step is to try to determine if the behavior is internally motivated (the child may be venting her frustration over trying to cope with some aspect of her environment), or if the tantrum is externally motivated (the child has learned that she will get something she wants, or avoid something she does not want to do, if she throws a tantrum). An externally motivated tantrum is generally a behavior learned by a child over the age of 3 years.

TAPVR

The abbreviation for total anomalous pulmonary venous return.

Target Behavior

The specific *behavior* (such as "Jacob will verbally request a push on the swing when given spoken and visual *prompts*") that a teacher or parent is planning to teach a child. A target behavior can also be a specific behavior that a parent or teacher intends to change, either by extinguishing it or strengthening it.

Tarsal (TAR-suhl)

Pertaining to the *tarsus*, or ankle.

Tarsus (TAR-suhs)

The seven bones that form the instep part of the foot and ankle.

Task Analysis

Dividing a task into steps. In this way it can be determined which steps toward task completion a child has mastered. For example, task analysis can be used to determine whether the infant can feed herself a cracker. The child will be observed as to which, if any, of the following steps she can perform: extend her arm, voluntarily *grasp* a cracker, bring the cracker to her mouth, gum or bite the cracker, swallow the cracker. Task analysis enables the caregiver or teacher to know which skills need to be taught.

Taste

The sense of perceiving and distinguishing between different flavors (sweet, salty, sour, and bitter) that come in contact with the tongue. (The sense of smell is needed to *discriminate* between subtle variations of the four flavors.) When the taste receptor *cells* (*taste buds*, which are found mainly on the tongue) receive taste sensations, they send *nerve impulses* to special taste centers in the *brain*.

Taste Buds

The small *cells* found primarily on the tongue that detect different flavors (sweet, sour, bitter, and salty). The taste buds that are sensitive to sweet *tastes* are located at the center of the tip of the tongue; the taste buds that are sensitive to salty tastes are located on the sides of the tongue, at the front; the taste buds that are sensitive to sour tastes are located on the sides of the tongue, in the middle and toward the back; and the taste buds that are sensitive to bitter tastes are located across the back of most of the tongue.

tax-
A prefix meaning arrange or order.

Tay-Sachs Disease (tay-SAKS)
An *autosomal recessive brain disorder* characterized by *failure to thrive, blindness, seizures,* and progressive *paralysis.* These *symptoms* begin by the time the infant is 6 months old, and are caused by a deficiency of the *enzyme* hexosaminidase A, which results in an accumulation of a chemical called a *ganglioside* that damages the brain. Tay-Sachs is a fatal *disease* that usually results in death by 4 years of age. It is most prevalent in Jewish families of Eastern European descent.
Also known as **Infantile Cerebral Sphingolipidosis.**

TB, tb
The abbreviation for tuberculosis.

TBI
The abbreviation for traumatic brain injury.

T Cell
A *lymphocyte* that is important to the body's *immune system. Killer T cells* and helper T cells are two types of T cells.
Compare **B Cell.**
Refer to **Lymphocyte.**

TEACCH
A state-funded research, teacher training, and direct service program, based at the University of North Carolina at Chapel Hill, that was developed to educate children with *autism spectrum disorders (ASDs).* TEACCH stands for Treatment and Education of Autistic and Related Communication-Handicapped Children. As a teaching method, the TEACCH Program emphasizes the relative strengths of the child with an ASD in visual processing over verbal processing and incorporates parent-professional collaboration. It uses schedules consisting of objects, pictures, or written plans (depending on the child's *developmental* level) that the child can understand and follow independently to complete tasks. It utilizes a work system that helps the child organize, manage time and sequencing, and finish tasks.

TEF
The abbreviation for tracheoesophageal fistula.

Tegretol™ (TEG-ri-tahl)
Refer to **Carbamazepine.**

Telangiectatic Nevus (tuh-lan-jee-ek-TAT-ik NEE-vuhs)

A common skin condition of newborn infants characterized by flat, deep pink areas on the back of the neck, the base of the head, the upper eyelids, upper lip, and bridge of the nose. The pink areas of color are caused by *capillary* dilation that disappears by about 2 years of age.

Also known as a **Stork Bite.**

Telecanthus (tel-uh-KAN-thus)

Increased distance between the inner corners of the eyelids, resulting in eyes that look more widely spaced than usual.

Temperament

The child's characteristic emotional response. Temperament is an important consideration for planning appropriate learning experiences and discipline techniques. For example, for some children, a high level of activity is normal (and does not mean the child has *hyperactivity*). Other examples of temperaments that are normal for some children include poor adaptability to change or an increased sensitivity to *sensory stimulation* (loud noise, bright lights, etc.).

Temper Tantrum

Refer to **Tantrum.**

Temporal Lobe (TEM-por-uhl)

Refer to **Cerebral Hemisphere.**

Temporal Lobe Seizure (TEM-por-uhl)

Refer to **Complex Partial Seizure, Partial Seizure,** *and* **Epilepsy.**

Tendo-Achilles Lengthening (TAL) (TEN-doe uh-KIL-eez)

Refer to **Achilles Tendon Lengthening.**

Tendon

The fibrous cord of *connective tissue* in which the fibers of a muscle end and by which a muscle is attached to a bone or other structure.

Tendon Lengthening

A surgical procedure to release muscle *contractures*. An example of a tendon lengthening procedure is heel cord (*Achilles tendon*) lengthening.

Tenex™ (TEN-eks)

Refer to **Guanfacine Hydrochloride.**

Tenormin™ (ten-OR-min or Ten-or-min)

Refer to **Atenolol.**

Tenotomy (tuh-NOT-uh-mee)

A surgical procedure that involves cutting a *tendon* to correct a muscle imbalance. For example, it may be done to release muscle *contractures* or to lengthen shortened muscles, allowing for better movement of a *joint,* or to correct *strabismus* of the eye.

Tension
The *state* of being stretched.

Tent
A tent erected over the patient's bed into which humidified air and/or *oxygen,* vaporized drugs, or a cool mist of water is passed to treat certain *respiratory* conditions. An *oxygen tent* is an example.
Also known as **Mist Tent.**

Teratogen (tuh-RAT-uh-juhn or TER-uh-tuh-juhn)
An agent that affects normal *embryonic* and *fetal* development, when the pregnant mother is exposed. This disruption may cause *abnormalities* in the *fetus.* Examples of teratogens include certain drugs, the *rubella virus,* and *x-rays.* The various teratogens cause a wide range of *congenital anomalies,* including *brain damage,* missing or malformed *limbs, heart* anomalies, and *blindness.*

Terbutaline Sulfate (ter-BYOO-tuh-leen SUL-fayt)
A drug that relaxes the *uterus* in order to prevent premature *labor.* It is also a *bronchodilator drug* used to treat *asthma.* Brethine™ is the brand name of this drug.

Term Infant
Any newborn infant born between the beginning of the 38th week and the end of the 42nd week of *gestation.* Term infants usually measure from 48-53 centimeters (approximately 19-21 inches) in length, and weigh between 2700 and 4000 grams (approximately 5 pounds, 15 ounces to 8 pounds, 13 ounces).
Compare **Premature Infant.**

Testes (TES-teez)
Plural of *testis.*

Testis (TES-tis)
One of a pair of male *gonads,* or sex *glands,* which forms *sperm cells,* necessary for reproduction. The *testes* are normally situated in the scrotum.
Compare **Ovary.**

Tetanus (TET-uh-nuhs)
A potentially fatal *neurological disease* caused by infection of a wound with the *bacterium* Clostridium tetani. Tetanus is characterized by painful muscle *spasms,* stiffness of the jaw, (which is why tetanus is sometimes referred to as "lockjaw"), and stiffness in other muscle groups. Tetanus can be prevented with a *vaccine* (it is the "T" part of the *DTaP* vaccine) given during infancy and childhood. To maintain *immunity* in individuals who have not been wounded, a *booster injection* (shot) is necessary every 10 years. Individuals with burns or cuts should have a booster if one has not been given in the last 5 years.
Refer to **Trismus.**

Tetracycline Hydrochloride (tet-ruh-SIE-kleen hie-droe-KLOR-ied)
An *antibiotic drug* used to treat many conditions. It should not be given to children under 8 years of age or to pregnant women because tetracycline hydrochloride may discolor developing teeth and affect developing bone.

Tetralogy of Fallot (te-TRAL-uh-jee of fal-OE)
A *congenital heart defect* that is made up of four *anomalies*: a narrowed *pulmonary valve*, a hole in the ventricular *septum* (*ventricular septal defect*), malposition of the *aorta*, and enlargement (thickened wall) of the right ventricle. Tetralogy of Fallot results in insufficiently *oxygenated* blood being pumped from the *heart* to the rest of the body, which causes *cyanosis* (a blue color to the skin caused by a lack of oxygen in the bloodstream). Surgery is necessary to correct these heart defects.

Textual Script
A written word, phrase, or sentence provided to a child with the intention of encouraging him to initiate and expand language use and pursue social interaction. The adult provides the child appropriate scripted comments (often reflecting his preferences and interests) in written form and the child is encouraged to use them to speak about what he has done or is planning to do. Using scripts allows the child to engage others in his activities and to share and receive information.
    Compare **Auditory Script.**

Thalamus (THAL-uh-muhs)
A part of the *diencephalon* of the *brain* that functions as a relay station for most *sensory* impulses going to the brain.

Thalassemia (thal-uh-SEE-mee-uh)
A group of *autosomal recessive disorders* of abnormal *hemoglobin* production rate or synthesis that leads to *anemia*. If a child inherits the defective *gene* that causes thalassemia from one parent, the condition is called thalassemia minor, and the *symptoms* are few, if any. If a child inherits defective genes from both parents, the condition is called thalassemia major, and the symptoms include anemia, *jaundice, failure to thrive, spleen* enlargement, lack of normal growth, and, if left untreated, death. The symptoms of thalassemia major appear during the first 3 to 6 months of life. Treatment is with blood transfusions. Thalassemia major is also known as *Cooley's Anemia.*

thel-
A prefix meaning nipple.

Theophylline (thee-OF-uh-lin or thee-oe-FIL-een)
A *bronchodilator drug.* Somophyllin-CRT™ is the brand name of this drug.

Theory of Mind (ToM)
A *cognitive* skill that develops around 4 years of age in which the child is able to have an understanding of other people's perspective. The inability to recog-

nize that other people have personal feelings and needs is a characteristic of some children with an *autism spectrum disorder.*

Therapeutic Blood Level (ther-uh-PYOO-tik)
The level at which a drug is most effective but not *toxic.* For example, the dose of an *antiepileptic drug* is adjusted so that a level that provides effective protection against seizures, but a minimum of adverse *side effects,* is maintained.

Therapy Roll
Refer to Roll.

therm-, thermo-
Prefixes meaning heat.

Thermogenesis (thur-moe-JEN-uh-sis)
The production of heat by the *cells* of the body.

Thermoregulation (thur-moe-reg-yuh-LAY-shuhn)
The body's control of heat production and heat loss (maintenance of normal body temperature).

Theta Wave (THEE-tuh or THAY-tuh)
One of the four types of *brain waves* creating the rhythm of electrical activity as seen on an *EEG.* Theta waves are seen when the child is awake but relaxed and sleepy. Theta waves are characterized by a low voltage and a relatively low *frequency* of 4 to 7 *Hz.*
>Compare **Alpha Wave, Beta Wave,** *and* **Delta Wave.**
>*Refer to* **Brain Wave.**

Thimerosal (thie-MER-uh-sal)
A *mercury*-based preservative previously used in certain *immunizations* (e.g., the vaccine against *measles, mumps, and rubella,* or *MMR*) believed by some people to produce mercury poisoning and to trigger *symptoms* of *autism spectrum disorder* (*ASD*) in young children. Although the majority of research indicates there is no cause-effect relationship between immunizations and the *incidence* of ASDs, in 1999 it was determined that thimerosal should no longer be used in routine childhood vaccines.

Thioridazine Hydrochloride (thie-oe-RID-uh-zeen hi-droe-KLOR-ied)
An *antipsychotic drug* sometimes used in the treatment of *hyperactivity.* Mellaril™ is the brand name of this drug.

Thiothixene (thie-oe-THIKS-een)
An *antipsychotic drug.* Navane™ is the brand name of this drug.

Thomas Heel™
A shoe modification (a piece added to the heel of the shoe) that helps keep the foot in correct alignment and body weight centered while walking.

Thoracic Cavity (thuh-RAS-ik)
The chest cavity.

thoraco-
A prefix meaning chest.

Thoraco-Lumbar-Sacral Orthosis (TLSO)
(THOR-uh-koe LUM-bahr SAK-ruhl or SAY-kruhl or-THOE-sis)
A *brace* that supports the *spine* and is worn to prevent spinal deformities, such as *scoliosis*, from worsening. The TLSO is often a molded plastic shell that keeps the spine in a straightened position.
　　Refer to **Orthosis.**

Thorax (THOR-aks)
The chest.

Thorazine™ (THOR-uh-zeen)
　　Refer to **Chlorpromazine.**

Three-Day Measles
　　Refer to **Rubella.**

Three Point Position
Positioned on three *limbs*.

thromb-, thrombo-
Prefixes meaning clot or lump.

Thrombocyte (THROM-boe-siet)
　　Refer to **Platelet.**

Thrombocytopenia (throm-boe-sie-tuh-PEE-nee-uh)
An *abnormal* blood condition characterized by a reduced number of *platelets* (due to a decreased production of the platelets or an increased rate of destruction of the platelets) that results in bleeding and easy bruising. While the underlying cause is often unknown, thrombocytopenia may be associated with another *disease*, result from a drug reaction, or occur as a response to a severe infection in which platelets are consumed as part of the process of coagulation.

Thrush
Infection of the oral cavity with the *fungus Candida Albicans.*
　　Refer to **Candida Albicans.**

Thymic (THIE-mik)
Related to the *thymus gland.*

Thymic Alymphoplasia (uh-lim-foe-PLAY-zee-uh)
A *disorder* in which the *thymus gland* fails to develop. It is one of the main characteristics of *Di George syndrome.*
　　Refer to **Di George Syndrome.**

Thymic Parathyroid Aplasia (THIE-mik per-uh-THIE-roid uh-PLAY-zhuh)
Refer to Di George Syndrome.

Thymus Gland (THIE-mus)
An organ important to the *maturation* of *T cells,* which are essential to the body's *immune system.* The thymus is also important in the development of the newborn's immune response.

Thyroid Gland (THIE-roid)
The *gland* located in the front of the neck, below the *larynx.* The thyroid gland, under control by the *pituitary gland, secretes hormones* that play an important part in controlling body *metabolism.*

TIA
The abbreviation for transient ischemic attack.

Tiagabine Hydrochloride (tie-AG-uh-been hie-droe-KLOR-ied)
An *antiepileptic* drug. Gabatril™ is the brand name of this drug.

Tibia (TIB-ee-uh)
The shin bone. (The other bone of the lower leg is the *fibula.*)

Tic
A repetitive, uncontrolled movement of a muscle or small muscle group caused by muscle *contraction.* Tics most often occur in the facial, shoulder, or arm muscles. Purposeless blinking is an example of a tic. Tics that occur on a *transient* basis are common in young and school-aged children. Tics are also characteristic of *Tourette syndrome.* Tics are usually distressing to a child who has them, in contrast to a *stereotypic behavior* that a child may find pleasurable or neutral.

tid
The abbreviation for the Latin words meaning three times a day.

Time-Out
A method of disciplining the child who is behaving in an unacceptable manner. Time-out is an opportunity for the child to regain control over her actions, so she can resume playing or interacting with others in appropriate ways. Time-out is accomplished by removing the child to a quiet place (always the same place, if possible) where she won't be distracted. It is important that the child does not become frightened by time-out and that she is not left alone. Time away from playing with peers, or from adult interaction, need not be long; under 1 minute is usually enough time for an older toddler and up to 5 minutes for a 5-year-old (or until the child is calm and appears ready to rejoin the group).

Tinea Capitis (TIN-ee-uh KAP-i-tis)
A *fungal* infection of the scalp commonly referred to as ringworm. A child may be infected with tinea capitis via direct contact with another person. It causes severe itching and scaling of the scalp and sometimes temporary hair loss.

Tissue (TISH-oo)
A collection of similar *cells* working together to fulfill a specific function.

Titubation (tich-uh-BAY-shun)
Unsteady *posture*, possibly the result of *disease* of the *cerebellum*. A child experiencing titubation may stumble or stagger while walking, and her head or trunk may sway while sitting.

TLSO
The abbreviation for thoraco-lumbar-sacral orthosis.

TM
The abbreviation for tympanic membrane.

TNR
The abbreviation for tonic neck reflex.

Tocolytic Drug (toe-koe-LIT-ik)
Any drug used to stop premature *labor*.

Toddler
A child between 1 and 3 years of age.

Toe Grasp
The *grasping* (curling under) movement of the toes in response to pressure to the sole, such as by touching the floor.

Toeing In
A turning inward of the foot caused by the foot, *tibia* (shin bone), and/or *femur* (thigh bone) turning inward.
> *Also known as* **Pigeon-Toed** *and* **Intoeing**.
> *Compare* **Metatarsus Varus** *and* **Toeing Out**.

Toeing Out
A turning outward of the foot caused by the foot, *tibia* (shin bone), or *femur* (thigh bone) turning outward, or by *pes planus* (*flatfeet*).
> *Also known as* **Duck Feet** *and* **Outtoeing**.
> *Compare* **Toeing In**.

Toe-Off
The action of the foot when, during walking, it points downward, pushing off from the floor.

Toe Walking
Walking up on the toes rather than on the whole foot. Toe walking may be used by the child who develops *contractures* in the calf muscles and *tendons* and cannot place the whole foot on the floor. It can also be a *sign* of *muscular dystrophy*. Some children with *autism spectrum disorders* tend to walk on their toes (with varying frequency).

Tofranil™ (to-FRA-nil)
>*Refer to* ***Imipramine Hydrochloride.***

ToM
The abbreviation for Theory of Mind.

Tomography (tuh-MOG-ruh-fee)
>*Refer to* ***CT Scanning.***

-tomy
A suffix meaning cutting or surgical incision.

Tone
1. A sound of distinct pitch, quality, or duration, as with a musical note or with voice. Adjusting the tone of voice helps convey the meaning of spoken words.
2. Pertaining to *muscle tone.*
>*Refer to* ***Fluctuating Tone, Hypertonia, Hypotonia, Muscle Tone,*** *and* ***Tonus.***

Tongue Protrusion Reflex
>*Refer to* ***Tongue Thrust.***

Tongue Thrust
The strong, involuntary (*reflexive*) protrusion of the tongue. Tongue thrust interferes with eating because food is pushed out of the mouth. It also creates dental problems because the tongue pushes against the back of the upper teeth. Children with some forms of *cerebral palsy* may exhibit this reflex. (The child with *Down syndrome* may have a protruding tongue, too, but this is not always due to a tongue thrust. It is likely due to having a smaller mouth size with a more shallow roof, and/or due to having *low muscle tone*; it is not the result of the child having a too-large tongue. The child can learn to bring/keep her tongue in her mouth.)
>*Also known as* ***Tongue Protrusion Reflex.***

Tongue-tie
>*Refer to* ***Ankyloglossia.***

Tonic (TON-ik)
Having continuous muscular *contraction.*
>*Compare* ***Atonic.***

Tonic-Clonic Seizure (TON-ik KLON-ik)
A form of *generalized seizure* that is named after the two phases involved in the seizure: the *tonic* phase and the clonic phase. Before a tonic-clonic seizure begins, the child may experience a warning called an *aura.* During the tonic phase there is usually loss of consciousness and the child falls to the floor. Her body stiffens, and she may breathe irregularly, drool, and lose *bladder* control. The tonic phase usually lasts 10 to 30 seconds and is followed immediately

by the clonic phase. It is characterized by alternating *rigidity* and relaxation (jerking) of the muscles. After the clonic phase, the child is usually sleepy or disoriented, and may have a headache or other discomfort.

Formerly known as a **Grand Mal Seizure.**
Refer to **Generalized Seizure** *and* **Epilepsy.**

Tonic Labyrinthine Reflex
(TON-ik lab-uh-RIN-thin or lab-uh-RIN-theen or lab-uh-RIN-thien)
A normal *reflex* in the first 4 months of life that is elicited by a change in position of the *labyrinth* inside the *inner ear*. (The labyrinth position is changed when the neck flexes or extends and the head moves.) Testing for the presence of this *primitive reflex* in an older child can be done while the child is lying on her back or on her stomach. While lying on her back with her neck in an extended position, the reflex is seen when the child's arms and legs extend and her shoulders pull back toward the surface on which she is lying (her shoulders *retract*). When the child is lying on her stomach with her neck in a flexed position, the reflex is seen when the child's arms, legs, and hips bend and the shoulders move forward (her shoulders protract). In either position (lying on the back or on the stomach), an involuntary increase in *muscle tone*, even if there is no actual movement of the arms or legs to a new position, indicates that the reflex is present. A positive response beyond the age at which the reflex is normally present may be a *sign* of *brain damage*, such as occurs with *cerebral palsy*.

Refer to **Primitive Reflex.**

Tonic Neck Reflex (TNR)
Refer to **Asymmetrical Tonic Neck Reflex** *and* **Symmetrical Tonic Neck Reflex.**

Tonsil
One of two *tissue* masses located at each side of the back of the throat. The tonsils provide the first defense against *microorganisms* capable of producing *respiratory disease*.

Tonsillectomy
Surgical removal of the *tonsils*.

Tonus (Tone) (TOE-nuhs)
The slight, continuous balanced *contraction* of muscles. In skeletal muscles, tonus is involved in the ability to maintain *posture* and to return blood to the *heart*.

Topamax™ (TOE-puh-maks)
Refer to **Topiramate.**

Topiramate (toe-PIER-uh-mayt)
An *antiepileptic drug*. Topamax™ is the brand name of this drug.

TORCH-S
Refer to STORCH Infections.
tors-
A prefix meaning twist.

Torsion (TOR-shuhn)
The process of twisting or being turned.

Torticollis (tor-ti-KOL-is)
A condition in which the head tends to tilt to one side as a result of the muscles contracting on that side of the neck. An infant can be born with torticollis, with the condition tending to be worse in a baby who is born in *breech presentation*. Torticollis can also be an *acquired* condition. It is believed that a birth trauma can cause damage to a neck muscle resulting in that muscle healing at a shorter length. It can be caused by injury to the *nerves* or muscles of the neck or be the result of a muscle *spasm*, a *tumor* at the base of the skull, infections of the *pharynx* or ear, surgical removal of the *adenoids*, a high degree of *astigmatism*, or eye muscle *palsy* (partial *paralysis*). Treatment to correct torticollis may include *physical therapy*, bracing, or surgery.
*Also known as **Wryneck**.*

Total Anomalous Pulmonary Venous Return (TAPVR)
(uh-NOM-uh-luhs PUL-muh-ner-ee VEE-nuhs)
A *congenital heart defect* in which the *pulmonary veins* are unable to bring *oxygenated* blood back to the left side of the *heart* (and thus to the rest of the body) from the lungs.
*Also known as **Anomalous Pulmonary Venous Return**.*

Total Communication
A method of communicating by using a combination of any of the existing forms of *communication*, including facial expression, *gesture, sign language, fingerspelling, lipreading,* speech, writing, and *augmentative and alternative communication* devices.

Total Parenteral Nutrition (TPN) (puh-REN-tuhr-uhl)
The process of feeding a child fluids via an *intravenous catheter* (such as a *central line* [*central venous nutrition*], which is threaded through a *vein* to the *heart*, or *peripheral* lines, which are inserted into peripheral *blood vessels* such as those in the hands, feet, or scalp). The catheter is left in place (not removed and then replaced at each feeding), and an *infusion pump* regulates the flow of the fluids. Feeding (continuous infusion) may take place over 10 to 24 hours. The *intravenous* solution is called *hyperalimentation* and it can include sugar, *amino acids, electrolytes, minerals, vitamins,* and fats. TPN is used when the intestines are not able to absorb food adequately.

Touch Screen
An electronic screen placed on a computer monitor to assist the young child in activating software.

Tourette Syndrome (TS) (too-RET)

A *developmental disability* that usually starts between 2 and 15 years of age, characterized by *motor tics* (for example, eye blinking or foot stomping) and vocal tics (for example, coughing or *echolalia*). Children with Tourette syndrome typically have *normal intelligence*. Some children experience *attention-deficit/ hyperactivity disorder*, *learning disabilities* (in 50 percent of children), *obsessive-compulsive behavior*, and *coprolalia* (in approximately one-third of affected children). The cause of Tourette syndrome is unknown, but research suggests that it is an *autosomal dominant disorder* in about one-third of cases. An imbalance of *neurotransmitters* is also being investigated as a possible cause.

Also known as Gilles de la Tourette Syndrome.

Toxemia of Pregnancy (tok-SEE-mee-uh)

Refer to Pre-eclampsia.

Toxic

Poisonous.

Toxicology Screen (tok-si-KOL-uh-jee)

A test of urine or blood samples to determine the presence of drugs or alcohol.

Refer to Prenatally Exposed to Drugs.

Toxin

A poison produced by a plant, animal, or *bacteria*.

Toxoplasmosis (tok-soe-plaz-MOE-sis)

A common infection caused by the *microorganism* Toxoplasma gondii. The infection is harmless in an immunologically intact individual, except when transmitted by the pregnant woman to her *fetus* through the *placenta* (especially early in the pregnancy). This condition, known as *congenital* toxoplasmosis, may result in *miscarriage* or *stillbirth*. The infant who survives may have a premature birth, *low birth weight*, *jaundice*, an enlarged *liver* and *spleen*, *brain damage*, *hydrocephalus*, *seizures*, *blindness*, *microcephaly*, and *mental retardation*. Congenital toxoplasmosis can be fatal to the infant. Toxoplasmosis is also a serious infection in people who have an *immune system disorder*, such as *AIDS*. Toxoplasmosis may be contracted by eating undercooked meat or eggs of animals containing the microorganism, or by coming in contact with an infected cat or with animal *feces*.

TPN

The abbreviation for total parenteral nutrition.

TPR

The abbreviation for temperature, pulse, respiration.

Trach (trayk)

An informal word for *tracheostomy* or *tracheal tube*.

Trachea (TRAY-kee-uh)

The tube that extends from the *larynx* (voice box) downward toward the lungs, dividing into the two *bronchi* of the lungs. The trachea functions as the passageway for air in and out of the body for breathing.

Also known as the **Windpipe.**

Tracheal (TRAY-kee-uhl)

Pertaining to the *trachea.*

Tracheal Catheter (TRAY-kee-uhl)

A *catheter* used to remove *mucus* from the *trachea* by a machine that applies suction.

Tracheal Tube

A tube placed into the opening created by a *tracheostomy.*

Refer to **Tracheostomy.**

tracheo-

A prefix meaning *windpipe.*

Tracheobronchial Tree

Refer to **Bronchoscopy.**

Tracheoesophageal Fistula (TEF)
(tray-kee-oe-ee-sof-uh-JEE-uhl FIS-chuh-luh)

A *congenital anomaly* in which the baby is born with an *abnormal* passage that connects the *trachea* (the windpipe) and the *esophagus* (the tube that carries food from the throat to the stomach). The *fistula* causes the baby to cough and become *cyanotic* (develop a blue color to the skin due to a lack of *oxygen* in the bloodstream) when attempting to swallow saliva. It also causes the baby to *regurgitate* food. Food may also enter the infant's lungs, causing her to develop *aspiration pneumonia.* This type of congenital anomaly can be corrected surgically.

Refer to **Fistula.**

Tracheomalacia (tray-kee-oe-muh-LAY-shee-uh)

A condition in which the *tracheal cartilage* is softened and inadequate for maintaining an open airway. It can be a *congenital* condition, occurring alone, or with other defects (such as *tracheoesophageal fistula*), or an *acquired* condition, which has been associated with long-term *ventilator* use (such as a *premature infant* might need). Sometimes tracheomalacia improves without treatment, but if other defects are present, or if the condition is severe, treatment, including surgery, may be required.

Tracheostomy (tray-kee-OS-tuh-mee)

A surgical procedure in which an opening is made through the base of the throat and into the *trachea* to create an airway. A *tracheal tube* (the tube through which the child breathes) is inserted into the opening and the child will then either breathe room air, or, if she cannot breathe without assistance, have her tube connected to a *ventilator*.

Compare **Tracheotomy.**
Refer to **Tracheal Tube.**

Tracheotomy (tray-kee-OT-uh-mee)

Cutting into the *trachea* to create an airway, usually below a blockage in the trachea.

Compare **Tracheostomy.**

Tracking

The ability to follow moving objects with the eyes. Tracking develops initially at 2 to 6 weeks, and the skill is refined over the first 8 months of life as the infant's ability progresses from tracking with head movement to tracking without head movement.

Traction (TRAK-shuhn)

A pulling force to hold two body parts in the correct position relative to each other, or to correct their alignment. Traction involves the use of *tension* to immobilize the body parts being treated.

Tranquilizer Drug

A drug that has a sedative (calming) effect.

trans-

A prefix meaning across or through.

Transdisciplinary Team

A group of professionals who each represent areas of expertise useful in planning and implementing the educational, therapeutic, and/or medical treatment program of children with *special needs*. The team gathers periodically to evaluate the child, share their expertise, and, with the child's parents, determines the child's areas of strength and *deficit*. Based on the evaluation, a plan for addressing the child's needs is developed, and the professionals who will implement the plan are designated. Members of the transdisciplinary team may include the *service coordinator, infant educator, physician, psychologist, physical* or *occupational therapist, speech-language pathologist,* and *social worker,* in addition to the child's parents. Professionals on the transdisciplinary team may provide *assessments,* recommendations, and treatments that overlap other team members' activities. For example, both the speech-language pathologist and the occupational therapist may address a young child's *oral tactile defensiveness,* and then share their activities with the child's parents, infant educator, and child care provider. Transdisciplinary team members also provide training to other team members and jointly share the responsibility of implementing the child's plan.

Compare **Interdisciplinary Team** and **Multidisciplinary Team.**

Transfer
1. To move an object held in one hand to the other hand. The ability to transfer an object from one hand to the other emerges around 6 to 7 months of age.
2. To move from one position to another, such as from a *wheelchair* to bed.

Transient (TRAN-shuhnt or TRAN-zhuhnt or TRAN-zee-uhnt)
Pertaining to a condition that is temporary, such as a *transient ischemic attack*.

Transient Ischemic Attack (TIA)
(TRAN-shuhnt or TRAN-zee-uhnt is-KEE-mik)
A smaller *stroke*, usually lasting a few minutes, that can be mistaken for a *seizure*.

Transition
The purposeful, organized process of helping children who are *at-risk* or have a *developmental disability* move from one program to the next, such as from the hospital to home or from an *infant development program* to a preschool program. The child's parents and *interdisciplinary team* are involved in the process of selecting the program/class that will best meet the child's needs and in preparing for the change. Preparation should include the development of a formal, written plan (a transition plan) that details the steps necessary for a smooth transition.

Transition Object
On object such as a blanket or stuffed animal that a young child habitually uses to comfort herself.

Transition Plan
Refer to Transition.

Translocation (tranz-loe-KAY-shuhn)
Refer to Chromosomal Translocation.

Translocation Trisomy 21
The attachment of an extra (a third) *chromosome* 21 to another chromosome. *Refer to Down Syndrome.*

Transplacental (tranz-pluh-SEN-tuhl)
Referring to the crossing of a substance (for example, a drug), from the mother's bloodstream to the *fetus's* bloodstream (or from the fetus's to the mother's) via the *placenta*. *Refer to Placenta.*

Transposition of the Great Vessels (tranz-poe-ZI-shuhn)
A *congenital heart anomaly* in which the *aorta* and *pulmonary artery* are attached to the wrong ventricles, resulting in an insufficient amount of *oxygenated* blood being delivered to the body and oxygenated blood returning to the lungs. This anomaly must be repaired surgically. Once corrected, the child should be able to live an active life.

Tranxene™ (TRAN-zeen)
Refer to **Clorazepate.**

Trauma (TRO-muh)
A physical injury caused by external force (such as a car accident or an act of violence) or a severe emotional *shock*.

Traumatic Brain Injury (TBI)
Physical damage to the *brain* or to brain function due to a head injury, such as from an automobile accident, a fall, or physical abuse, including *shaken baby syndrome*. A *brain injury* that is *acquired* during the birth process, or caused by a lack of *oxygen* to the brain or due to poisoning, is not considered a TBI. A mild injury may not cause permanent damage, but a moderate or severe injury may cause a life-long *disability*.

Treacher Collins Syndrome
An *autosomal dominant disorder* characterized by a flattening of the cheek bones, an underdeveloped jaw, *external ear* malformation, *congenital auditory impairment*, downslanting *palpebral fissures*, lower eyelid *coloboma* (a space, or *cleft*, of part of the eyelid), *cleft palate*, scalp hair growth on the cheek, and *respiratory* problems. The child usually has *normal intelligence*, but may have a *learning disability*. Treacher Collins syndrome is the incomplete form of *mandibulofacial dysostosis*. (*Franceschetti syndrome* is the complete form.)

Tremor
Involuntary, rhythmic, quivering movements caused by the *contraction* and relaxation of a group of muscles.

tri-
A prefix meaning three.

Triad (TRIE-ad)
A group of three, such as three *symptoms* or three major areas of concern. For children with *autism spectrum disorders*, the triad of symptoms include: 1) qualitative impairments in *social skills*; 2) qualitative impairments in *communication*; and 3) the presence of ritualistic, repetitive activities and interests.

Triceps (TRIE-seps)
The muscle on the back of the upper arm. The triceps straightens the elbow.

tricho-
A prefix meaning hair or hairlike.

Tricuspid Atresia (trie-KUS-pid uh-TREE-zhuh)
A *congenital heart anomaly* in which the *tricuspid valve* (the *valve* between the right *atrium* and the right ventricle) has failed to develop. This leaves no opening from the right atrium to the right ventricle. Without the valve, blood cannot flow through the normal route to the lungs to become *oxygenated*. Surgery is required to repair this condition.

Tricuspid Valve (trie-KUS-pid)

One of four *valves* in the *heart* that open and close with each heartbeat to control the flow of blood. Blood exits each chamber of the heart through one of the valves. The tricuspid valve is located between the right *atrium* and the right ventricle of the heart. The three cusps (small flaps) of the tricuspid valve close during each heartbeat to prevent blood from flowing back into the right atrium.

> *Compare* **Aortic Valve, Mitral Valve,** *and* **Pulmonary Valve.**

Tridione™

> *Refer to* **Trimethadione.**

Trifluoperazine Hydrochloride
(trie-floo-oe-PER-uh-zeen hie-droe-KLOR-ied)

An *antipsychotic drug*. Stelazine™ is the brand name of this drug.

Trimester (TRIE-mes-tuhr or trie-MES-tuhr)

One of the three periods into which pregnancy is divided. Each trimester is approximately three months long.

> *Refer to* **Gestation.**

Trimethadione (trie-meth-uh-DIE-oen)

An *antiepileptic drug*. The brand name of this drug is Tridione™.

Trimethoprim (trie-METH-uh-prim)

An *antibacterial drug*. The brand name of this drug is Trimpex™.

> *Refer to* **Septra™.**

Trimpex™

> *Refer to* **Trimethoprim.**

Triplegia (trie-PLEE-jee-uh)

Weakness or *paralysis* in three *extremities* of the body caused by *disease* or injury to the *nerves* of the *brain* or *spinal cord* that stimulate the muscles, or by disease to the muscles themselves.

> *Refer to* **Paralysis** *and* **Pyramidal Cerebral Palsy.**

Triple Screen

A *prenatal* test to measure the levels of three substances (including *alpha-fetoprotein*) in the blood *serum* of a pregnant woman. The test is called a screen because it can indicate that the *fetus* may be at a higher risk for certain *congenital disorders*, such as *Down syndrome* or *spina bifida*, but the test does not diagnose (prove the presence of a disorder). The triple screen is usually performed during the second *trimester* of pregnancy.

Triploid (TRIP-loid)

Having three sets of *chromosomes*.

> *Compare* **Diploid** *and* **Haploid.**

Trismus (TRIZ-muhs)
A prolonged involuntary muscle *contraction* of the jaw.
> *Also known as* **Lockjaw.**
> *Refer to* **Tetanus.**

Trisomy (TRIE-soe-mee)
The presence of an extra (a third) of a particular numbered *chromosome* within the body's *cells*. (Normally, there is a pair of each numbered chromosome.) A trisomy can occur if there is an extra chromosome in either the egg or *sperm* cell that is involved in fertilization. A trisomy can also occur as a result of a *translocation* of *genetic* material that is passed on from parent to child. The most common trisomy is Trisomy 21 (*Down syndrome*).
> *Compare* **Monosomy.**

Trisomy 8 Syndrome
A *chromosomal disorder* caused by an extra chromosome 8 (sometimes with part of it missing) in some of the body's *cells*. It is characterized by variable degrees of *mental retardation, joint contractures* and other skeletal malformations, deep creases on the soles of the feet and palms of the hands, *cleft palate, heart* and *kidney* malformations, deep set and widely spaced eyes, and prominent *external ears*.

Trisomy 13
The presence of a third *chromosome* number 13 in the *cells* of the body. This results in a child with a *genetic disorder* characterized by severe *brain* malformation, *microcephaly, seizures, deafness, cleft lip* and/or *cleft palate, mental retardation, polydactyly*, and *heart defects*. Fewer than 20 percent of children with Trisomy 13 live beyond 1 year of age.
> *Also known as* **Patau Syndrome.**
> *Refer to* **Trisomy.**

Trisomy 18
The presence of a third *chromosome* number 18 in the *cells* of the body. This results in a child with a *genetic disorder* characterized by *failure to thrive*; growth deficiency; *hypertonia*; skull, facial, hand, and feet *anomalies; severe mental retardation; heart defects*; and *kidney* anomalies. Only about 10 percent of children with Trisomy 18 live beyond 1 year of age.
> *Also known as* **Edward Syndrome.**
> *Refer to* **Trisomy.**

Trisomy 21
> *Refer to* **Down Syndrome** and **Trisomy.**

trop-, tropi-
Prefixes meaning turning toward, or affinity.

-trophic
A suffix meaning nourishment.

Trophic (TROF-ik)
Pertaining to *nutrition* or food.

-trophy
A suffix meaning nurture or *nutrition*.

Trunk Rotation
The ability to turn and twist the trunk. Trunk rotation is a necessary skill for walking.

TS
The abbreviation for Tourette syndrome.

Tuberculosis (TB, tb) (too-bur-kyoo-LOE-sis)
An infectious *disease* caused by the *bacterium* Mycobacterium Tuberculosis, which is transmitted by airborne droplets. Tuberculosis causes scarring of, or damage to, the lungs, and, if the primary infection is not healed, can spread to the *lymph nodes* or other organs. Because the lungs are typically affected, *symptoms* of the infection typically include coughing and lung disease, and can be fatal. Tuberculosis can be prevented by administering a *vaccine* and by monitoring people who have had contact with someone who has the disease. A test to check for the presence of TB (administered by injection) is recommended at 12 months, before starting school, or as needed (if there has been a possible or known exposure.)
*Refer to **Mantoux Test.***

Tuberous Sclerosis (TOO-bur-uhs skluh-ROE-sis)
An *autosomal dominant disorder* characterized by *lesions* on the skin and of the brain, eyes, *kidneys*, and, rarely, *heart*; *seizures*; and often *mental retardation*. The lesions and seizures tend to develop during the early childhood years.
*Also known as **Bourneville Disease** and **Epiloia**.*
*Refer to **Adenoma Sebaceum**.*

Tumor (TOO-muhr)
1. An *abnormal* growth of new *tissue* that may be *benign* or *malignant*. A tumor is characterized by a progressive and uncontrolled increase of *cells*. Some tumors remain *localized* and some spread to other parts of the body.
2. Tissue swelling or enlargement due to *inflammation*.

Tunnel Vision
A condition affecting the eyes in which the *visual field* is constricted, giving the impression of looking through a tunnel (only straight-ahead vision is possible). Tunnel vision may be caused by *glaucoma*, a *disorder* of the *brain* and *optic nerve*, or *retinitis pigmentosa*.

Turbinate Bone (TUR-bi-nayt)
*Refer to **Concha**.*

Turner Syndrome

A *chromosomal disorder* caused by the absence of an *X chromosome* in all or some of a girl's body *cells*. Turner syndrome is characterized by *short stature*, *webbing* of the skin of the neck, a broad chest with underdeveloped breasts and widely spaced nipples, infertility, eye *abnormalities* such as *ptosis* (drooping of the eyelid) and *strabismus* (a condition in which the eyes do not work together), bone abnormalities, including deformity of the elbow in which it deviates away from the *midline* of the body (as seen when the arm is extended and the palm is facing forward), and occasionally *mental retardation, kidney abnormalities,* and *coarctation of the aorta* (a *heart defect* that causes the *heart* to work harder than normal). Turner syndrome only affects females.

> Also known as **Bonnevie-Ullrich Syndrome, XO Syndrome, Monosomy X,** and **45, X Syndrome.**

Turribrachycephaly (tur-i-brayk-ee-SEF-uh-lee)

> *Refer to* **Hypsibrachycephaly.**

Turricephaly (tur-i-SEF-uh-lee)

> *Refer to* **Oxycephaly.**

Twin

> *Refer to* **Dizygotic Twins** *and* **Monozygotic Twins.**

Twister Cables

Cable-type devices that extend from a *pelvic band* to the child's shoes or short leg *braces* to assist the child with walking. The cables help control leg rotation, a problem common to some *neurological disorders*.

Two-Way Communication

The ability to have an emotional interaction, such as when a parent shows interest in her child (and the activity in which her child is engaged), and the child responds with *gestures* or words.

Tylenol™

> *Refer to* **Acetaminophen.**

Tympanic Membrane (TM) (tim-PAN-ik)

The fibrous *membrane* that carries sound vibrations to the *inner ear* via the bones of the *middle ear*. It is located at the innermost end of the *auditory canal* (the auditory canal leads inward from the outer ear) and separates it from the middle ear.

> Also known as **Eardrum.**

Tympanic Membrane Temperature

The body's temperature when measured with a device placed in the ear (the external portion of the *auditory canal*).

> Compare **Axillary Temperature, Oral Temperature,** *and* **Rectal Temperature.**

Tympanometer (tim-puh-NOM-uh-tuhr)
An electrical instrument that measures changes in the pressure and mobility of the *tympanic membrane* to detect *middle ear* fluid.
Refer to Immittance Audiometry.

Tympanometry (tim-puh-NOM-uh-tree)
Refer to Immittance Audiometry.

Tympanostomy Tube (tim-puh-NOS-tuh-mee)
Refer to Ear Tube.

Tympanum (TIM-puh-nuhm)
The cavity of the *middle ear*.

Type I Crigler-Najjar Syndrome
Refer to Crigler-Najjar Syndrome.

Type II Crigler-Najjar Syndrome
Refer to Crigler-Najjar Syndrome.

Typically Developing
Describing the development of an infant or child that includes *behaviors* and skill acquisition that are demonstrated within the expected time frames.

Tyrosine (TIE-roe-seen or TIE-roe-sin or tie-ROE-sin)
An *amino acid*. When the body is unable to convert *phenylalanine* (another amino acid) to tyrosine (due to a defective *enzyme*), the *disorder PKU* results.

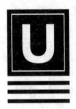

UAC
The abbreviation for umbilical artery catheter.
> *Refer to* **Umbilical Catheter.**

UAL
The abbreviation for umbilical artery line.
> *Refer to* **Umbilical Catheter.**

UE
The abbreviation for upper extremity.

Ulcer (UL-suhr)
An open sore on the skin or on a *mucous membrane*. An ulcer may be small and shallow or deep and crater-like. Ulcers are caused by *tissue* death resulting from an *inflammation*, infection, decreased blood supply (usually to a *limb*), constant pressure to an area, or *malignancy*.

Ulegyria (yoo-lee-JIE-ree-uh)
A *brain lesion* of the *cerebral cortex*. It is usually the result of scar *tissue* forming from injuries such as when there is a sudden drop in systolic *blood pressure*. The condition is most common in newborns and can cause *brain damage*.
> *Refer to* **Blood Pressure.**

Ulna (UL-nuh)
The long bone on the little finger side of the forearm, extending from the elbow to the wrist. It is the larger of the two lower arm bones. (The other bone is the *radius*.)

Ulnar (UL-nuhr)
Pertaining to the side of the hand and arm nearest the little finger (fifth finger).

Ulnar Palmar Grasp
Grasp of an object using the ring finger and little finger and the palm of the hand. The ulnar palmar grasp usually develops around 4 months of age.
> *Refer to* **Grasp.**

ultra-
A prefix meaning beyond or excess.

Ultrasonography (ul-truh-suh-NOG-ruh-fee)
*Refer to **Ultrasound Scanning**.*

Ultrasound Scanning
A *diagnostic* procedure in which echoes of high *frequency* sound waves produce a picture of internal organs or of a *fetus* in the *uterus*.
*Also known as **Ultrasonography** and **Sonography**.*

Umbilical
Of or referring to the *umbilicus*.

Umbilical Artery Catheter (UAC)
*Refer to **Umbilical Catheter**.*

Umbilical Artery Line (UAL)
*Also known as **Umbilical Artery Catheter**.*
*Refer to **Umbilical Catheter**.*

Umbilical Catheter (uhm-BIL-i-kuhl)
A *catheter* (tube) placed in a *blood vessel* in a baby's *umbilicus*. It is placed in an umbilical *artery* to collect blood samples and/or to feed a newborn who requires *total parenteral nutrition*. A catheter is placed in an umbilical *vein* for an *exchange transfusion* or the emergency administration of *drugs* or fluids.
*Refer to **Catheter**.*

Umbilical Cord
The flexible structure connecting the *placenta* within the pregnant woman's *uterus* to the *umbilicus* of her *embryo/fetus*.

Umbilical Hernia
A common condition in newborn infants in which there is a soft protrusion of *bowel* or *peritoneum* at the *umbilicus* caused by a weakness in the *abdominal* wall. Umbilical hernias usually disappear around 2 years of age, although sometimes they remain throughout life.

Umbilical Venous Catheter (UVC)
*Refer to **Umbilical Catheter**.*

Umbilical Venous Line (UVL)
*Also known as **Umbilical Venous Catheter**.*
*Refer to **Umbilical Catheter**.*

Umbilicus (um-BIL-i-kuhs or um-bi-LIE-kuhs)
The site on the *abdomen* where the *umbilical cord* was attached.
*Also known as **Navel** or **Belly Button**.*

Umbrella Stroller
A stroller that has a *hammock*-type seat. The umbrella stroller is useful with the child who stiffens into *extension* and needs to be in a more flexed position, as well as with the child who has *low muscle tone* and needs some support of his head and trunk.

un-
A prefix meaning not.

Underreactive
Refer to Hyporesponsive.

Underresponsive
Refer to Hyporesponsive.

Undescended Testes (un-di-SEND-id TES-teez)
A condition in which one or both of the *testes* have not moved down into the scrotum.
Also known as Cryptorchidism.

uni-
A prefix meaning one.

Unifactorial Disorder
A *disorder* caused by a defective *gene* or gene pair. Unifactorial *genetic disorders* are classified as either autosomal disorders (the defective gene is on one of the 22 pairs of *autosomes*) or X-linked (the defective gene is on the *sex chromosomes*).
Compare Multifactorial Disorder and Chromosomal Abnormality.
Refer to Autosomal Dominant Disorder, Autosomal Recessive Disorder, X-Linked Dominant Disorder, and X-Linked Recessive Disorder.

Unilateral
Affecting or occurring on only one side of the body.

Unilateral Hearing Impairment
Auditory impairment in only one ear.
Refer to Auditory Impairment.

Unilateral Reaching
Reaching with only one arm.

Uniparental Disomy (YOO-ni-puh-REN-tuhl DIE-soe-mee)
An unequal chromosomal *inheritance* in which a baby receives both *chromosomes* of a given pair (two of a specific numbered chromosome) from one parent. (Usually a baby receives one of a specific numbered chromosome from each parent to complete his chromosome pair.) The two chromosomes received from one parent can be identical copies or two different chromosomes.

UO
The abbreviation for of undetermined origin.

Upper Extremity (UE)
One of either arm.

Upper GI
Pertaining to the upper *gastrointestinal tract* (the *esophagus* through the *duodenum*). Upper GI is commonly used to refer to the *barium swallow* test.

Upper Respiratory Infection (URI)
A *cold*, or any infection affecting the nose, throat, *sinuses*, ears, and *larynx* (voice box).
> Compare **Lower Respiratory Tract Infection.**

ure-
A prefix meaning urine.

Urea (yoo-REE-uh)
A substance produced in the *liver*. It is the chief end-product of nitrogen *metabolism*.
> Refer to **Uremia.**

Uremia (yoo-REE-mee-uh)
A condition in which an excessive amount of *urea* is in the blood. It is a *sign* of *renal failure*.

Ureter (YOOR-uh-tuhr or yoo-REE-tuhr)
One of two tubes (one per *kidney*) that transport urine from the kidneys to the *bladder*. The ureters are located behind the *abdominal* organs.

Urethra (yoo-REE-thruh)
The tube leading from the *bladder* through which urine is *excreted* from the body.

uri-, uric-, urico-
Prefixes meaning *uric acid*.

URI
The abbreviation for upper respiratory infection.

-uria
A suffix meaning urine.

Uric Acid (YOOR-ik)
A crystalline compound found in urine.

Urinary (YOOR-i-ner-ee)
> Refer to **Bladder.**

Urinary Catheter
Refer to **Urinary Catheterization** *and* **Catheter.**

Urinary Catheterization
A procedure in which a *catheter* is inserted through the *urethra* into the *bladder* to drain urine.
Refer to **Catheter.**

Urinary Tract
All of the organs and ducts involved in the *secretion* and elimination of urine from the body (the *kidneys, ureters, bladder,* and *urethra*).

urino-, uro-
Prefixes meaning urine.

Urologist (yoo-ROL-uh-jist)
A doctor who specializes in the care of the *urinary tract* in males and females, and of the male genital tract. The urologist treats *urinary tract diseases.*

Urticaria (ur-ti-KAR-ee-uh)
A skin condition characterized by an itchy, white *rash* with central swelling, surrounded by red *inflammation*. It is usually caused by an *allergic* reaction, but often the cause is unknown. Attempts to pinpoint the cause should be made so that it can be avoided. Treatment with antihistamines often gives the best *symptomatic* relief.
Also known as **Hives.**

Usher Syndrome
A *genetic disorder* characterized by *auditory impairment* and *retinitis pigmentosa*, and sometimes *balance* problems. Depending on the type of Usher syndrome (Type 1, 2, or 3, with Type 1 being the most severe), a baby can be born with profound hearing loss and balance problems, and *visual impairment* by 9 to 10 years of age, or a baby can be born with moderate or later-developing *auditory impairment*, little or no balance problems, and loss of vision in the teenage years.

Uterine Contraction (YOO-tuh-rin kuhn-TRAK-shuhn)
A rhythmic tightening of muscles of the *uterus* when a woman is in *labor*. Uterine contractions decrease the size of the uterus and squeeze the *fetus* through the birth canal.
Also known as **Labor Contraction.**

utero-
A prefix meaning *uterus.*

Uterus (YOO-tuhr-uhs)
The female organ located in the *pelvis* between the *bladder* and the *rectum*. It is within the uterus that the *fetus* develops.
Also known as **Womb.**

UTI
The abbreviation for urinary tract infection.

UVC
The abbreviation for umbilical venous catheter.
> *Refer to* **Umbilical Catheter.**

UVL
The abbreviation for umbilical venous line.
> *Refer to* **Umbilical Catheter.**

Uvula (YOO-vyoo-luh)
The *tissue* hanging from the middle of the back of the mouth (from the edge of the *soft palate*). It assists in closing the nasal cavity during the production of certain speech sounds.

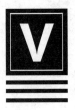

VAA
The abbreviation for verbal auditory agnosia.

Vaccination (vak-si-NAY-shuhn)
Refer to **Immunization.**

Vaccine (vak-SEEN)
A solution containing a killed or weakened *bacterium* or *virus*, given to boost the body's *immunity* (resistance) against an infectious *disease* caused by the bacteria or virus. Most vaccines are given by injection.
Refer to **Immunization** *and* **Inoculate.**

Vagal Stimulation (VAY-guhl)
Use of a medical device (a small *pulse* generator) that may suppress *seizures* caused by *refractory epilepsy*. The device is surgically placed in the chest underneath the skin with leads that run to the *vagus nerve* in the neck. The pulse generator is set to activate at regular intervals, but a person can manually trigger it and maybe stop a seizure. It works by stimulating the vagus nerve, which transmits an electrical signal to the *brain*. The signal adjusts brain chemical levels, which can stop a seizure from occurring.

Vagus Nerve (VAY-guhs)
One of the pair of the long cranial *nerves* that carry signals from four areas in the *brain* to the *heart* and many other internal organs.

Valgus (VAL-guhs)
A bending or twisting outward of a body part, such as the lower leg in *genu valgum* (knock knees).
Compare **Varus.**

Validity
The extent to which a test instrument measures what it is designed to measure.

Valium™
Refer to **Diazepam.**

Valproic Acid (val-PROE-ik AS-id)

An *antiepileptic drug*. Depakene™ and Depakote™ are both brand names for this drug.

Valsalva's Maneuver (val-SAL-vuhz)

An attempt to forcibly exhale when the airway is closed. It can occur naturally such as when lifting a heavy object or at the beginning of a sneeze. It can also be done deliberately by closing off the nose and keeping the mouth shut while breathing out, in order to "open" ears that have become blocked, such as during descent from a high altitude.

Valve

A structure in a passage or *vessel* that prevents a backward flow of the fluid contents passing through it.

> *Refer to* **Aortic Valve, Mitral Valve, Pulmonary Valve,** *and* **Tricuspid Valve.**

Valvuloplasty (VAL-vyoo-loe-plas-tee)

A surgical procedure to repair or reconstruct a *heart valve*.

Vancomycin (VAN-koe-mie-sin)

An *antibiotic drug* used to treat infections, primarily *staphylococcal* infections resistant to other antibiotics.

Varicella (var-i-SEL-uh)

> *Refer to* **Chicken Pox.**

Varicella-Zoster Virus (VZV) (var-i-SEL-uh ZOS-tuhr)

A type of *virus* that causes *chicken pox*.

> *Refer to* **Chicken Pox** *and* **Varicella-Zoster Virus Vaccine.**

Varicella-Zoster Virus Vaccine (VZVV)

An *immunization* against *Varicella-Zoster Virus* (to prevent illness with *chicken pox*). Children receive a single dose between 12 and 18 months of age. It is administered by injection.

> *Also known as* **Chicken Pox Vaccine.**

Varus (VAY-ruhs)

A bending or twisting inward of a body part, such as the lower leg in *genu varum* (bowleg).

> *Compare* **Valgus.**

vas-, vaso-

Prefixes meaning *vessel*.

Vascular (VAS-kyuh-luhr)

Pertaining to *vessels*.

VA Shunt
The abbreviation for ventriculoatrial shunt.

VCFS
The abbreviation for Velocardiofacial syndrome.

VCUG
The abbreviation for voiding cystourethrography.

VD
The abbreviation for venereal disease.
> *Refer to* **Sexually Transmitted Disease.**

Vein (VAYN)
A *blood vessel* carrying non-*oxygenated* blood from the body to the right side of the *heart*. The two exceptions to this are the *pulmonary veins*, which carry oxygenated blood from the lungs to the left side of the heart and the portal vein, which transports blood from the intestines to the *liver*.

Velocardiofacial Syndrome (VCFS) (vee-loe-kar-dee-oe-FAY-shuhl)
A *sporadic* or sometimes *autosomal dominant disorder* characterized by *cleft palate* and *velopharyngeal insufficiency*, resulting in speech delays; *cardiovascular anomalies* varying in severity; *mild* to *moderate mental retardation* or *learning disabilities;* and facial anomalies (a long, narrow face with a small jaw and mouth; a prominent nose; narrow, "squinting" eyes; and slightly malformed ears). Children with velocardiofacial syndrome can have a normal life span, depending on the type and severity of *cardiac* defect.
> *Also known as* **Shprintzen Syndrome** *and* **22q11.2 Deletion Syndrome.**

Velopharyngeal Insufficiency/Incompetence (VPI) (vee-loe-fer-IN-jee-uhl)
A condition caused by a *congenital defect* in which the *soft palate* doesn't completely seal off the oral cavity beneath the nasal passages (the passages that link the throat and the nostrils). During speech, air leaks through, resulting in *hypernasality*. Also, food may be *regurgitated* through the nose. VPI is common with *cleft palate*.

Velum (VEE-luhm)
> *Refer to* **Soft Palate.**

Vena Cava (VEE-nuh KAY-vuh)
One of two large *veins* that return *deoxygenated* blood from the body to the right *atrium* of the *heart*. The two venae cavae are called the inferior vena cava (which returns blood to the heart from the parts of the body below the *diaphragm*) and the superior vena cava (which returns blood to the heart from the diaphragm and the parts of the body above the diaphragm).

Venae Cavae
Plural of *vena cava.*

vene-
A prefix meaning *vein.*

Venereal Disease (VD) (vuh-NEER-ee-uhl)
> *Refer to* **Sexually Transmitted Disease.**

Venlafaxine Hydrochloride (VEN-lah-fax-een hie-droe-KLOR-ied)
An *antidepressant drug* sometimes used in the treatment of certain *behaviors* associated with *autism spectrum disorder.* Effexor™ is the brand name of this drug.

Venogram (VEE-nuh-gram)
An *x-ray* film of a *vein* that shows the *venous* pulse. The procedure is done by injecting dye into the veins.
> *Also known as* **Phlebogram.**

Venous (VEE-nuhs)
Of or pertaining to the *veins.*

Venous Catheter/Venous Line
A *catheter* placed in a *vein* to give nutrients, medication, or blood, or to withdraw blood.
> *Also known as* **Indwelling Venous Catheter/Line.**
> *Refer to* **Catheter.**

Vent
> *Refer to* **Ventilator.**

Ventilation
The part of *respiration* that includes inhalation and exhalation.

Ventilation Tube
> *Refer to* **Ear Tube.**

Ventilator
A mechanical device used to provide assisted breathing for the child who cannot breathe on his own. The ventilator pumps humidified air (with a measured amount of *oxygen*) into the lungs via an *endotracheal tube* or *tracheal tube.* The elasticity of the lungs allows the air to be expelled.
> *Also known as a* **Respirator** *or* **Life Support Machine.**

Ventral (VEN-truhl)
Relating to a position toward the front of the body.
> *Also known as* **Anterior.**
> *Compare* **Dorsal.**

Ventral Suspension

A position of holding an infant horizontally in the air (supporting her around the trunk) with her face downward. The infant is held in this position to observe the degree to which she can hold up her head, and, then later as she develops, her back, hips, and legs.

Ventricle

A small chamber, as in the ventricles of the *heart* or the ventricles of the *brain*. The heart has two ventricles, or pumping (lower) chambers. (The two upper chambers are the *atria*.) Blood flows from the atria to the ventricles, where it is then pumped to the lungs and the rest of the body. The brain has four ventricles. It is within the ventricles of the brain that *cerebrospinal fluid* is made and circulated.

Ventricular Septal Defect (VSD) (ven-TRIK-yuh-luhr)

A *heart defect* in which there is an *abnormal* opening in the wall (the *septum*) that separates the right and left ventricles. Depending on the size of the hole (which typically allows blood to leak through from the left ventricle to the right ventricle), the *heart* may ultimately be forced to work harder to pump blood to the rest of the body. A large hole may need to be corrected surgically, but a small hole may close on its own.

Ventriculitis (ven-trik-yuh-LIE-tuhs)

An infection of the ventricles in the *brain*, sometimes associated with *spina bifida*.

Ventriculoatrial Shunt (VA Shunt) (ven-trik-yuh-loe-AY-tree-uhl)

A diversion to drain excess *cerebrospinal fluid* from the ventricles of the *brain* via a *catheter* that runs from the ventricles through the skull, down the outside of the skull (under the scalp) to the *jugular vein* in the neck and into the right *atrium* of the *heart*, where it joins the bloodstream.

> *Compare* **Ventriculovenous Shunt** *and* **Ventriculoperitoneal Shunt**.
> *Refer to* **Shunt**.

Ventriculojugular Shunt (ven-trik-yuh-loe-JUG-yuh-luhr)

> *Refer to* **Ventriculovenous Shunt**.

Ventriculoperitoneal Shunt (VP Shunt)
(ven-trik-yuh-loe-per-i-toe-NEE-uhl)

A diversion to drain excess *cerebrospinal fluid* from the ventricles of the *brain* via a *catheter* that runs from the ventricles through the skull, down the outside of the skull (under the scalp), along the neck and chest (under the skin) and into the *abdomen*, where it is absorbed by the *peritoneum* (the *membrane* lining the *abdominal* cavity and covering the abdominal organs).

> *Compare* **Ventriculoatrial Shunt**.
> *Refer to* **Shunt**.

Ventriculovenous Shunt (ven-trik-yuh-loe-VEE-nuhs)

A diversion to drain excess *cerebrospinal fluid* from the ventricles of the *brain* via a *catheter* that runs from the ventricles through the skull, down the out-

side of the skull (under the scalp) to the *jugular vein* in the neck, where it joins the bloodstream.
>   *Also known as* **Ventriculojugular Shunt.**

Venule (VEN-yool)
One of many small *blood vessels* that join together to form *veins*. Venules receive *deoxygenated* blood from *capillaries* and carry it on to the veins.

Verbal Auditory Agnosia (VAA) (VUR-buhl AW-di-toe-ree ag-NOE-zhuh)
An inability to understand meaningful language even though *hearing* is intact. This type of *developmental language disorder* can be *congenital* or *acquired*. The cause of verbal auditory agnosia is unknown.
>   *Compare* **Auditory Agnosia.**

Verbalize
To express words vocally.
>   *Compare* **Vocalize.**

Vernix Caseosa (VUR-niks kas-ee-OE-suh)
The pale, fatty substance that protects the *fetus's* skin and insulates the baby *in utero*.

VERs
The abbreviation for visual-evoked responses.

Vertebra (VUR-tuh-bruh)
Any of the 33 bones that form the *spine* (*spinal column*). The first seven *vertebrae* form the *cervical* spine (in the neck area). The first cervical vertebra is called the *atlas* and the second cervical vertebra is called the *axis*. These two vertebrae enable the head to turn. The next 12 vertebrae form the thoracic spine (in the chest area). The next five vertebrae form the lumbar spine (in the lower back area). The next five vertebrae are fused together and form the *sacrum*. The last four vertebrae are fused together and form the *coccyx* (the tailbone). The vertebrae are separated by spongy disks called intervertebral disks.
>   *Refer to* **Spinal Column.**

Vertebrae (VUR-tuh-bray)
Plural of *vertebra*.

Vertebral Column
>   *Refer to* **Spinal Column.**

Vertebroauriculofacial Syndrome
(vur-tuh-broe-aw-rik-yoo-loe-FAY-shuhl)
>   *Refer to* **Goldenhar Syndrome.**

Vertex Presentation (VUR-teks)
The birth (delivery) of a baby in which the top of the head emerges first out of

the mother's *pelvis*. (The *fetus* is lying in the *uterus* with her head downward.)
>*Refer to* **Fetal Presentation.**

Vertical Talus (TAY-luhs)
Refer to **Congenital Rocker-Bottom Foot.**

Vertigo (VUR-ti-goe or vur-TIE-goe)
A feeling that one's surroundings, or one's own body, is spinning. Vertigo is caused by a disturbance of the *vestibular apparatus* contained in the *labyrinth* (*inner ear*).

Very Low Birth Weight Infant (VLBW)
A baby who weighs less than 1500 grams (approximately 3 pounds, 5 ounces) at birth.
>*Compare* **Birth Weight, Low Birth Weight Infant,** *and* **Extremely Low Birth Weight Infant.**
>*Refer to* **Premature Infant.**

Vesicle (VES-i-kl)
A small, fluid-filled sac. Vesicles are found within the body (such as the seminal vesicles in males that function as *reservoirs* for *sperm*), and on the skin (such as *chicken pox*).

vesico-
A prefix meaning *bladder*.

Vesicostomy (ves-uh-KOS-tuh-mee)
A surgically created opening of the *bladder* and *abdomen* through which urine can drain. This procedure is done if *urinary catheterization* is not useful in resolving the problem of a *neurogenic bladder*.
>*Also known as* **Cutaneous Vesicostomy.**

Vesicoureteral Reflux (ves-i-koe-yoo-REE-tuhr-uhl)
A condition in which urine flows back from the *bladder* into the *ureter* or ureters and sometimes up as far as the *kidney*. It may be due to blockage in the *urinary tract*, which may be a *congenital* condition, or may be caused by a urinary infection. It may occur due to an anatomic *abnormality* or secondary to infection not related to blockage. Persistent urinary *reflux* can cause kidney damage.
>*Refer to* **Reflux.**

Vesiculation (vuh-sik-yuh-LAY-shuhn)
The presence or formation of *vesicles* (small sacs that contain liquid).

Vessel (VES-uhl)
Any one of the small tubes that convey fluid throughout the body. The main types of vessels are the *arteries*, *veins*, and *lymphatic* vessels.

Vestibular (ves-TIB-yoo-luhr)

Pertaining to the *sensory* system (the *vestibular apparatus*), located in the *inner ear*, that responds to the position of the head in relation to gravity and to movement. This sensory system allows the body to maintain *balance* and to enjoyably participate in movement such as swinging and roughhousing.

Vestibular Apparatus

Refer to **Labyrinth.**

Vestibular Board

A large platform on rockers that may be used as a *vestibular stimulation* exercise to encourage the development of the child's *balance reactions*. The child is placed on her *abdomen* on the board, which is then tilted, changing the child's body position in space.

Vestibular Stimulation

An activity that stimulates the *vestibular apparatus* (the structures contained in the *inner ear* that provide the sense of *balance*) and helps the child develop awareness of her body position while moving in space, as well as her *balance reactions*. Examples of vestibular stimulation include rocking on a *vestibular board* and swinging.

Refer to **Labyrinth.**

Vestibulocochlear Nerve (ves-tib-yoo-loe-KOK-lee-uhr)

Refer to **Auditory Nerve.**

VIA

The abbreviation for Visual Interaction Augmentation.

Viable (VIE-uh-buhl)

Capable of sustaining life outside of the *uterus*.

Vibrotactile Hearing Aid (vie-broe-TAK-til)

A device used with children with *auditory impairment* that changes sound *stimuli* to vibratory stimuli. The vibration is transmitted to the inside of the wrist. This type of *hearing aid* helps the child who is totally *deaf* to feel the rhythm, or pattern, of speech. (The child with no measurable hearing does not benefit from regular hearing aids, which make sound louder.)

Compare **Hearing Aid.**

Refer to **Auditory Impairment.**

Vineland Adaptive Behavior Scales

A standardized *evaluation* tool used to assess the *communication* skills, daily living skills, socialization skills, *fine motor* skills, and *gross motor* skills of the birth to 30-year-old. Typically, the Vineland is administered by a professional with a minimum of a college degree. A parent interview format is used.

Previously known as the **Vineland Social Maturity Scale.**

Vineland Social Maturity Scale

*Refer to **Vineland Adaptive Behavior Scales.***

Viral Croup

*Refer to **Croup.***

Viral Meningitis

*Refer to **Meningitis.***

Virus/Viral (VIE-ruhs/VIE-ruhl)

The tiniest of known infectious *organisms* that is obligated to live inside body *cells*. Viruses invade the body in several ways, including: through airborne droplets which are inhaled, through contaminated food sources, through an insect or animal bite, through a needle, through the *conjunctiva* of the eye, and through direct contact with the *membranes* lining the genital tract during sexual intercourse. A virus may cause nuisance infections, such as the *common cold*, or serious infections, such as *AIDS*, or anything in between. For the most part, there is no treatment for viral infections, except to alleviate discomfort.

*Also known as **Germ.***

*Compare **Bacteria.***

Viscera (VIS-uhr-uh)

1. A term that collectively refers to the internal organs, especially the *abdominal* organs.
2. Plural of *viscus*.

Viscus (VIS-kuhs)

Any large internal organ, especially in the *abdomen*.

Vision

The sense of sight. Vision is a process involving both the eyes and the *brain*. For vision to occur, light waves from the object being viewed must enter through the *pupil* of the eye. The *cornea* and the *lens* make it possible to focus the light waves at precisely the right spot (thus forming an image) on the *retina*. The retina then transmits the visual data via the *optic nerves* to the brain. Lastly, the vision center of the brain analyzes the data in order to interpret a visual image. Because some of the optic nerve fibers cross over in the brain, both sides of the brain normally receive information from both eyes. The measurement of normal vision is 20/20, which means that the eye can see at a distance of 20 feet (this is the numerator, or first "20") what the normal eye is supposed to see at 20 feet (this is the denominator, or second "20"). *Visual impairment* may occur if there is damage to the eye, to the optic nerve or nerve pathways that connect the optic nerves to the brain, or to the brain.

*Refer to **Eye** and **Blindness.***

Vision Therapist

A specialist who works with people with *visual impairment* to help them learn to use their remaining vision as effectively as possible.

Visual Acuity

The ability of the eye to see clearly, specifically to perceive objects and to distinguish detail within central (straight-ahead) vision. It is expressed in 20/x terms, such as 20/20, 20/80, or 20/200 (meaning that at 20 feet, the eye can see as well as an eye with normal *acuity* can see at the distance expressed by the denominator).

Refer to **Vision.**

Visual-Evoked Potential

A procedure to test vision that involves recording the *brain's* response to visual *stimulation* via *electrodes* placed on the head. This procedure is useful for testing the vision of infants and nonverbal children.

Visual-Evoked Responses (VERs)

Refer to **Evoked Potential Studies.**

Visual Field

The total area that can be seen without moving the eyes or head. More area can be seen by the visual fields to either side of central vision than can be seen by the visual fields above and below central vision.

Visual Field Defect

A defect in an area of vision that moves with the eye, as the eye turns in different directions. A visual field defect may be caused by *brain damage, optic nerve* damage, injury to the eye, or *disease* of the eye.

Visual Impairment

Decreased *vision* caused by damage to the eye, the *optic nerve*, or nerve pathways that connect the optic nerve to the brain. Wearing eyeglasses may improve some forms of visual impairment.

Refer to **Eye, Vision,** *and* **Blindness.**

Visual Interaction Augmentation (VIA)

An approach to teaching *communication* skills to children with *autism spectrum disorders*. It emphasizes teaching the meaning of non-verbal communication (such as with eye-gaze, *gestures*, and facial expression) and uses *linguistic* features (such as vocal *tone* and simplified speech) as would be done with a typically-developing child of a similar *developmental* level. The VIA approach involves exchanging a picture of an item the child wants for the actual item (such as with the *Picture Exchange Communication System*), but with an emphasis on the exchange as being a very social interaction (i.e., a conversation) that may contribute to the development of the child's "*theory of mind.*"

Visual Learner

Refers to a person who learns best by what she sees, especially compared to what she hears. For example, the visual learner responds better to watching a demonstration of a task, such as stacking blocks, rather than to listening to an explanation of how it is done.

Visual-Motor Coordination
The ability to successfully engage in activity that involves both visual and *motor skills*, such as putting a puzzle piece into a puzzle board.

Visual Regard
The act of looking or gazing.
> *Refer to* **Prolonged Regard.**

Visual Response Audiometry (VRA) (aw-dee-OM-uh-tree)
A method of testing an infant's *hearing* in which a visual *reinforcer* (such as a toy that lights up) is activated each time the baby turns her head to sound *stimulation*. This type of hearing test can be used with infants as young as 6 months of age.
> *Also known as* **Conditioned Orientation Reflex.**

Visual Sequential Memory
The ability to remember a sequence of pictures or words that is seen.

Visual Tracking
Following a moving object with the eyes.
> *Refer to* **Tracking.**

Visuospatial Capacities (vi-zhoo-oe-SPAY-shuhl)
The ability to use the sense of sight to develop body awareness, including the location of the body in space and in relation to the environment (for example, objects and other people). Visuospatial capacities are important to the development of visual logical thinking and *representational* thought.

Vital Capacity
The volume of air one can take in with maximum inhalation.

Vital Signs
Body temperature, *heart rate*, *blood pressure*, and rate of breathing.

Vitamin
One of many complex chemical nutrients needed in small amounts for normal bodily functions and maintenance of health. Vitamins are obtained through the diet and sometimes through vitamin supplements. Vitamins are classified as either fat-soluble vitamins (these include vitamins A, D, E, and K), which are absorbed with *fats* and stored, or water-soluble (these include vitamins C, B12, and the B-complex vitamins), which are stored in the body for a short length of time and then *excreted* in the urine. (The exception is vitamin B12, which the body stores for a longer period of time.)

Vitrectomy (vi-TREK-toe-mee)
A procedure to remove the contents from the cavity of the eyeball that is situated behind the *lens* (the *vitreous chamber*), and then to refill the cavity with a sterile *saline solution*.

Vitreous Body (VIT-ree-uhs)
Refer to **Vitreous Humor.**

Vitreous Chamber
The part of the cavity of the eyeball behind the *lens*.

Vitreous Humor (HYOO-mor)
The gel-like substance of the eye located between the *lens* and the *retina* (the area within the inside of the eyeball).
Also known as **Vitreous Body.**
Refer to **Eye.**

VLBW
The abbreviation for very low birth weight infant.

VOCA
The abbreviation for Voice Output Communication Aid.

Vocalize
To produce *consonant* or *vowel* speech sounds, but not necessarily actual words.
Compare **Verbalize.**

Voice Disorders
Conditions that result in *abnormal phonation* (speech sounds), such as excessive hoarseness, a nasal voice, a high-pitched voice, or a too soft voice.

Voice Output Communication Aid (VOCA)
An electronic *communication* device with the capability of producing speech when specific buttons are activated. The speech may be digitized, recorded, or synthesized.
Also known as **Speech Generating Device.**

Voiding Cystourethrography (VCUG) (sis-toe-yoo-ree-THROG-ruh-fee)
Refer to **Cystourethrography.**

Volar (VOE-luhr)
Pertaining to the palm or the sole.

Vomer (VOE-muhr)
The bone that forms part of the nasal *septum* (wall) separating the two sides of the nose.

von Recklinghausen Disease (von REK-ling-hou-zen)
Refer to **Neurofibromatosis.**

Vowel
One of the letters of the alphabet that is not a *consonant*. The vowels include a, e, i, o, u. (Sometimes y functions as a vowel.) Vowels are produced when air

flows over the vocal cords and through the mouth. (Air flow is not obstructed as it is when producing consonant sounds.) Vowels are produced at the front of the mouth or at the back of the mouth, and are produced with the tongue in various (high and low) positions. Vowel sounds that are produced at the back of the mouth are the easiest (and thus the first) sounds a baby makes (other than crying). For example, the /o/ sound in "hot" is a low back vowel and the /i/ sound in "hit" is a high front vowel. Vowels are also described as being open vowel sounds (such as "aah") or closed vowel sounds (such as "ee"). *Diphthongs* are the last vowel sounds a baby produces.

Compare **Consonant.**

VPI
The abbreviation for velopharyngeal insufficiency and velopharyngeal incompetence.

VP Shunt
The abbreviation for ventriculoperitoneal shunt.

VRA
The abbreviation for visual response audiometry.

VSD
The abbreviation for ventricular septal defect.

VZV
The abbreviation for Varicella-Zoster Virus.

VZVV
The abbreviation for Varicella-Zoster Virus Vaccine.

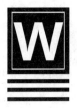

Waardenburg Syndrome (VAHR-den-buhrg)
An *autosomal dominant disorder* characterized by a wide bridge of the nose; eye *anomalies*, including *lateral displacement* of the inner *canthi* (the angle at the inner end of the opening between the upper and lower eyelids), more than one color of the *iris* of the eyes (or eyes of different colors), and white eyelashes; a white *forelock* of hair; loss of skin pigment in small areas; and sometimes *congenital sensorineural hearing impairment*.

WAGR Syndrome
A *congenital disorder* resulting from a *deletion* of the short arm of *chromosome* 11. WAGR is an acronym for W̲ilms Tumor (a *cancerous tumor* of the *kidney*), A̲niridia (absence of an *iris* of the eye at birth, resulting in some degree of *visual impairment*), G̲enitourinary anomalies, and *mental r̲etardation*. Children with WAGR syndrome also have facial dysmorphism, and may have other eye problems, such as *cataracts* and *ptosis*.
     Also known as **Aniridia-Wilms Tumor Association.**

Walker
An ambulation (walking) aid used with children who can *balance* independently while in a standing position. Walkers come with or without wheels and are either pushed or lifted and placed.

Walking Reflex
     Refer to **Stepping Reflex.**

Wall-Eye
     Refer to **Exotropia.**

Water on the Brain
An outdated phrase referring to *hydrocephalus*.
     Refer to **Hydrocephalus.**

Waterston Shunt™
A type of *shunt* placed between the ascending *aorta* and the right *pulmonary artery*. It functions to allow increased *pulmonary circulation* in *cyanotic heart disease* such as *tetralogy of Fallot*, which involves a narrowed *pulmonary valve*.
     Refer to **Shunt.**

WBC
The abbreviation for white blood cell.

WDWN
The abbreviation for well-developed, well-nourished.

Weaver Syndrome
A rare *syndrome* characterized by *congenital macrosomia* (an excessively large body size) and advanced bone *maturation*; *macrocephaly* with a broad, protruding forehead; facial *anomalies*, including widely-spaced eyes and/or increased distance between the inner angles of the eyelids, a prominent or long *philtrum*, a small jaw, large ears, and a depressed nasal bridge; hand and foot anomalies; *umbilical* and *inguinal hernias*; excessive and loose skin of the neck or *extremities*; *undescended testes*; a deep, hoarse voice; *strabismus*; *hypertonia* with *motor* delay; and, frequently, *mental retardation* that is usually mild, but can be profound. Weaver syndrome is caused by a *genetic mutation*.

Webbing
A *congenital anomaly* in which there is a *membrane* or flap of skin between two or more adjoining fingers or toes. Webbing can also occur on the neck.

Weider, Dr. Serena
> *Refer to* Developmental, Individual-Difference, Relationship-Based (DIR®) Model, Following the Child's Lead, *and* Interdisciplinary Council on Developmental and Learning Disorders (ICDL).

Wechsler Preschool and Primary Scale of Intelligence™-Third Edition (WPPSI™-III)
A *standardized test* used to evaluate the *intelligence* (verbal and performance skills) of the 2- to 6½-year-old. This test may be used as an indicator of academic readiness. Typically, it is administered by a professional who holds a doctoral degree and/or has significant experience and training.

Wedge
A wedge-shaped platform, usually made of foam, that assists the child in maintaining correct *positioning* while *prone*. The child is placed on the wedge on his *abdomen* with his head and arms over the thicker (higher) end. In this position he is able to work on his *head control* and his *weight bearing* on his hands and arms.

Weight Bearing
Supporting some or all of the weight of the body while in various positions, such as on the hands while *prone*, or on the feet while standing.

Weight Shifting
Moving the placement of weight from one body part to another. Examples include shifting weight from one hand to the other while in *prone* in order to *grasp* a toy, or shifting weight from one foot to the other while walking. Weight shifting involves movement that changes the body's center of gravity.

Welfare
Refer to **Aid to Families with Dependent Children** *and* **Department of Public Social Services.**

Werdnig-Hoffmann Disease (VERD-nig HOF-muhn)
The most severe form of *spinal muscular atrophy* (a *neuromuscular disorder*), characterized by increasing weakness and floppiness, lack of stretch *reflexes*, and *paralysis*, especially of the trunk and *limbs*. The lack of muscle control associated with Werdnig-Hoffmann disease results from *degeneration* of the *motor* neurons in the *spinal cord*. It is an *autosomal recessive disorder* that usually results in death in early life, most often due to *pneumonia* and *respiratory failure*.
Also known as **Infantile Muscular Atrophy** *or* **Infantile Spinal Muscular Atrophy.**
Refer to **Spinal Muscular Atrophy.**

Wernicke's Aphasia (VER-ni-keez uh-FAY-zee-uh)
A type of *aphasia* affecting *receptive language* in which the child may be able to articulate words correctly but the speech is incoherent due to substitute words and grammatical errors.
Refer to **Aphasia.**

Wernicke's Center
An area of the *brain* involved in comprehension of spoken and written words.

West Syndrome Epilepsy
A serious type of *epilepsy*, characterized by *infantile spasms*. Two main causes of West syndrome epilepsy are *brain* infections and brain *tumors*, although sometimes a cause is not identified. It is also frequently associated with *Sturge-Weber syndrome* and *tuberous sclerosis*. West syndrome epilepsy typically first appears in babies under 1 year of age and continues through life, resulting in *cognitive* impairment. West syndrome epilepsy more commonly affects males than females.

Wheelchair
A chair with large wheels that assists an individual with mobility. Wheelchairs are either manually operated or electronically powered.

Wheezing
A whistling, rattling, noisy sound made during breathing, caused by air flowing through narrowed airways.

White Blood Cell (WBC)
One of three types of *blood cells*. They protect the body by destroying harmful or foreign substances such as *bacteria*, *viruses*, and *fungi*.
Also known as a **Leukocyte.**
Compare **Platelet** *and* **Red Blood Cell.**

White Matter/Substance
The white *tissue* of the *central nervous system*. It is responsible for transmitting information related to *sensory*, *motor*, and other brain functions.
Compare **Gray Matter/Substance.**

Whooping Cough (HOOP-ing kof)
> *Refer to* **Pertussis.**

WIC
The abbreviation for the Women, Infants, and Children Program.

Wilbarger Deep Pressure and Proprioceptive Technique (DPPT)
A method of *stimulation*, used to help the brain organize *sensory* information, wherein a specific pattern of massage is provided using a soft, plastic surgical brush, followed by *joint compressions*. DPPT has been found in some cases to be beneficial for children with *sensory integration dysfunction*, decreasing *tactile defensiveness*, increasing *self-regulation*, and improving attention and the ability to use sensory information. DPPT was developed by Dr. Patricia Wilbarger, an *occupational therapist* and *clinical psychologist*. The technique should only be done by an individual who has been properly trained.
> *Refer to* **Brushing** and **Compression.**

Williams-Beuren Syndrome
> *Refer to* **Williams Syndrome.**

Williams Syndrome
A *congenital disorder* caused by a *microdeletion* on the long arm of one of the child's *chromosome 7s*. It is characterized by *heart anomalies*; small size; distinct facial features, including a short, upturned nose, long *philtrum*, broad forehead, full cheeks, puffiness under the eyes, and prominent earlobes; *strabismus*; *low muscle tone* and *hyperextensible joints*; occasional *hypercalcemia*; *hyperacuity*; and *mild mental retardation*.
> *Also known as* **Elfin Facies Syndrome** and **Williams-Beuren Syndrome.**

Wilms' Tumor (VILMS)
A *cancerous tumor* of the *kidney*.

Windpipe
> *Refer to* **Trachea.**

Withdrawal Position
Simultaneous *flexion* (bending and bringing together) of the arms and legs while *supine* (lying on the back) or side lying.

WNL
The abbreviation for within normal limits.

Wolfe-Parkinson-White Syndrome
A *disorder*, most likely present at birth, in which the infant experiences *arrhythmias* (changes in the rhythm or rate of the heartbeat). Affected children may have some form of structural *heart disease* and *paroxysmal tachycardia* (excessively rapid *heart rate*), which can lead to *heart failure*, *angina*, *cerebral* insufficiency, and even death. Wolfe-Parkinson-White can occur as an isolated

problem, but it is also associated with other *heart defects*. Treatment in children usually includes medication for the tachycardia.

Wolf-Hirschhorn Syndrome (WOOLF HURSH-horn)
Refer to 4p- Syndrome.

Womb (WOOM)
Refer to Uterus.

Women, Infants, and Children Program (WIC)
A federally funded program that provides pregnant women, new mothers, infants, and young children who qualify with food vouchers, *nutrition* counseling, and referrals to health care.

Worms
A common term for *parasites* that live in the *gastrointestinal tract*, blood, or other organs of the body. Infestation occurs by eating undercooked or infected meats, by ingesting contaminated water, or by coming in contact with contaminated soil, and may cause *acute illness* or may not be recognized for years. An example of a type of worm is the *pinworm*, which causes itching of the skin around the *anus* where the pinworm eggs are laid.

WPPSI™-III
The abbreviation for Wechsler Preschool and Primary Scale of Intelligence™-Third Edition.

Wryneck (RIE-nek)
Refer to Torticollis.

"W" Sitting Position
Sitting on the buttocks between the heels of the feet. (The knees are bent, forming a "W.") Children with *hypertonia* (stiffness in the muscles) often assume this position, but it should be discouraged because it hinders *motor development* and increases *spasticity*. It also encourages hip *joint* malformation and structural strain on the knee and ankle.

Wt
The abbreviation for weight.

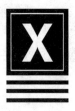

X Chromosome
A *sex chromosome* that in humans is present in both sexes. Females have two and males have one in the *cells* of their body.

Xeroderma Pigmentosum (XP)
A rare, *inherited* skin condition in which the skin is very dry, rough, wrinkled, freckled, and prematurely aged (by about 5 years of age), due to extreme sensitivity to UV (ultraviolet) rays in sunlight. *Inflammation* of the *cornea* and *tumors* on the eyelids and cornea can develop and may result in *blindness*. Exposure to sunlight must be avoided.

X-Linked Dominant Disorder
A *disorder* transmitted by an *abnormal dominant gene* on the *X chromosome*. Children who inherit the abnormal *gene* from an affected parent are always born with the traits of the condition; however, children of an affected parent who receive a normal chromosome are not affected. Normal children of an affected parent have normal offspring. X-linked dominant disorders appear to primarily affect females. It is theorized that males conceived with X-linked dominant disorders may be miscarried soon after conception since they do not have a second, normally functioning X chromosome. An example of an X-linked dominant disorder is *Rett's disorder*.
    *Refer to **Sex-Linked Disorder**.*

X-Linked Recessive Cutis Laxa Syndrome (KYOO-tuhs LAX-uh)
    *Refer to **Occipital Horn Syndrome**.*

X-Linked Recessive Disorder
A *disorder* transmitted by an *abnormal recessive gene* on the *X chromosome*. The mother usually does not have the disorder, but is a *carrier*. This is because females have two X chromosomes, and when one of the X chromosomes carries an abnormal *gene*, the other one usually does not. X-linked recessive disorders primarily affect males. The sons of a carrier mother have a 50 percent chance of being affected and her daughters have a 50 percent chance of carrying the gene (but not having the disorder themselves). In rare instances a female child of an affected father and a carrier mother might be affected. Ex-

amples of X-linked recessive disorders include *Duchenne muscular dystrophy* and *hemophilia*.

> *Refer to* **Sex-Linked Disorder.**

XO Syndrome
> *Refer to* **Turner Syndrome.**

XP
The abbreviation for Xeroderma Pigmentosum.

X-ray
A radiological technique that produces images of internal body structures by passing low doses of x-rays (high-energy, invisible electromagnetic waves) through the body to strike an x-ray film or fluorescent screen. X-ray radiation may also be used to destroy *diseased tissue*.

XX
The normal *sex chromosome* complement in females.

XXY Syndrome (XXXY Syndrome, etc.)
> *Refer to* **Klinefelter Syndrome.**

XY
The normal *sex chromosome* complement in males.

XYY Syndrome
A *chromosomal abnormality* in which affected males have an extra *Y chromosome*. Often XYY syndrome is not *diagnosed* because the features of the *disorder* are subtle: accelerated growth beginning around 5 or 6 years of age, resulting in tall stature; a thin build with less-developed chest and shoulder musculature; a long head with long ears; relative weakness; poor *fine motor* coordination; *learning* and/or speech *disabilities*; low-normal *IQ scores*; and *behavior* problems including *distractibility, hyperactivity*, and *temper tantrums*. The behaviors may be expressed as antisocial behaviors as an adult.

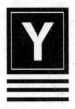

Y Chromosome
A *sex chromosome* that in humans is present only in the male.

Yeast
A microscopic *fungus* that can cause infection. An example of a yeast is *Candida Albicans*.

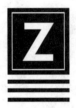

Zarontin™ (zuh-RON-tin)
Refer to **Ethosuximide.**

Zellweger Syndrome (ZEL-weg-uhr)
A rare *autosomal recessive disease* caused by a significant reduction or lack of a *peroxisomal enzyme*. Zellweger syndrome results in *brain abnormalities*, including *lissencephaly*; *seizures*; severe *hypotonia* (that may make the infant unable to move, suck, and/or swallow); *liver* enlargement; *heart disease;* vision problems (in some cases); and *mental retardation*. This disease is usually fatal within the first 6 months of life.
Also known as **Cerebrohepatorenal Syndrome.**

Zero Reject
The principle that no child with a *disability* should be refused a free, appropriate, education if other children the same age are being served.

Zero to Three: National Center for Infants, Toddlers, and Families
A national resource organization dedicated to promoting the healthy development of infants and young children. Zero to Three conducts research and

training institutes, publishes literature, and aims to strengthen the roles of parents, professionals, and policymakers who want to give children the best possible start in life.

Zinc
An essential nutrient in the body. Zinc is necessary for healing, cellular *immunity*, and normal growth.

Zoloft™ (ZOE-loft)
Refer to **Sertraline Hydrochloride.**

Zygomatic Bone (zie-goe-MAT-ik)
The cheekbone.
Also known as **Malar.**

Zygote (ZIE-goet)
The *cell* produced when a *sperm* (male sex cell) fertilizes an *ovum* (egg, or female sex cell). The zygote contains all the *genetic* information about the new individual that will develop.

Zyprexa™ (zie-PREKS-uh)
Refer to **Olanzapine.**

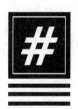

4p- Syndrome
A *chromosomal disorder* in which part of the short arm of *chromosome* number 4 is deleted. This disorder is characterized by *microcephaly* (an *abnormally* small head size), usually *profound mental retardation*, *seizures*, growth deficiency, *hypotonia* (decreased *muscle tone*), eye *anomalies*, *strabismus* (a condition in which the eyes do not work together), *cleft lip* and/or *palate*, cranial and facial abnormalities, *clubfoot*, genital abnormalities, and *heart* anomaly. Children with 4p- syndrome often do not survive beyond early childhood.
Also known as **Wolf-Hirschhorn Syndrome.**

5p- Syndrome
A *genetic disorder* that primarily occurs when part of the short arm of *chromosome* 5 is deleted. It is characterized by *microcephaly*, wide-spaced eyes, a

catlike cry in infancy (possibly due to a small *larynx* or associated with *central nervous system* dysfunction), *short stature*, and *mental retardation*.

Also known as **Cri du Chat Syndrome** (the French words meaning "cry of the cat").

13q- Syndrome

A *chromosomal disorder* that occurs when part of the long arm of a *chromosome* number 13 is deleted. This *syndrome* is characterized by *mental retardation* and growth deficiency and sometimes *microcephaly*; a high nasal bridge; eye *anomalies*, including *hypertelorism* (an *abnormally* wide space between the eyes), *ptosis* (drooping of the upper eyelid), *epicanthal folds* (a vertical skin fold at the inner corner of the eyes), abnormally small eyeballs, and *retinoblastoma* (a *malignant tumor* of the *retina*); a small lower jaw, low-set ears; a webbed and short neck; *clubfoot*; small or absent thumbs; *heart defect*; and genital anomalies, including *hypospadias* and *undescended testes*. Children with 13q- syndrome usually die before reaching adulthood.

20/20 Vision

Refer to **Vision** *and* **Visual Acuity.**

22q11.2 Deletion Syndrome

Refer to **Velocardiofacial Syndrome.**

45, X Syndrome

Refer to **Turner Syndrome.**

47, XXY Syndrome

Refer to **Klinefelter Syndrome.**

Appendices

APPENDIX I—GROWTH CHARTS

CDC Growth Charts: United States

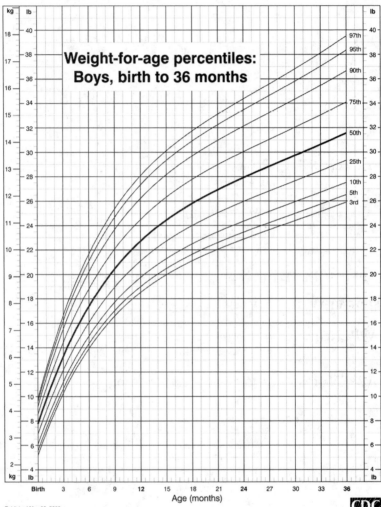

Weight-for-age percentiles: Boys, birth to 36 months

Age (months)

Published May 30, 2000.
SOURCE: Developed by the National Center for Health Statistics in collaboration with
the National Center for Chronic Disease Prevention and Health Promotion (2000).

CDC
SAFER · HEALTHIER · PEOPLE

CDC Growth Charts: United States

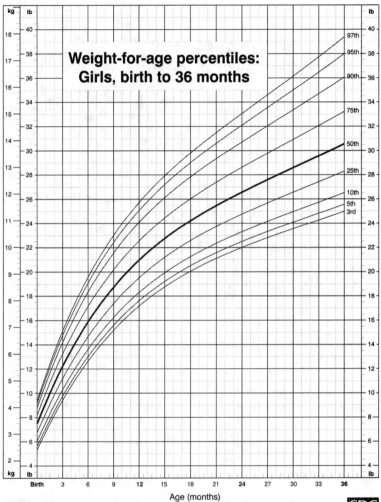

Weight-for-age percentiles: Girls, birth to 36 months

Age (months)

Published May 30, 2000.
SOURCE: Developed by the National Center for Health Statistics in collaboration with the National Center for Chronic Disease Prevention and Health Promotion (2000).

CDC
SAFER · HEALTHIER · PEOPLE

CDC Growth Charts: United States

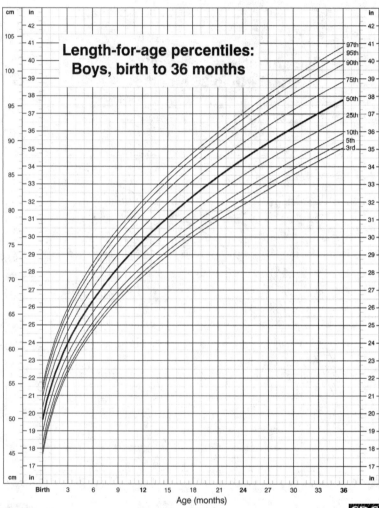

Length-for-age percentiles: Boys, birth to 36 months

Age (months)

Published May 30, 2000.
SOURCE: Developed by the National Center for Health Statistics in collaboration with
the National Center for Chronic Disease Prevention and Health Promotion (2000).

CDC
SAFER · HEALTHIER · PEOPLE

CDC Growth Charts: United States

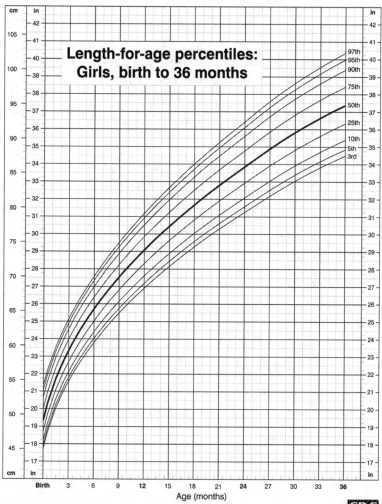

Length-for-age percentiles:
Girls, birth to 36 months

Age (months)

Published May 30, 2000.
SOURCE: Developed by the National Center for Health Statistics in collaboration with
the National Center for Chronic Disease Prevention and Health Promotion (2000).

CDC

SAFER·HEALTHIER·PEOPLE

CDC Growth Charts: United States

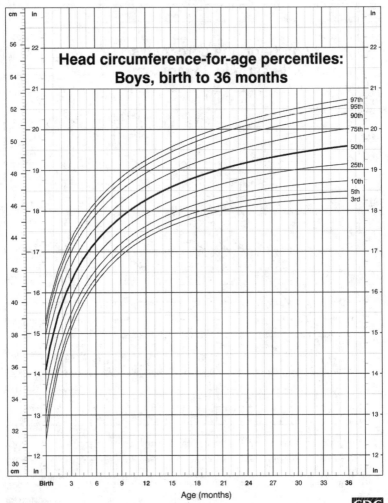

Head circumference-for-age percentiles: Boys, birth to 36 months

Age (months)

Published May 30, 2000.
SOURCE: Developed by the National Center for Health Statistics in collaboration with
the National Center for Chronic Disease Prevention and Health Promotion (2000).

CDC Growth Charts: United States

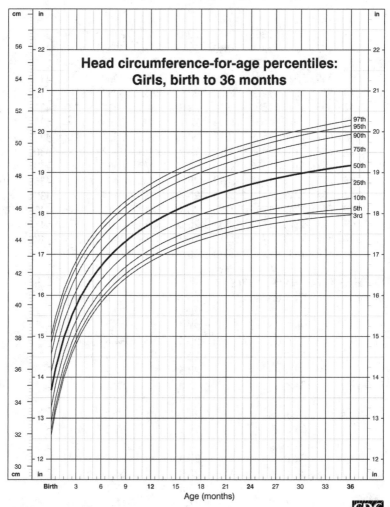

Head circumference-for-age percentiles: Girls, birth to 36 months

Published May 30, 2000.
SOURCE: Developed by the National Center for Health Statistics in collaboration with
the National Center for Chronic Disease Prevention and Health Promotion (2000).

CDC
SAFER·HEALTHIER·PEOPLE

APPENDIX II

CONVERSION CHARTS: POUNDS and OUNCES TO GRAMS

		Pounds										
		0	1	2	3	4	5	6	7	8	9	10
	0	—	454	907	1361	1814	2268	2722	3175	3629	4082	4536
Oz.	1	28	482	936	1389	1843	2296	2750	3203	3657	4111	4564
	2	57	510	964	1417	1871	2325	2778	3232	3685	4139	4593
	3	85	539	992	1446	1899	2353	2807	3260	3714	4167	4621
	4	113	567	1021	1474	1928	2381	2835	3289	3742	4196	4649
	5	142	595	1049	1503	1956	2410	2863	3317	3770	4224	4678
	6	170	624	1077	1531	1984	2438	2892	3345	3799	4252	4706
	7	198	652	1106	1559	2013	2466	2920	3374	3827	4281	4734
	8	227	680	1134	1588	2041	2495	2948	3402	3856	4309	4763
	9	255	709	1162	1616	2070	2523	2977	3430	3884	4337	4791
	10	283	737	1191	1644	2098	2551	3005	3459	3912	4366	4819
	11	312	765	1219	1673	2126	2580	3033	3487	3941	4394	4848
	12	340	794	1247	1701	2155	2608	3062	3515	3969	4423	4876
	13	369	822	1276	1729	2183	2637	3090	3544	3997	4451	4904
	14	397	850	1304	1758	2211	2665	3118	3572	4026	4479	4933
	15	425	879	1332	1786	2240	2693	3147	3600	4054	4508	4961

INCHES TO CENTIMETERS

Inches	Centimeters	Inches	Centimeters
10	25.4	20.5	52.1
10.5	26.7	21	53.3
11	27.9	21.5	54.6
11.5	29.2	22	55.9
12	30.5	22.5	57.2
12.5	31.8	23	58.4
13	33.0	23.5	59.7
13.5	34.3	24	61.0
14	35.6	24.5	62.2
14.5	36.8	25	63.5
15	38.1	25.5	64.8
15.5	39.4	26	66.1
16	40.6	26.5	67.4
16.5	41.9	27	68.7
17	43.2	27.5	69.9
17.5	44.4	28	71.2
18	45.7	28.5	72.5
18.5	47.0	29	73.8
19	48.3	29.5	75.1
19.5	49.5	30	76.4
20	50.8	30.5	77.6

APPENDIX III

APGAR SCORING CHART

Test	0 points	1 point	2 points
Activity (Muscle Tone)	absent, limp	some flexion of extremities	active motion, well flexed
Pulse (Heart Rate)	absent	below 100 beats per minute (bpm)	above 100 beats per minute (bpm)
Grimace (Reflex Irritability) 1. when a catheter is placed in a nostril	1. absent	1. grimace	1. sneeze, cough
2. when foot is flicked	2. absent	2. movement, crying	2. vigorous crying and withdrawal of foot
Appearance (Skin Color)	blue-grey, pale all over	hands and feet blue, body pink	completely pink all over
Respiration (Breathing Effort)	absent	irregular, slow, weak cry	good strong cry

APPENDIX IV
NUTRITIONAL INTAKE & STAGES OF STANDARD FEEDING DEVELOPMENT

AGE	FOOD	FEEDING STYLE/ POSITIONING
0-4 months	Breast milk or formula	Child held by parent or caretaker in semi-reclined position
4-6 months	Breast milk or formula Smooth solids (strained or pureed foods)	Child held by parent or caretaker in more upright manner Child fed with feeder spoon (small, narrow spoon with long handle)
8 months	Breast milk or formula Finger foods (baby cookies, crackers) Lumpy solids (ground junior foods or mashed foods)	Child seated in high chair or other feeder chair Given choice of bottle so child can hold independently Cup drinking introduced
12 months	Milk Meat sticks, fruit, vegetables Coarsely chopped table food	Child seated in high chair or other feeder chair Child is now active participant in feeding process Uses fingers to feed and is introduced to spoon feeding (child-sized spoon) Drinks mealtime liquid from cup
18 months	Coarsely chopped table food Most meats	Child seated in high chair or youth chair at table Independent spoon feeding (messy) Drinks all liquid from cup

(Elaine Geralis, ed., *Children with Cerebral Palsy: A Parent's Guide*, 2nd ed. Bethesda, MD: Woodbine House, 1998, p. 129)

APPENDIX V

RECOMMENDED IMMUNIZATION SCHEDULES

Immunization/Test	Recommended Age
Hepatitis A (HepA)	Between 12-23 months of age, with 2 doses separated by 6-12 months or 6-18 months, depending on the formulation
Hepatitis B (HepB)	Shortly after birth with a total of 3 doses by 18 months of age
Diptheria, Tetanus, Pertussis [DTaP-diptheria and tetanus toxoids (a toxin that has been treated to decrease its poisonous effect but keep its power to stimulate the formation of antibodies) and acellular pertussis vaccine]	2, 4, 6, and between 15-18 months, with a booster before starting school (4½-6 years of age)
Hemophilus Influenzae type b (Hib)	2, 4, 6 months (depending on the particular vaccine used), and a booster at 15 months of age
Pneumococcal Conjugate Vaccine (PVC7)	2, 4, 6, and between 12-15 months
Polio (IPV-E - Inactivated Poliovirus Vaccine of Enhanced Potency)	2, 4, and between 6-18 months, and again before starting school (4½-6 years of age)
Measles, Mumps, Rubella Viruses (MMR)	Between 12-15 months and again before starting school (4½-6 years of age)
Varicella-Zoster Virus (VZV)	Between 12-18 months of age
Tuberculosis (tuberculin test - TB)	12 months, before starting school, or as needed (if there has been a possible or known exposure)

About the Author

Since 1984, **Jeanine G. Coleman, M.Ed.**, has been the Program Director for Advance Infant Development in La Verne, California, a program for infants from birth to three years of age who are at-risk or developmentally disabled. Her responsibilities include training and supervising a staff of infant educators, and working with various state, therapy, and educational agencies. Coleman also teaches child development and early intervention courses, and speaks at seminars and conferences and to child development center staffs on such topics as inclusion of children with special needs, identifying developmental delays, effective behavior management techniques, and early intervention terminology. She lives with her husband, Dale, and son, Jacob in La Verne, California.